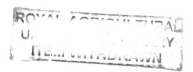
Becoming a Reflective Practitioner

Becoming a Reflective Practitioner

Second edition

Christopher Johns

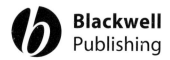

Blackwell Publishing

Editorial offices:
Blackwell Publishing Ltd, 9600 Garsington Road, Oxford OX4 2DQ, UK
  Tel: +44 (0) 1865 776868
Blackwell Publishing Inc., 350 Main Street, Malden, MA 02148-5020, USA
  Tel: +1 781 388 8250
Blackwell Publishing Asia Pty Ltd, 550 Swanston Street, Carlton, Victoria 3053, Australia
  Tel : +61 (0)3 8359 1011

First edition published by Blackwell Science Ltd 2000
Reprinted 2001, 2002, 2003
Second edition published by Blackwell Publishing Ltd 2004
Reprinted 2005

Library of Congress Cataloging- in-Publication Data

Johns, Christopher.
  Becoming a reflective practitioner / Christopher Johns.—2nd ed.
     p. ; cm.
  Includes bibliographical references and index.
  ISBN 1–4051–1833–4 (pbk. : alk. paper)
  1. Nursing—Philosophy. 2. Holistic nursing.
  [DNLM: 1. Philosophy, Nursing. 2. Holistic Nursing. 3. Models, Nursing.
WY 86 J65b 2004] I. Title.

  RT84.5.J636 2004
  610.73'01—dc22   20004000126

ISBN-10: 1-4051-1833-4
ISBN-13: 978-14051-1833-0

A catalogue record for this title is available from the British Library

Set in 10/12.5pt Palatino
by Graphicraft Ltd, Hong Kong
Printed and bound in India
by Gopsons Paper Ltd, Noida

For further information on Blackwell Publishing, visit our website:
www.blackwellnursing.com

Contents

Foreword

Jean Watson

And just what are we to make of becoming a reflective practitioner? Are we to learn? Are we to change? Are we to work toward transformation of self and other?

This work by Christopher Johns brings us face to face with the human elements and human dilemmas, the deep level of humanity that clinicians encounter daily, moment by moment, the blessings and challenges of living, suffering, changing, evolving, dying, leading us to nothing less than a rebirthing of self and work. And how are we to live this practice of reflection? How are we to be? To become? To evolve? To alter? To repattern? To rethink?

We do so by stepping into practice moments; we do so by honouring our own inner humanness; we do so by stopping, being present, listening to stories, life narratives, filled with inner meanings, myths, metaphors and by reflecting on one's own presence of being and becoming in the moment. It is through the reflective moment that we both seek and gain insights, dynamics of wisdom and depth of meanings revealed whole to us but only when we stop, pause and are present to such profound human mystery and wisdom that is already contained on the margin, in the shadows, in the distant haze of our own existence.

It is here, when we are still, witness to our own openness, that we connect with self and other in shared moments of human being and becoming. A multifaceted jewel, the diamond net of refracted light contained within each human moment of human encounter . . . a clue, a coloured hue, contributing to a human canvas, a human studio of caring moments, each one a possibility for hope, for movement through pain, suffering, loss, challenge, while being present to the joy; the aesthetic, the paradox, the dilemma, the eternal, uncovered from the journey toward wholeness. In the nurse's presence, in listening to and becoming part of another's story, life drama, myth for meaning and hope, we are able to promote health or become true instruments of timeless healing that transcend self, other and system alike.

Reflective stories in this text offer models of insight; they reveal the hidden subtext of paradox, inner drama, unaddressed questions, unknowns, that lead to ethical grids and maps on the reflective journey – a reflective journey, into context, discovery, relationships, non-objectivist, non-formulaic notions and moods that guide not by convention and rationalistic principles but rather by intentional consciousness, by awakening. Awakening to presence, relationships, being and becoming part of the connections, patterns and processes that mirror human-to-human caring and healing. This reflective subtext of nursing invites us into and through informed, reflective, appropriate skilled action of human connectivity, creativity and intuition. Through internal and external existential dialogue and story and guidance we journey into the spiritual, the aesthetic, the ethical, the arts, that touch and celebrate the non-quantifiable, that once again reunite the profession and the practitioner alike, with the compassion and passion of nursing's life and work.

It is here through the Johns reflective practice model and its evolving process for self-reflection and guidance that we discover, once again, that the 'personal becomes the professional'. It is here that we learn to grow in caring by becoming instruments of healing, first by learning about our own inner healing and health processes and needs that flow from self to other. These lessons transcend yet inform each caring moment, consciously or unconsciously. It is through reflective practice that nurses and nursing learn about nursing as never known before. It is here, in honouring the whole, in gleaning and seeking meaning from parts and particles of light in the institutional and often individual darkness, that we find new hope for transforming nursing and nurses alike.

Finally, it is through reflective practice, as continually explored and explicated by Johns and colleagues, that we are offered a method, a mode, a mood, a model of being and becoming that allows us to face and live through, if not be blessed by, our own woundedness. This model is a guide that informs and invites us, in uniquely individual ways, to engage in authentic caring and become part of a process of healing and wholeness that is required for a new era in human history and futuristic nursing.

In the past nurses and nursing have tried to escape the inner learning and healing that is required for the practice journey; we have done this by succumbing to medical science, medical-nursing tasks, industrial-system demands. It has turned out that these routes to nursing have been a detour from our human caring practices and commitment to processes of wholeness and healing that have motivated, inspired and informed individuals and communities across time.

It is through the breakdowns of conventional practices, combined with breakthroughs of reflective practice, which can now be integrated with the most up-to-date knowledge and skills, philosophies and theories, that we enter a new world of professional care practices that embrace, encompass and more fully actualise the paradigm of hope spread before and behind nursing in its history and traditions. It is only by stopping, pausing and reconsidering our encounters and relationships with self and other that we mature as a distinct caring, healing and health profession.

However, it is the reflective practice processes and approaches that may be the most threatening, yet at the same time offer the greatest hope for growth, maturity and personal and professional maturity. If nursing turns its back on reflection, it is turning its back on its woundedness and core humanity, which is the ground of being and becoming. In not pausing to consider reflection, we remain technical assistants, trying to defend ourselves from our own wounds and suffering, forever stranded on the shoreline as humanity and health care itself sets out to pursue new horizons of possibilities contained within the depths of our shared humanity and the oceanic changes possible for human evolution and growth.

Will we choose reflection and human transformation as a path to the future or succumb to robotic mutation? Which route will we take? Reflect upon it and choose but do so with passion and purpose. As we individually and collectively ponder the future, this text offers a holistic lesson that will serve us well into the next millennium.

Preface

Welcome to the second edition of this book. The major aim of the book remains the same as the first edition; to pose and respond to the question, 'What does it mean to be a reflective practitioner?'

The book takes the general view that reflective practice is essentially a way of being, an active way of engaging practice towards realising desirable practice, in whatever way that is known and understood. As such, reflective practice is fundamental to professional practice, because I assume that all professionals are fundamentally concerned with knowing and realising desirable and effective practice, yet work in conditions where, for one reason or another, such realisation is difficult. I shall argue that reflective practice *is* holistic practice and perhaps the only way holism can be embraced within each unfolding practice moment.

Reflective practice is holistic practice because:

- It focuses on the whole experience and then seeks to understand its significance within the whole.
- It is grounded in the meanings the individual practitioner gives to the particular experience and seeks to facilitate such understanding.
- It acknowledges that the practitioner is ultimately self-determining and responsible for his or her own destiny and seeks to facilitate such growth.

Newman (1994) commented that to view the world from a different perspective requires a paradigm shift which incorporates the old paradigm and transforms it (p. 13). In transcending our own boundaries as nurses and health care practitioners, we have to move beyond these boundaries and embrace new ideas and new language. Because we tend to probe things with our minds rather than with our hearts, we tend to reject certain ideas that are framed in complex language and do not fit in with our existing conceptualisation of the world. If we aspire to become holistic then the language of holism and reflection must not intimidate us otherwise we fail ourselves and the people we aspire to care for and work with.

This book is extensively rewritten from the first edition although many of the exemplars of practice remain intact. To commence I have used Jean Watson's postscript from the first edition as a foreword as a way of connecting between the two editions. Jean's words are a beacon for the spirit of reflective practice and the evolution of health care into new dimensions. Chapter 1 offers an introduction to reflective practice theory. As in the first edition I have generally taken a cognitive view of reflective theories although I am ever more conscious of more holistic influences on the nature of reflection through Buddhist philosophy and Native American ritual. However, I needed to draw a line somewhere and have left these more esoteric influences to forthcoming work.

I extend the first edition by considering reflection as humanities, the therapeutic benefits of reflective writing and evaluating reflection. Chapter 2 offers a reflective model for clinical practice based on the Burford NDU Holistic model: Caring in Practice. At the core of a reflective model is a *valid* vision for practice that gives meaning and direction to practice and poses the question, 'If we hold these values, what abilities do we need to realise them as a lived reality?' In response I assert the 'Being Available' template as a skills framework. The remainder of the book can be viewed as a reflective path toward realising the vision as a lived reality and developing the practitioner's ability to be available.

Chapter 3 is an exposition on guiding reflection and clinical supervision to enable the reader to appreciate the pattern of guidance within the exemplars and theories to frame their own clinical supervision work.

Chapters 4 to 7 each focus on the development of specific attributes of the Being Available template. In Chapter 4, I focus on knowing the person and compassion. I set out a reflective lens to view the person, arguing that traditional assessment models are redundant for the reflective and holistic practitioner. Indeed, the concept of assessment is replaced by the idea of 'pattern appreciation.' At the core of knowing the person is the empathic ability to connect with the experience of the person. Compassion is a healing energy, yet an energy that needs to be nurtured and focused. In Chapter 5, I explore the idea of the 'aesthetic response', which is essentially the ability to make effective clinical judgement, and on this basis to respond with appropriate, effective and ethical action and reflect on its impact. In particular I reflect on the use of touch. In Chapter 6 I reflect on the significance of knowing and managing self within relationships. It is the flip-side of compassion and empathy, to tune into and flow with the person in ways that our own 'stuff' does not get in the way. Chapter 7 explores the significance of creating and sustaining an environment where it is possible for the practitioner to be available and places the nurse–patient relationship into its organisational context and an understanding of those factors that may constrain the practitioner's ability to be available: issues of tradition, authority and embodiment. It deals with issues such as managing change, assertiveness, managing conflict, and stress and support.

Chapter 8 considers reflective communication, both verbal and written. The core value of communication is that it must be both practical and meaningful. The nursing process is critiqued and exposed as an absurd model for the reflective practitioner. Instead I assert the movement towards narrative forms.

Chapter 9 is concerned with managing quality and responding to the clinical governance agenda through reflective techniques such as clinical audit and standards of care to get valid feedback that our visions of practice are indeed realised as a lived reality. I assert that quality must be the responsibility of each practitioner intrinsic to everyday practice rather than something abstract and imposed.

Chapter 10 is an exposition of transformational clinical leadership through exemplars of students on the masters of clinical leadership programme at the University of Luton. Transformational leadership is reflective leadership dedicated to establishing the learning organisation, yet can it shift the prevailing transactional culture of health care or is it just another example of rhetoric? I also review how I have incorporated reflective practice into curriculum.

I have endeavoured to write the book in a reflective style, in contrast with a more traditional text style, incorporating the extensive use of stories taken from my reflective journal or those shared with me in guided reflection or clinical supervision. The beauty of story is the way it can illuminate the contextual meaning of complex theory in ways the reader can sense in relation to their own experiences. Story illuminates the complexity of caring as a whole. It draws out the subtlety and nuances of caring from its apparent mundaneness and its significance within health care. As the reader will note, the stories are emotional, reflecting the intimacy, anguish and beauty of the human caring encounter. In this respect, story is a way of honouring caring work.

Writing in a more traditional style would be a contradiction with what I view as the essential nature of reflective practice. It would only reinforce the idea that reflective practice was a technology with specific techniques to apply. Perhaps as novices we need techniques to access the artistry of reflective practice yet I urge the reader to keep this point in perspective, because as you develop expertise the techniques can become a burden, constraining, rather than liberating, the self.

The reflective practitioner has an open and curious mind in order to be receptive to what the text has to say. As a consequence I have not always drawn out the significance of the stories. Where I have, these are only my view. I do intend to impose these. Indeed as a 'reflective reader' the reader will relate to the stories in terms of their own experiences, and make their own interpretations. This is the value of 'reflective texts': it is possible to relate to the stories because they are deeply subjective and contextual.

Christopher Johns

While this book uses 'she' to indicate 'the nurse' this is for descriptive ease only, and the author recognises the contribution of both male and female nurses to the profession.

Acknowledgements

My thanks and love to Jean Watson who constantly inspires my work and encourages me to move beyond boundaries. She is truly a beacon to help others see.

My thanks to all the practitioners and patients who are the focus of the stories within the book given pseudonyms to obscure their identity. Thanks to Simon Lee for his story in Chapter 5. Simon wrote this story whilst a student undertaking the 'Becoming a Reflective Practitioner' course at the University of Luton. Thanks to Moira Vass who requested that I publish her account of living with motor neurone disease in Chapter 4 that offers valuable insight into the therapeutic benefits of journaling. Thanks to Susan Brooks and 'Sally' who share their leadership stories from assignment work on the masters in clinical leadership programme at the University of Luton.

The story *Stephen* in Chapter 4 is taken from my book *Being Mindful, Easing Suffering: Reflections on Palliative Care* published by Jessica Kingsley Publishing, London.

Finally, my thanks to Beth Knight and the team at Blackwell Publishing.

Chapter 1

Becoming Reflective

What does it mean to be a reflective practitioner? Is reflection something I write in a journal after work or perhaps it is something I do in clinical supervision? Is reflection a technology I might be exposed to on an educational course? Is it simply a form of thinking that I do anyway? Or is it a way of being within everyday practice that makes me more mindful of the ways I think, feel and respond to situations? Is it a particular style of leadership? Perhaps it is all of these things and more? In response to these questions, I am going to suggest a typology of reflective practices that moves from *doing* reflection towards reflection as a *way of being* within everyday practice (Box 1.1).

I suspect that many practitioners consider reflection as reflection-on-experience or reflection-on-action (Schön 1987): looking back at 'an experience' or some event that has taken place. The idea of an 'experience' is difficult to grasp: where does one experience begin and another end? Is experience not the endless flow of life? Is anticipating a forthcoming event an experience in itself? Simply put, an experience can be thinking, feeling or doing something.

Schön (1983, 1987) distinguished reflection-*on-action* with reflection-*in-action* as a way of thinking about a situation whilst engaged within it, in order to reframe and solve some breakdown in the smooth running of experience. Schön's thinking was influenced by Heidegger's idea of breakdown. Heidegger (1962, cited in Plager 1994) describes three inter-related modes of involvement or engagement with practical activity we have in day-to-day life:

- *Ready-to-hand*: In the ready-to-hand mode of engagement, equipment and practical activity function smoothly and transparently. The person is involved in an absorbed manner so that the activity is for the most part unnoticed.
- *Unready-to-hand*: In the unready-to-hand mode, some sort of breakdown occurs in the smooth functioning of activity; becoming conspicuous to the user.
- *Present-to-hand*: In the present-to-hand mode, practical everyday activity ceases, and the person stands back and reflects on the situation.

The practitioner can adjust to minor interruptions to the smooth flow of experience without having to overtly think about it, because the body has embodied knowing. Sometimes the practitioner is faced with situations that do not go smoothly. In order to move on the practitioner must stand back

Box 1.1   Layers of reflection

Reflection-on-experience: Reflecting on a situation or experience after the event with the intention of drawing insights that may inform my future practice in positive ways.

Reflection-in-action: Pausing within a particular situation or experience in order to make sense and reframe the situation proceeding towards desired outcomes.

The internal supervisor: Dialoguing with self whilst in conversation with another in order to make sense.

Reflection-within-the-moment: Being aware of the way I am thinking, feeling and responding within the unfolding moment and dialoguing with self to ensure I am interpreting and responding congruently to whatever is unfolding. It is having some space in your mind to change your ideas rather than being fixed to certain ideas.

Mindful practice: Being aware of self within the unfolding moment with the intention of realising desirable practice (however desirable is defined).

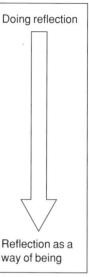

Doing reflection

Reflection as a way of being

and consider how best to proceed. This is Schön's reflection-in-action, a type of problem-solving whereby the problem is considered, re-framed and ways of resolving the problem contemplated and tested to move on with the experience. It is easy to misunderstand reflection-in-action as *merely* thinking about something whilst doing it. Schön drew on examples from music and architecture, situations of engagement with inanimate forms. His example of counselling is taken from the classroom not from clinical practice. The classroom is a much easier place to freeze and reframe situations in contrast with clinical practice grounded within the human encounter.

Casement (1985), a psychoanalyst, offers a more satisfactory concept of reflection as the ability to dialogue with self whilst dialoguing with a client. He calls this dialogue with self the *internal supervisor* – paying attention to the way the self interprets what the other is saying and weighing up how best to respond. However, like reflection-in-action, it is a technique used in a particular situation.

The idea of paying attention to self within the unfolding moment defines *reflection-within-the-moment*; the exquisite paying attention to the way the self is thinking, feeling and responding within the particular moment, and those factors that are influencing the way self is thinking, feeling and responding. Such self-awareness moves reflection away from techniques to apply to a way of being.

Reflection-within-the-moment is developed through reflecting-on-experience: the more reflective I am after the event the more reflective I become within practice itself. Although I cannot prove this point in conventional research terms, most practitioners I have taught demonstrate this ability. As a consequence normal everyday practice becomes alive and dynamic. The mundane becomes profound.

Mindful practice

Mindful practice is, in essence, the same level of awareness as reflection-within-the-moment but distinguished by the conscious intent to realise a vision of practice. For example, as a complementary therapist and palliative care practitioner, my vision is *to ease suffering and nurture growth through the health–illness experience*. The idea of vision is further developed in Chapter 2. To realise this vision I must help the person appreciate their own suffering and envision a place where they might rather be – a place free from suffering, whether the suffering is physical, emotional, psychological, social or spiritual (Johns 2004).

Being mindful is fundamental to wisdom: the ability to make best judgements about situations by seeing the big picture for what it is. Within the complex and often indeterminate world of clinical practice, the ability to make good judgements would seem most significant, together with a deep compassion for the experience of the patient and family.

Defining reflection

Definitions of reflection are characterised as learning through experience toward gaining new insights or changed perceptions of self and practice (Boud *et al.* 1985; Boyd and Fales 1983; Mezirow 1981). I describe reflection (adapted from the first edition) as being mindful of self, either within or after experience, as if a window through which the practitioner can view and focus self within the context of a particular experience, in order to confront, understand and move toward resolving contradiction between one's vision and actual practice. Through the conflict of contradiction, the commitment to realise one's vision, and understanding why things are as they are, the practitioner can gain new insights into self and be empowered to respond more congruently in future situations within a reflexive spiral towards developing practical wisdom and realising one's vision as a lived reality. The practitioner may require guidance to overcome resistance or to be empowered to act on understanding.

From this description, the core characteristics of reflection can be elicited:

- practical wisdom
- reflexivity
- becoming mindful
- commitment
- contradiction
- understanding
- empowerment

Practical wisdom

The reflective effort is towards enabling practitioners to develop practical wisdom: the practitioner's knowing within the particular situation. Much has been written and debated about the distinction between art and science in nursing knowledge. Science is seen as the hard evidence whilst artistry is viewed as what nurses actually do. The work of Carper (1978) helps to visualise the wholeness of practical wisdom and the way types of knowledge integrate to inform practical wisdom woven together in unique patterns of knowing in response to each particular situation.

Carper's fundamental ways of knowing in nursing

At the core of Carper's work is the *aesthetic* way of knowing (Jchns 1995) or what I now describe as practical wisdom. Practical wisdom is reflected in the way the practitioner grasps, interprets, envisages what is to be achieved and responds to the unfolding moment. In essence this is practical wisdom: clinical judgement and response.

As I set out in Box 1.2, practical wisdom or aesthetics is influenced by *the empirical, the ethical, the personal patterns of knowing* and what I term *reflexivity*, that together weave the unique pattern of knowing reflected in the practitioner's practical wisdom of each particular experience. Carper describes the empirical as:

> 'Knowing knowledge that is systematically organised into general laws and theories for the purpose of describing, explaining and predicting phenomena of special concern to the discipline of nursing'. (p. 14)

I would extend this empirical view of knowledge to include all sources of extant knowledge that might inform the practitioner within the particular clinical moment. Practitioners draw on different types of knowledge, both subjective and objective, each with its own rules for determining its truth claims (Johns 2002; Wilber 1998). *Reflexivity* acknowledges both the influence of previous experience on clinical judgement and response, and the impact of applying new insights about practice through reflection on future experience.

Reflexivity

My description of reflection states that *the practitioner can gain new insights into self and be empowered to respond more congruently in future situations within a reflexive spiral towards realising one's vision as a lived reality.* Such words reflect the purposefulness of reflection: it is action oriented towards the development of practical wisdom and realisation of vision. Reflexivity is a looking back and reviewing self's development over time: the way insights have emerged and influenced future experience. In this sense, reflection is like a drama unfolding over time, a systematic and disciplined pursuit towards realising desirable practice however that is known. As I shall explore, the practitioner can utilise markers to plot the reflexive journey of development.

Box 1.2   Carper's fundamental pattern of knowing in nursing (1978) (reproduced from Johns 1995a)

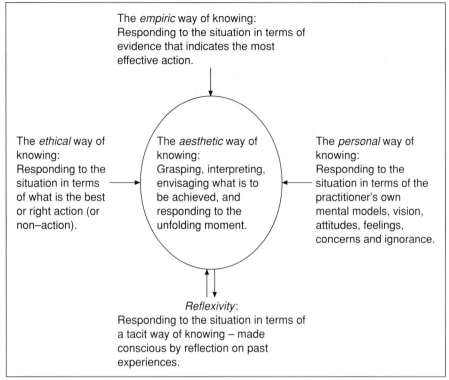

The *empiric* way of knowing:
Responding to the situation in terms of evidence that indicates the most effective action.

The *ethical* way of knowing:
Responding to the situation in terms of what is the best or right action (or non–action).

The *aesthetic* way of knowing:
Grasping, interpreting, envisaging what is to be achieved, and responding to the unfolding moment.

The *personal* way of knowing:
Responding to the situation in terms of the practitioner's own mental models, vision, attitudes, feelings, concerns and ignorance.

Reflexivity:
Responding to the situation in terms of a tacit way of knowing – made conscious by reflection on past experiences.

Becoming mindful

The idea of *a window* is to look inside at self, to understand the way I am thinking (head), feeling (heart) and responding (hand) to situations as I do, and also use a window to look out at practice, in particular the way the environment influences the way I am thinking, feeling and responding. I shall assume that the effective practitioner seeks congruence between head, heart and hand (Cope 2001).

There is a beautiful complexity of growth through reflection. Extending *window* as a metaphor, O'Donohue (1997) notes the way:

'many people remain trapped at the one window, looking out every day at the same scene in the same way. Real growth is experienced when you draw back from that one window, turn and walk around the inner tower of the soul and see all the different windows that await your gaze. Through these different windows, you can see new vistas of possibility, presence and creativity. Complacency, habit and blindness often prevent you from feeling your life. So much depends on the frame of vision – the window through which we look.' (pp. 163–64)

The image of practitioners opening shutters to see themselves and practice is a powerful visualisation of mindfulness – the antidote to complacency, habit and blindness that O'Donohue poetically captures.

Commitment

In my definition of reflection I suggested that commitment was necessary for reflection. Fay (1987) considers that commitment, or what he terms wilfulness, besides the qualities of openness, curiosity and intelligence, are prerequisites for reflection – I pay attention to something because it matters to me. Why else would I pay attention to it except to relieve my anxiety? I pay attention to my 'experience' because I constantly strive to become a more effective practitioner and realise my vision of practice.

This commitment is the very heart of what it means to be caring. Because I pay attention to my practice I am open to what is unfolding. Being open I am not defensive, but curious and ready to consider new possibilities. Every situation becomes an opportunity for learning. Curiosity is being mindful – Why do I feel that way? Why do I think that way? Why do I respond that way? Why are the walls green? Does music help patients relax? Why is Jim unhappy – would a SSRI anti-depressant work better than a tricylic? Etcetera. Everything enters into the gaze of the curious practitioner on her quest to realise desirable and effective practice. From this angle it is perhaps easy to see the scope of reflection. As Gadamer (1975) noted:

> 'The opening up and keeping open of possibilities is only possible because we find ourselves deeply interested in that which makes the question possible in the first place. To truly question something is to interrogate something from the heart of our existence, from the centre of our being.' (p. 266)

If things are not cared for they wither and die. When those things are people then the significance of commitment becomes only too apparent. Commitment harmonises or balances conflict of contradiction, it is the energy that helps us to face up to unacceptable situations. As Carl Rogers (1969) notes, the small child is ambivalent about learning to walk; he stumbles and falls, he hurts himself. It is a painful process. Yet the satisfaction of developing his potential far outweighs the bumps and bruises. As I know only too well through years of guiding practitioners to learn through experiences, nurses reflect on painful situations. Practice is not always a pretty sight. Yet with commitment, even in the darkest moments, the glimmer of caring shines through. The realisation of caring within such moments is profoundly satisfying and sustaining, it nourishes commitment and reaffirms our beliefs. No words express this senti-ment better than Van Manen (1990):

> 'Retrieving or recalling the essence of caring is not a simple matter of simple etymo-logical analysis or explication of the usage of the word. Rather, it is the construction of a way of life to live the language of our lives more deeply, to become more truly who we are when we refer to ourselves [as nurses].' (p. 58)

Perhaps many practitioners have had their commitment numbed or blunted through lack of attention or working in uncaring environments. It is a tough world out there where it can be very difficult to realise one's caring ideals in the pressure to get through the work with limited resources. Perhaps satisfac-tion is making it through to the end of the shift with minimal hassle rather than fulfilling caring ideals. Often when things get overly familiar we no longer pay attention to them. As O'Donohue (1997) notes:

> 'People have difficulty awakening to their inner world, especially when their lives become familiar to them. They find it hard to discover something new, interesting or adventurous in their numbed lives.' (pp. 122–3)

Practitioners who have become numb will not enjoy reflection. Indeed they will turn their heads away from the reflective mirror because it is too painful or do not want to face themselves and the responsibility to care. On the other hand, reflection offers the practitioner a way to re-kindle commitment and reconnect to caring ideals.

Contradiction

Contradiction is the *creative tension* that exists between our visions of practice and our current reality (Senge 1990). This tension is the learning opportunity. For people concerned with doing what is best, this tension can feel uncomfortable or like a gnawing ache. Reflection is often triggered by negative feelings such as anger, guilt, sadness, frustration, resentment or even hatred. Such feelings create anxiety within the person and bring the situation that caused these feelings into the conscious mind. The practitioner may *naturally* reflect either consciously or subconsciously to try and defend against this anxiety in order to try and bring self back into a harmonious state. The practitioner may distort, rationalise, project or even deny the situation that caused the feelings. They may take action to relieve the tenseness anxiety causes by attacking the source of the negative feeling or taking it out on someone else. They may more quietly talk it through with someone willing to listen, or, more vigorously, take some exercise. We all have our own tactics for such moments. We may even write in a journal.

On the other hand, the practitioner may reflect on positive feelings such as satisfaction, joy and love. However this is less likely because we are more likely to accept such feelings. Experiences that arouse no strong feelings are simply taken for granted, that is until the practitioner becomes *mindful*, in which case all experience becomes available for reflection.

Reflection is cathartic in encouraging the expression and understanding of strong feelings. In this process, negative feelings or energy can be converted into positive energy for taking future action based on an understanding of the situation and appropriate ways of responding. Lydia Hall (1964) puts this succinctly:

> 'Anxiety over an extended period is stressful to all the organ functions. It prepares people to fight or flight. In our culture however, it is brutal to fight and cowardly to flee, so we stew in our own juices and cook up malfunction. This energy can be put to use in exploration of feeling through participation in the struggle to face and solve problems underlying the state of anxiety.' (p. 151)

Reflection offers a path for the exploration of feeling. Yet to do this may require guidance because of learnt responses to anxiety. The nature of guidance and clinical supervision as a particular form of guidance is developed in Chapter 3.

The idea of contradiction resonates with critical social science concerned as it is with the liberation of individuals and groups from states of oppression to realise practitioners' own best interests. Whether you view nurses or nursing as oppressed makes for interesting debate. Fay (1987) views reflection as a critical process moving three stages of enlightenment, empowerment and emancipation towards overcoming the forces that constrain practitioners from realising desirable practice. Each stage represents a significant level of learning:

Enlightenment (understanding)	Understanding why things have come to be as they are in terms of frustrating self's realisation of desirable practice.
Empowerment	Creating the necessary conditions within self whereby action to realise desirable practice can be undertaken.
Emancipation (transformation)	A stable shift in practice congruent with the realisation of desirable practice.

Understanding

Understanding is the basis for making good judgement and taking action congruent with realising desirable practice. It is only when practitioners understand themselves and the conditions of their practice that they can begin to realistically plan how they might respond differently. Yet we do not live in a rational world. There are barriers that limit the practitioner's ability to respond differently to practice situations even when they know there is a better way of responding to situations in tune with desirable practice. These barriers blind and bind people to see and respond to the world as they do.

People are not radically free to act on rationality but are bound by social norms (tradition), by power relationships with others (authority) and by previous learning that has become embodied (embodiment). By embodiment I mean I do not have to think about how to do something because my body has learnt to do it, for example driving a car. Of course, this makes learning to do something differently difficult because what is embodied has to be unlearnt. Because of the forces of tradition and authority, practitioners' freedom to act is a relative freedom in terms of the limits imposed by normal society. Change is always a process of social change because of the way change disrupts the status quo. As such, there is always a built-in resistance to change in order to maintain the status quo even by those who may benefit from change. In exploring the nature of contradiction, the practitioner must inevitably explore the conditions that bind her to normal ways of being. The effort is to un-bind in order to move on.

Empowerment

Returning to my definition of reflection, I suggested that it is the force of conflict, commitment and understanding that empowers the practitioner to take action based on insights. Kieffer (1984) noted that the process of empowerment involved:

> 'Reconstructing and re-orientating deeply engrained personal systems of social relations. Moreover they confront these tasks in an environment which historically has enforced their political oppression and which continues its active and implicit attempts at subversion and constructive change.' (p. 27)

Kieffer's words are very powerful and may not rest comfortably with many readers. Yet the truth of the situation is stark; if practitioners truly wish to realise their caring ideals then they have no choice but to become political in working towards establishing the conditions of practice where that is possible.

Yet, the health care agenda has shifted considerably in recent years, opening up the possibilities for practitioners to expand their roles. On the other hand, it might be argued that the health care agenda has become increasingly concerned with productivity rather than care processes. In response practitioners may feel frustrated, leading to low morale, increased dissatisfaction and burnout. Practitioners may respond by shifting things on the surface but real change is much deeper.

Developing voice

The emergence of *voice* is a powerful metaphor for empowerment, as exemplified through the work of Belenky *et al.* (1986). Belenky and her co-researchers, in examining women's ways of knowing, describe five different perspectives from which women view reality and draw conclusions about truth, knowledge and authority: silence, received knowing, subjective knowing, procedural knowing, and constructed knowing. These different voices offer a pathway to plot increasing levels of empowerment. I use the pathway to guide practitioners to appreciate and develop what voices they are using within specific situations. The pathway also works for men although the tendency of men towards a morality based on justice rather than a morality based on responsibility and care may result in a different pattern of men's knowing; an assumption drawn from Gilligan's work (1993) *In a Different Voice*.

Silence

At the level of silence practitioners have no voice. They are not lost for words so much as have no words to say. It is the position of the subordinate and powerless practitioner. Perhaps you can remember being silenced, not so much by others but by yourself. Practitioners often say 'I wish I had said something but . . .'.

Is it fear of repercussion or humiliation? Either way, it is a reflection of knowing your place to be silent in a situation. Think of a recent experience when you would have liked to say something. Write it down and ask yourself why you were silent. What would you liked to have said? How did you feel? What do you imagine the response of others to be?

Cumberlege observed at meetings concerned with the discussion of her report on community nursing that doctors sat in the front rows and asked all the questions, whilst nurses sat in the back rows and kept silent. She commented how nurses needed to find a voice so they could be heard, otherwise they would have no future in planning health care services.

Received knowing; the voice of others

At the level of received knowing, practitioners listen and speak with the voices of others that they have embodied. They conceive themselves as capable of receiving, even reproducing, knowledge from the all-knowing external authorities but not capable of creating knowledge of their own.

When I read these words I am reminded of my 'nurse training' and how I was filled with this type of knowledge usually copied verbatim from the all-knowing external authorities. I have no sense of being enabled to develop critical thinking skills, and even if I had, the all-knowing authorities within clinical practice would have soon put me in my place. Despite the rhetoric of developing the practitioner as a critical thinker, the weight of tradition and authority continues to suppress her emergence.

So when I ask a nurse, 'Why do you do it like that?' she is likely to reproduce knowledge from an external authority that has been unquestioned. When I ask her how else she might do it, she may struggle to think laterally, locked into habitual patterns of response. The reflective perspective at this level is to simply challenge the taken for granted and veracity of received knowledge.

Subjective: the inner voice

At the level of subjective knowing, the practitioner is engaged on a quest for self: listening to, valuing and accepting her own voice as a source of knowing. This may mean rejecting the authoritative voice that has dominated the way the practitioner views, thinks about and responds to the world. It is like waking up and seeing yourself as a person in your own right. The subjective voice may be confusing, because it is competing with received voices, hence it is easy to discount one's own subjective voice as being unsubstantiated, even ridiculed by more 'knowing' others. Listening to self, the self may see an uncanny stranger on display, a self that has been censored (Cixous 1996).

This is the voice that reflective practice seeks to surface in the first place. Yet it can also be a tentative voice, vulnerable in its uncertainty, and hence may need to be nurtured in a community of like-minded people. Belenky *et al.* (1986) note:

> 'During the period of subjective knowing, women lay down procedures for systematically learning and analysing experience. But what seems distinctive in these women is that their strategies for knowing grow out of their very embeddedness in human relationships and the alertness of everyday life. Subjectivist women value what they see and hear around them and begin to feel a need to understand the people with whom they live and who impinge on their lives. Though they may be emotionally isolated from others at this point in their histories, they begin to actively analyse their past and current interactions with others.' (p. 85)

Reflection encourages the practitioner to pay attention to self within the context of human relationships and encourages this alertness to everyday life. The idea that practitioners are isolated is intriguing, many nurses talk of chatting with others, but to what purpose? Does such chat reinforce prejudices and discontent or does it enable the growth of knowing?

Procedural knowing: the connected and separate voices

I suggested that the subjective voice was largely unsubstantiated and, as such, at risk of being dismissed. At the level of procedural voice, the voice becomes increasingly substantiated because it is grounded in techniques of knowing the world.

The connected voice
Connected knowing is the ability to connect with the experiences of others through empathy. What is the other experiencing? What meanings do others give to their experience? Empathy is a dispassionate view, because in order to sense what is it like for the other, the practitioner must first know and clean her viewing lens to see the other's experience in the other's own terms rather than her own distorted interpretation. I shall pick this point up in Chapter 4 when considering the significance of knowing the person, but we can see that at this level, knowing the other is not simply opinion but grounded in connection. When the practitioner is skilled and confident at this level her voice becomes powerful in challenging the perceptions of others and ensuring that the other's voice is indeed heard within decision-making loops. The connected voice is the feminine voice grounded in morality of responsibility and care.

The separate voice
In contrast with the connected voice, the separate voice is dispassionate in its ability to critique and reason. It is the rational voice that seeks to understand things in terms of logic and procedures. It is the antithesis of received knowledge: no longer is knowledge accepted on face value but now challenged for its validity and appropriateness to inform the particular situation. This voice is the dominant voice within organisations, thirsting for the 'facts' and reasoned argument, even though most decisions are made in terms of authority and subjectivity. The separate voice is the masculine voice grounded in rules for justice.

Constructed knowing

At the level of constructed knowing, the practitioner weaves the subjective and procedural voices into an informed, connected to self and others, passionate and assertive voice. There is no longer any dualistic thinking between art and science as they are woven into practical wisdom. From the perspective of constructed voice practitioners view all knowledge as contextual, experience themselves as creators of knowledge and value both subjective and objective strategies for knowing. Virginia Woolf (1945) considered that the great mind was androgynous, having found the balance between masculine and feminine. Knowing is deeply embodied and expressed in intuitive ways. However, to close the circle, even practitioners capable of speaking with this level of voice may be silenced:

> 'Even among women who feel they have found voice, problems with voice abound. Some women told us, in anger and frustration, how frequently they felt unheard and unheeded – both at home and work. In our society which values male authority, constructivist women are no more immune to the experience of feeling silenced than any other group of women.' (Belenky *et al.* 1986, p. 146)

Writing as agentic action

Picking up the sentiment expressed in Belenky *et al.*'s quote, another way to view empowerment is in terms of realising and sustaining agency. Agentic people are clear on what they want to accomplish, understand how intended actions will contribute to their accomplishments and are confident that they can complete the intended actions and attain their goals. In contrast, the practitioner may perceive herself as a victim, feeling powerless to take action to realise her vision of practice.

The reflective effort is to move from the victimic position to become agentic (Polkingthorne 1996). To view self as a victim is to experience a loss of person-hood and to project the blame for this loss onto others rather than take responsibility for self. Loss theory (Marris 1986) highlights the need for people to connect between the past (traumatic) event and the present. Indeed it is this search for meaning that characterises this phase of life. Marris (1986) suggests that until people have made this connection it is difficult for them to move positively into an optimistic future.

In the victimic role the person is passive and receptive. Victimic people depict their lives as being shaped by events beyond their control. Others' actions and chance determine life outcomes, and the accomplishment or failure to achieve life goals depends on factors they are unable to change. Bruner (1994) notes that persons construct a victimic self by:

> 'reference to memories of how they responded to the agency of somebody else who had the power to impose his or her will upon them, directly or indirectly by controlling the circumstances in which they are compelled to live.' (p. 41)

Bruner's words highlight that the construction of life plots is always in relation to others. They are oriented towards avoiding negative possibilities rather than to actualising positive possibilities. In contrast, Cochran & Laub (1994) (as cited in Polkingthorne 1996), considered that the change from a victimic to agentic identity consisted of two correlative movements: the progressive construction of a new agentic life story, and the destruction and detachment from the victimic life story. The victimic plot does not simply fade away; it must be actively confronted, which can generally be seen moving within four phases:

Phase 1:   This first phase is dominated by the person's sense of entrapment or incompleteness, being controlled, helplessness – described as 'trapped in a world in which most of what makes life worthwhile is gone, and threatened by the possibility that this bleak existence might extend indefinitely.' (p. 90)

Phase 2:   In phase 2, people become involved in activities that will assist in (re)gaining an agentic life. Escape from phase 1 begins with the formation of a goal that is worthwhile and attainable (vision). The person takes ownership of their practice, and can see that their efforts make a difference and affect outcomes. The person monitors her progress and establishes standards for success in achieving progressively more difficult goals. Experiences of success in achieving their goals are crucial to validate the person's capacity to make a difference and fuel their optimism for a better future and produce a sense of freedom and control.

Phase 3:   In phase 3, people engage in activities more closely related to their goals in more self-directed ways – what Cochran & Laub (1994) describe as actually playing the game, whereas phase 2 was practising the game. The person becomes aware that the remaining major barriers to fuller and more agentic life reside as much in their own beliefs and attitudes; rather than outside themselves.

Phase 4:   In phase 4, people experience a liberating sense of completing their goals. Cochran & Laub (1994) note: 'Now one lives with a sense of life being on course, full, open to possibilities unrestricted' (p. 94). The person has achieved a sense of wholeness that is no longer threatened by former recollections. They have become authors of their own lives and taken control of their existence.

Reflection and writing would enhance the core ingredients of personal agency: self-determination; self-legislation; meaningfulness; purposefulness; confidence; active–striving; planfulness; and responsibility (Cochran & Laub, cited in Polkingthorne 1996). The person's work is to create a plot out of a succession of actions as if to direct the actor in the midst of action. Locating ourselves within an intelligible story is essential to our sense that life is meaningful (p. 812). Being an actor at all means trying to make certain things happen, to bring about desirable endings, to search for possibilities that lead in hopeful directions. As actors, we require our actions to be not only intelligible but to get us somewhere. We act because we intend to get something done, to begin something which we hope will lead us along a desirable route. And we act with what Kermode (1966, cited in Mattingly 1994) calls the 'sense of an ending':

> 'Because we act with the sense of an ending, we try to direct our actions and the actions of other relevant actors in ways that will bring the ending about.' (p. 813)

The significance of reflective practices for professional practice

Schön (1987) in his book *Educating the Reflective Practitioner* opens with these words:

> 'In the varied topography of professional practice, there is the high, hard ground overlooking the swamp. On the high ground, manageable problems lend themselves to solution through the application of research-based theory and technique. In the swampy lowland, messy, confusing problems defy technical solution. The irony of this situation is that the problems of the high ground tend to be relatively unimportant to individuals or society at large, however great their technical interest may be, while in the swamp lie the problems of greatest human concern. The practitioner must choose. Shall he remain on the high ground where he can solve relatively unimportant problems according to prevailing standards or rigor, or shall he descend into the swamp of important problems and non-rigorous inquiry?' (p. 1)

Schön's *swampy lowlands* draws attention to the type of knowing that practitioners need in order to respond to the problems of everyday practice that defy technical solution. Perhaps this is no more true than in nursing, where the nurse faces issues of distress and conflict within the unique human–human encounter on a daily basis. Having no solutions to apply, the practitioner must draw on her intuition, tuned through previous experience, to inform her response. Schön's distinction between the swampy lowland and the hard high ground reflects the dualism between art and science. The dualism is unhelpful and needs to be firmly pushed aside and replaced with the idea of practical wisdom.

Schön (1983, 1987) describes empirics as 'technical rationality' and notes that this type of knowledge has traditionally been the most valued type of professional knowledge above the type of knowing necessary to effectively navigate the swampy lowlands. Schön challenges this value hierarchy, suggesting that swampy lowland knowledge is most significant because it is the knowledge practitioners need to practice. Such knowledge is subjective and contextual. Subjective knowing has often been denigrated as a lesser form of knowing, even dismissed as 'anecdotal' by those who inhabit the hard high ground of technical rationality. It is as if people get locked into a paradigmatic view of knowledge and become intolerant of other claims because such claims fail the technical rationality rules for what counts as truth.

Benner (1984) and Benner *et al.* (1996), in determining the pathway from *novice to expert*, drew heavily on Dreyfus & Dreyfus's model of skill acquisition (1986), to consider the nature of expertise (see Box 1.3 for a comparison of novice and expert characteristics). In contrast with novices, experts intuit and respond appropriately to a situation as a whole without any obvious linear or reductionist thinking. These experts intuit by drawing on a reservoir of embodied or tacit knowing especially in situations of existential caring and coping skills akin to Schön's swampy lowlands. The novice simply does not have this tacit knowledge accumulated from past experiences. Reflection as a learning process,

Box 1.3 Comparison of novice–expert characteristics

NOVICE ←——————————————→	EXPERT
Linear thinking and acting	Intuitive
View parts in isolation from whole	Holistic or gestalt vision
Reliance on external authorities	Reliance on internal authority
See self as separate from situation	See self as integral to the situation
Application of knowledge	Wisdom

enables the practitioner to surface, scrutinise, and develop her intuitive processes and, *ipso facto*, to develop her tacit knowing. As Holly (1989) notes:

> 'It [keeping a reflective journal] makes possible new ways of theorizing, reflecting on and coming to know one's self. Capturing certain words while the action is fresh, the author is often provoked to question why . . . writing taps tacit knowledge; it brings into awareness that which we sense but could not explain.' (pp. 71, 75)

As a consequence, the practitioner may, on subsequent experiences, respond differently although still on an intuitive level. This is subliminal learning, only revealed in light of reflection on subsequent experiences. Of course, learning through reflection also takes place on a deliberative level. Indeed, through reflection, the practitioner will become more mindful and increasingly sensitive to her intuitive responses.

Cioffi (1997) draws on the work of Tversky & Kahneman (1974) to suggest that judgements made in uncertain conditions are most commonly heuristic in nature. Such processes are servants to intuition. The heuristics intend to improve the probability of getting intuition right by linking the current situation to past experience, being able to see the salient points within any situation, and having a baseline position to judge against. Without doubt, the majority of decisions practitioners make are intuitive. King & Appleton (1997) and Cioffi (1997) endorse the significance of intuition within decision making and action following their reviews of the literature and rhetoric on intuition; they note that reflection accesses, values and develops intuitive processes. The measured intuitive response is wisdom, another key quality of expertise.

Studies have been undertaken in an attempt to understand why research is not used in practice by practitioners (Armitage 1990; Hunt 1981). These authors suggest that blame lies with the practitioners because of their failure to access and apply research. However, Schön (1987) argues that little research has been done to address the real problems of everyday practice and that research always needs to be interpreted by the practitioner for its significance to inform the specific situation. The decontextualised nature of most research with its claims for generalisability makes this a difficult, if not impossible, task. Any claim for generalisability *must* be treated with extreme caution within unique human–human encounters. Such encounter is essentially unpredictable. The insensitive application of technical rationality is likely to lead to stereotyping: fitting the patient to the theory rather than using the theory to inform the situation. Schön exposes the illusion that research can simply be applied.

Technical rationality (or evidence-based practice) has been claimed as necessary for nursing's disciplinary knowledge base because it can be observed and verified (Kikuchi 1992). Historically, professions such as nursing have accepted the superiority of technical rationality over tacit or intuitive knowing (Schön 1983, 1987). Visinstainer (1986) notes that:

> 'Even when nurses govern their own practice, they succumb to the belief that the "soft stuff", such as feelings and beliefs and support, are not quite as substantive as the hard data from laboratory reports and sophisticated monitoring.' (p. 37)

The consequence of this position in nursing has been the repression of other forms of knowing that has perpetuated the oppression of nurses and of their clinical nursing knowledge (Street 1992). Since the Briggs Report (DHSS 1972) emphasised that nursing should be a research-based profession, nursing has endeavoured to respond to this challenge. However, the general understanding of what 'research-based' means has followed an empirical pathway reflecting a dominant agenda to explain and predict phenomena. This agenda has been pursued by nurse academics seeking academic recognition that nursing is a valid science within university settings. Whilst such knowledge has an important role in informing practice it certainly cannot predict and control, at least not without reducing the patient and nurses to the status of objects to be manipulated like pawns in a chess game.

Schön's notion of the hard high ground and the swampy lowlands reflect two types of knowing. However, I will take issue that the practitioner must choose which land to inhabit. Because of the very nature of everyday practice the practitioner must dwell in the swampy lowlands, and yet be comfortable with visiting the high hard ground for information to inform and assimilate into practice. Perhaps the reader can sense the swampy lowland as the world of the connected voice, and the high hard ground as the world of the separate voice. The reflective effort is to integrate these different ways of knowing in becoming a constructed voice.

Accessing reflection

People often say to me, 'Isn't it natural to reflect?', 'Don't we all do it anyway?', 'So what's the fuss?'. People think that reflection is just thinking about something and don't we all think? Well perhaps we do but that does not mean we reflect with the intention of learning through our thinking to develop new insights or perceptions of self and to shift the way we view and feel about the world.

Someone approaching reflection for the first time might ask certain questions:

- What is reflection?
- How do I do it?
- How do I know if I am doing it properly?
- How do I learn through reflection?

Numerous frameworks for facilitating reflection have been developed. In particular I introduce practitioners to four models that the practitioner can consider for their usefulness. These are Gibbs's reflective cycle (1988) (Box 1.4), Boyd and Fales's stages of reflection (1983) (Box 1.5), Mezirow's levels of consciousness (1981) (Box 1.6), and my own model for structured reflection

Box 1.4   Gibbs's reflective cycle (1988)

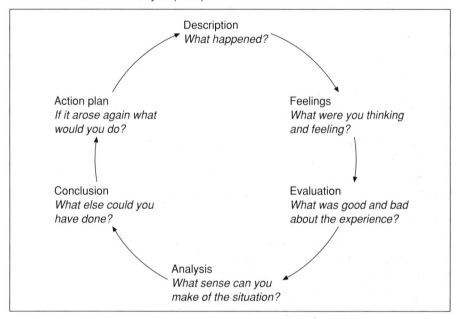

Box 1.5   Boyd and Fales's stages of reflection (1983)

- a sense of inner discomfort
- identification or clarification of concern
- openness to new information from external and internal sources
- resolution
- establishing continuity of self with past, present and future
- deciding whether to act on the outcome of the reflective process

Box 1.6   Mezirow's levels of reflectivity

Consciousness level
Affective reflectivity: becoming aware of how we feel about things.
Discriminant reflectivity: perceiving the relationships between things.
Judgmental reflectivity: becoming aware of how we make value judgements.

Critical consciousness level
Conceptual reflectivity: questioning the adequacy and morality of concepts.
Psychic reflectivity: recognising one's own prejudices and the impact of these on judgement and action.
Theoretical reflectivity: understanding self in the context of desirable action.

Box 1.7   Model for structured reflection – 14th edition

Reflective cue	Way of knowing
• Bring the mind home	
• Focus on a description of an experience that seems significant in some way	Aesthetics
• What particular issues seem significant to pay attention to?	Aesthetics
• How were others feeling and what made them feel that way?	Aesthetics
• How was I feeling and what made me feel that way?	Personal
• What was I trying to achieve and did I respond effectively?	Aesthetics
• What were the consequences of my actions on the patient, others and myself?	Aesthetics
• What factors influenced the way I was feeling, thinking or responding?	Personal
• What knowledge did or might have informed me?	Empirics
• To what extent did I act for the best and in tune with my values?	Ethics
• How does this situation connect with previous experiences?	Reflexivity
• How might I respond more effectively given this situation again?	Reflexivity
• What would be the consequences of alternative actions for the patient, others and myself?	Reflexivity
• How do I NOW feel about this experience?	Reflexivity
• Am I more able to support myself and others better as a consequence?	Reflexivity
• Am I more able to realise desirable practice monitored using appropriate frameworks such as framing perspectives, Carper's fundamental ways of knowing, other maps?	Reflexivity

(Box 1.7). This list is not exclusive; other models exist, which may have value for the practitioner.

Gibbs's reflective cycle takes the reflective practitioner through six stages. At each stage the practitioner considers a cue to help them reflect on experience. From the very outset, practitioners need to be encouraged to write vivid and spontaneous descriptions of their experiences. The emphasis on feelings is very significant because most reflection is triggered by feelings and decision is influenced by feelings (Callahan 1988). Gibbs's stages of *What was good or bad about the experience* and *Making sense* confront the practitioner to consider their normal way of thinking and responding within the situation toward gaining insights into self and practice. Boyd and Fales describe this perspective shift as *Changed perceptions* whilst Mezirow describes it as *Perspective transformation*. Gibbs's stages of *What else could you have done?* and *If it arose again what would you do?* focuses the practitioner on anticipating, fantasising and rehearsing other ways of responding with a view on future practice.

Boyd and Fales's (1983) six stages for reflection share much in common with Gibbs's model, which is reassuring for the would-be reflective practitioner wondering which model to use. Boyd and Fales's last stage *Deciding whether to act on the outcome of the reflective process* suggests that acting on perceptions and insights gained through reflection is deliberative. Perhaps on one level it is, but on another, altogether deeper intuitive level, changed perceptions of self must inevitably lead to changed actions.

Mezirow viewed reflection as emancipatory action, strongly influenced by the critical social science perspective. Mezirow's work suggests the depth of reflection through a number of processes spanning from consciousness: the way we might think about something, to critical consciousness: where we pay attention and scrutinise our thinking processes. This is a very significant idea, because it acknowledges that the way we think or feel about something may, itself, be problematic. I explore this idea more deeply in considering the nature of dialogue in Chapter 3.

Guarding against a prescriptive legacy

I am wary of cyclical or stage models because they suggest that reflection is an orderly step-by-step progression. There may be some value for stage models for novice practitioners in helping them grasp the essence of reflection, although I think the model for structured reflection does this adequately without the need for stages. My caution is that stage models immediately present reflection as some technical linear task. In a technology-driven society the risk exists that reflective models will be grasped as a technology and used in concrete ways. From a technological perspective, as opposed to a reflective perspective, the risk is that practitioners will fit their experience to the model of reflection rather than use the model creatively to guide them to see self within the context of the particular experience (I make the same point about models of nursing in Chapter 2). I have even seen the Model for Structured Reflection converted, or rather distorted, into a cyclical form (for example, see Bond & Holland 1998).

I must emphasise that all models of reflection are merely devices to help the practitioner access reflection, they are not a prescription of what reflection is. In other words, models are heuristic, a means toward an end, not an end in itself. From a reflective perspective, the practitioner will view all models for their value, rather than accepting the authority of the model on face value. Rather like the skilled craftsman, the practitioner will choose the tool that is most helpful.

Reflect on Rinpoche's words (1992):

> 'Largely because of our Western technological culture people tend to be absorbed by what I would call "the technology of meditation" [reflection]. The modern world, after all, is fascinated by mechanisms and machines, and addicted to purely practical formulae. But by far the most important feature of meditation [reflection] is not the technique, but the spirit: the skilful, inspired, and creative way in which we practice [reflect], which could also be called the "posture".' (pp. 64–5)

The model for structured reflection – MSR

The model for structured reflection is a technique to guide practitioners to access the depth and breadth of reflection necessary for learning through experience. The MSR was first designed in 1991 through analysing the pattern of dialogue that took place in guided reflection relationships and then framed within Strauss and Corbin's grounded theory paradigm model (Johns 1998a). Since then the MSR has been reflexively developed culminating in the 14th edition (Box 1.7). The cues within the MSR are arranged in a logical order, enabling a progression of thought through each cue. As I have noted, the cues are merely cues; the model is not intended to be prescriptive.

Bring the mind home

This first MSR cue is not so much a reflective cue but a preparatory cue, to put the person in the best position to reflect. The idea of bringing the mind home was inspired by Sogyal Rinpoche, from his book *The Tibetan Book of Living and Dying*. He states (I have replaced his meditation with reflection):

> 'We are fragmented into so many different parts. We don't know who we really are, or what aspects of ourselves we should identify with or believe in. So many contradictory voices, dictates, and feelings fight for control over our inner lives that we find ourselves scattered everywhere, in all directions leaving no one at home. *Reflection then helps to bring the mind home* (p. 59). . . . Yet how hard it can be to turn our attention within! How easily we allow our old habits and set patterns to dominate us! Even though they bring us suffering, we accept them with almost fatalistic resignation, for we are so used to giving into them.' (p. 31, cited in Johns 2002, pp. 10–11)

Do you recognise yourself in Rinpoche's words? The focus on bringing the mind home helps to shift the balance of seeing reflection as a cognitive activity to a more meditative activity; a time of quiet contemplation to pay attention to the self: the way I think, feel and respond to situations, mindful of the gusts that will blow us off course, and skilled to hold the rudder fast when the currents would take us elsewhere.

Yet can we create this space within ourselves to bring the mind home? Although I carry a reflective journal about with me from day to day, I find I am too easily caught up in my busy day to pause and write. Maybe there are moments when I can scribble a few words. It is in the evening that I can take some time out to reflect. Perhaps some breathing exercises – following the breath in and following the breath out – will help to bring the mind home and release the tension that has accumulated during the day. After a few breaths, your mind may be crowded with thoughts. If so, don't resist them but let them come and go . . . it is clearing the debris of the day. Maybe some thoughts will linger, especially if associated with some feeling and perhaps that is what you need to reflect on and write about.

Description

Some people like to tell their stories whilst others prefer to write them. Indeed many practitioners get stuck between telling their story and writing it. It is as if they hit a mental block. Perhaps the oral telling is more spontaneous whilst writing is more considered, more cognitive, more self-conscious. I sense the presence of an internal censor at work in writing that tries to fit the description into learnt ways of writing that dismisses or denigrates feelings and imagination. For whatever reason, some people struggle to write. Perhaps telling stories is essentially a creative right-brain act whilst writing is essentially a left-brain activity and between the two sides of the brain the connections are fuzzy and censored. If so, the practitioner may need guidance to release the imaginative and creative power into her writing.

Schön (1983) suggests a difficulty even in saying what we know, that much of our knowing is tacit and not easily explainable:

'When we go about the spontaneous intuitive performance of the actions of everyday life, we show ourselves to be knowledgeable in a certain way. Often we cannot say what it is we know. When we try to describe it we find ourselves at a loss, or we produce descriptions that are obviously inappropriate. Our knowing is ordinarily tacit, implicit in our action and in our feel for the stuff with which we are dealing. It seems right to say that our knowing is in our doing.' (p. 49)

So, how might you write? Here is an example from my shift on Friday, written on Sunday morning.

Friday 25th April, 2003
A message on my mobile phone from Kay, the senior nurse at the hospice: could I do a late shift this afternoon; her words 'as you can tell I'm desperate.' I feel ambivalent about this request, part of me says 'yes' because I enjoy working at the hospice and want to help. Another part of me is uncertain: I want to work on this book! I am at a meeting with Jenny and share my dilemma. She laughs and says I am feeling guilty if I don't say yes. She's right. Am I caught in the 'caring trap' that Dickson (1982) describes? I phone the hospice and say I will come in to discuss it.

When I arrive Kay is interviewing. Phyllis, the unit administrator explains the situation – there is no registered nurse cover. So I agree to do it on the proviso that Susan, my wife, has no arrangements this evening. But I still feel ambivalent, not helped by the fact I have to borrow a uniform.

I join the shift report. Kay joins us. The unit is quiet. Ray died yesterday evening. I had spent Wednesday looking after him and his family. Meeting and talking with Mary, his wife was particularly poignant – her sense of emptiness that Ray was not at home. She had spent so much time looking after him, and now she was alone in the house and didn't know what to do. She said how she reached out in bed and his side was empty. Yesterday was also their wedding anniversary, adding to the poignancy. But dying and death spares nobody. Yet I feel okay. I had only touched the surface of this family.

Later I phone Susan. She is going out this evening but offers to cancel, 'needs must.' Now my guilt spirals . . . I ask her to decide for me but she refuses. I sense the chaos of the unit and its fragile covering arrangements. The unit is quiet but . . . I decide to stay and Susan will cancel her evening out. An ironic twist for Kay, who is also going out. 'Now I feel guilty!' she laughs.

So much guilt, we dwell in a sea of guilt . . . trapped by our caring ethic . . . and yet it is because we care deeply and accept a responsibility as part of a caring community. It is the poignancy of talking with Mary; a release of spirit and love. I feel okay about my guilt and know I would respond in the same way again, yet with more certainty.

This was a very mundane event that I am sure many people can easily relate to. Yet within this description are very profound issues about myself and practice. Using the reflective cues I can now explore the situation more deeply if I feel it is significant. Some of the cues are already apparent within the description, reflecting that description has no boundaries but flows seamlessly within unfolding levels of reflection in the quest for understanding.

How was I feeling and what made me feel that way?

To re-iterate, reflection is most often triggered by negative or uncomfortable feelings (Boyd & Fales 1983). It seems natural to focus on negative experiences because these situations present themselves to consciousness. In general, practitioners are less likely to pay attention to experience that is normal simply because the experience does not project itself into conscious thought, or as Heidegger suggested, there is no breakdown. As practitioners become increasingly mindful of self within practice, then more experience becomes available for reflection, for example my own description above. I have also noted a shift of pattern as practitioners become more reflective: they reflect less on situations that show themselves as problematic and more on experiences that are self–affirming. Perhaps you have noted that within your own reflection?

A first year student nurse suggested to me that students always focused on negative experiences for two reasons; first, that was what teachers expected, and second, how can you reflect on a positive experience? He gave an example of a male patient thanking him for giving him a bath: 'What is there to reflect upon?'

For a moment I paused before this challenge and then a number of questions tumbled out:

- How did that make you feel?
- Is it important to feel like that?
- Why is it important to feel like that?
- How do you feel if patients don't thank you?
- Does it make you feel differently towards them (than those who do thank you)?
- If you feel negative towards the patient, are you less available?
- Do male patients like being bathed or touched by male nurses?
- How do you feel about bathing female patients?
- What theory might inform this discussion (for example the unpopular patient literature)?

It is like getting into a groove, tuning into the experience that appears, on the surface, as unproblematic. Scratch the surface and see what lies underneath. This example illustrates the need for guidance from another person perceptive enough to pose these types of questions, especially for practitioners who lack reflective or clinical experience, who have yet to develop their connected or separate voices. Yet what a rich teaching opportunity stemming from one line: *'A male patient thanked me for helping him bathe.'*

What was I trying to achieve?

This cue guides the practitioner to consider the purpose and meaning of her actions in terms of the way she grasped, interpreted and responded within the experience. The cue cuts across habitual action; so much of practice seems to be on auto-pilot: 'So why did I say that?' The cue brings one's personal and collective visions into focus.

Did I respond effectively?

Once the practitioner has clarified what she is trying to achieve, she can then consider whether her actions were effective. The cue challenges the practitioner to become mindful of her responses: how does she know whether her responses were effective or not? What criteria are used to make this judgement?

It is this cue that penetrates and surfaces any contradiction between our actions and our values. Yet what are our values? Are they valid? Are they shared by the patient?

What were the consequences of my actions on the patient, others and myself?

All actions have consequences for which the practitioner accepts responsibility. This cue guides the practitioner to contemplate the consequences of her actions on others and herself. It helps put the particular response (explored in the previous cue) into a wider perspective.

How were others feeling? What made them feel that way?

This cue guides the practitioner to appraise and develop their empathic connection with the other person, whether patient, family member or colleague. It challenges the practitioner to consider why the person felt as they did. So such questions as 'Why was she so angry?' 'Did I read her glance correctly?' 'Did she want me to do that?' might be in play.

What factors influenced the way I was feeling, thinking or responding?

This cue guides the practitioner to consider why she acted as she did. What factors influenced her? This always seems a difficult cue to respond to because so many factors that influence are deeply embodied and hence, not easily perceived. Yet it is an essential cue because unless we gain access to this self-understanding, it is difficult to bring about change in the way we think, feel and respond within particular situations. This is also quite a scary cue because it can require the person to look deep within themselves, unearthing, revealing influences that stem from social and cultural practices or past experiences that have left a scar in some way.

Box 1.8   Grid for considering 'What factors influenced my action?'

Expectations from self about how I should act? Conforming to normal practice?	Negative attitude towards the other?	Expectations from others to act in certain ways? Need to be valued by others?
Information/theory/research to act in a certain sort of way?	What factors influenced my actions?	Doing what was felt to be right? Guilty?
Emotional entanglement/over-identification? Strong feelings? Wrapped up in self-concern?		Misplaced concern? Loyalty to staff versus loyalty to patient?
Limited skills/discomfort to act in other ways? Stressed? Lack of confidence? Passive?	Time/priorities?	Anxious about ensuing conflict? Fear of sanction?

I have explicated common influencing factors into an influences grid (Box 1.8) as a guide for the practitioner to consider their impact within the particular experience, each of which leads the practitioner into a deeper reflection on the conditions of practice that may, on the surface, be taken for granted as normative.

What knowledge did or might have informed me?

This cue challenges the practitioner to identify, assess and critique appropriate theory or research for its value to inform the particular experience being reflected upon. Undoubtedly, the effective practitioner is an informed practitioner and must take responsibility for ensuring her practice reflects 'best practice'. Clearly this is a mighty onus on the individual practitioner given the vast amount of 'knowledge' and 'evidence' out there. An organisational response is required, for example developing standards of care and protocols (see Chapter 10). The relationship between practice and theory is developed further under theoretical framing.

To what extent did I act for the best and in tune with my values? (Ethical mapping)

This cue prompts the practitioner to pay attention to the ethical basis of her practice. To guide the practitioner to explore this cue I developed ethical mapping (Johns 1998b), shown in Box 1.9.

The ethical map trail

(1)   *Frame the dilemma*: most ethical issues can be reduced into a dilemma. For example, in Chapter 7 I use ethical mapping to consider whether Cathy should attend a patient's funeral or attend a management meeting.

Box 1.9   Ethical mapping (Johns 1998b)

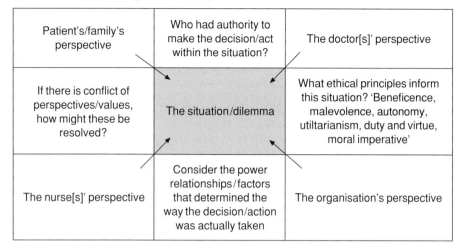

Patient's/family's perspective	Who had authority to make the decision/act within the situation?	The doctor[s]' perspective
If there is conflict of perspectives/values, how might these be resolved?	The situation/dilemma	What ethical principles inform this situation? 'Beneficence, malevolence, autonomy, utiltarianism, duty and virtue, moral imperative'
The nurse[s]' perspective	Consider the power relationships/factors that determined the way the decision/action was actually taken	The organisation's perspective

(2)   *Consider the perspective of different people commencing with the nurse[s]' own perspectives*: by considering the perspectives of people involved within the experience the practitioner is challenged to see and understand other peoples' perspectives and to confront her own partial perspective. It is rather like a fish bowl: depending on where you are coming from, you will see something different from other positions; each perspective is a partial view. These perspectives are not necessarily motivated by what's best but by personal, professional or organisational interests. Ethical mapping encourages the practitioner to move from her own partial view to gain a global or helicopter view of the whole. Only then is she in a position to negotiate in terms of what's best. Understanding the perspectives of others will help the practitioner develop empathic skills, which is the basis for all therapeutic relationship (this point is developed in Chapter 2).

(3)   *Consider which ethical principles apply in terms of the best (ethically correct) decision*: having gained an understanding of different and partial perspectives, the practitioner can then consider the way ethical principles might inform the situation. The major ethical principles are those concerned with professional autonomy – beneficence and malevolence, the idea of doing good and avoiding harm that forms the basis of the professional relationship. The professional will always have the patient's best interests at heart and will act accordingly. The other side of this ethical coin is patient autonomy: the idea that the patient's right to be self-determining is respected. From this perspective, the role of the professional is to enable the person or patient to make the best decision. One common dilemma is truth-telling. Natural tension exists between these two ideas of autonomy along which most dilemmas can be framed:

professional autonomy   ◄————————►   patient autonomy

Another key ethical principle is utilitarianism: the idea of greatest good whereby the needs of the individual are secondary to the needs of society as a whole. This principle involves the use of resources, justice and equity. Common issues are the use of time and appreciating priorities. From this perspective we can draw another natural tension along which many dilemmas can be framed:

needs of the individual   ←————————————→   needs of society

A further ethical principle is the idea of virtue or duty: the way the practitioner should conduct themselves befitting of the profession. An obvious example of this is that a nurse should always act in a caring manner. Nurses have a code of conduct that sets out the nurses' duty. Yet another ethical principle is Kant's moral imperative: 'do as you would be done for.' In other words imposing your own values into the situation – 'if that was my mother. . . .' The problem with this principle is that the patient is not your mother and that imposing such values may be misguided.

(4) *Consider what conflict exists between perspectives/values and how these might be resolved*: having considered the different perspectives and ethical principles, the practitioner can consider if conflict exists and if so, how it might be best resolved considering the ethical principles. I have previously noted (Johns 2002):

   'The map guides the practitioner(s) to view these competing perspectives from diverse ethical principles and to review the interface between ethical principle and the ethics of the situation (Cooper 1991).' (p. 15)

However, these principles are not prescriptive, they merely inform the thinking and counter the more subjective perspectives of the professionals involved. In an ideal world, professionals come together, including the patient as appropriate, to dialogue and find the best solution in terms of the patient's best interests.

(5) *Consider who had the authority for making the decision/taking action*: this part of ethical mapping challenges the practitioner to consider her autonomy, authority and accountability for making and acting on decisions. According to Batey & Lewis (1982), autonomy has two dimensions; legitimate autonomy as set out in the person's job description, and discriminant authority – the autonomy the person believes she has. However, job descriptions are often vague and working in bureaucratic organisations seems to diminish discriminant autonomy, especially for groups of workers such as nurses who may perceive themselves as a subordinate workforce, which may also distort their perception of responsibility. Reflection always seeks to empower practitioners to expand their field of autonomy and counter any sense of oppression.

(6) *Consider the power relationships/factors that determined the way the decision/action was actually taken*: in the real world, decisions are not necessarily made in terms of what's best for the patient or family, but in terms of power and fear of sanction. I explore the nature of power in relation to managing conflict in Chapter 7.

How does this situation connect with previous experiences?

An experience is not an isolated moment in time. It is part of a continuous stream of unfolding experiences. The cue challenges the practitioner to consider that if the experience being reflected on is linked to past experiences, how has the practitioner handled similar experiences in the past? Is there a pattern of response that the practitioner is locked into?

How might I respond more effectively given this situation again?

Besides linking the experience being reflected on with past experiences, this cue guides the practitioner to anticipate how they might respond to a similar situation in the future, challenging the practitioner to think laterally and imaginatively to see other options of response, even when they think they responded effectively. It is opening the shutters to other possibilities.

What would be the consequences of alternative actions for the patient, others and myself?

This cue follows on from the previous cue by challenging the practitioner to consider the possible consequences of responding in different ways within the particular situation. It helps the practitioner make judgements between different approaches. Considering each alternative way of responding is like planting a seed for responding in similar future situations (Margolis 1993). I develop this idea in Chapter 3 in relation to guiding reflection.

How do I NOW feel about this experience?

This cue draws the practitioner's attention to her feelings as a consequence of reflection. Is the practitioner left frustrated or angry or has she been able to work through the feelings in a positive way? What more does she need to do to mop up emotional mess and harness the residual bits of energy dissipated within the reflective space? How can she focus this energy for taking positive action based on insight gained? This work may be difficult to do without guidance from another person, another point I pick up in Chapter 3.

Am I now more able to support myself and others better as a consequence?

The penultimate cue challenges the practitioner to review their emotional and coping responses to the situations, and to reflect on the adequacy of their support systems within practice. As I have noted (Johns 2002):

> 'This cue often exposes impoverished support systems and challenges the practitioner to develop more effective systems.' (p. 17)

Stress depletes our energy, and it is our individual responsibility to keep ourselves in good shape to be available for therapeutic work. Yet so many of us carry loads of residual stress on our backs pulling us down, depleting our energy. Creating a therapeutic environment for practitioners as well as patients and families is explored in Chapter 7.

Before exploring the final cue – 'Have I learnt from this experience?' – consider the MSR cues in relation to my reflection concerning Ralph and Maisey I wrote one evening following a shift at the hospice.

REFLECTIVE EXEMPLAR 1.1 – RALPH AND MAISEY

I am very tired this evening but my head is full of thoughts of Maisey and Ralph, so I decide to write . . . Ralph is 68. He has SVC obstruction secondary to cancer of his bronchus. His condition is precarious. He quickly goes blue if laid flat. Because of this a scan to ascertain the extent of the blockage was cancelled. (But then I ask myself, why was the scan booked anyway – the urge for certainty?) There is no treatment except the 16 mg dexamethasone he has been having over the past three days that has made no difference to his condition. At the review meeting today, I feel certain we will begin to reduce the dexamethasone. Ralph wants to go home to die to be amongst the familiar surroundings of his life. Shandra is arranging his discharge this morning, ensuring the district nurses are well prepared.

I follow Shandra down the corridor towards Ralph's room. Ralph's wife, Maisey greets us by the door. She has just had a jacuzzi bath after sleeping in the room next to Ralph. She says she is refreshed – sleep is not easy. Ralph is asleep so Shandra leaves the medication on the side for a while. He has difficulty taking the 8 small dexamethasone tablets besides his other pain relieving tablets, gabapentin and diclofenac. He has a fentanyl patch and takes oromorph to diminish his anxiety with breathlessness. Perhaps another route would be an idea for the dexamathasone? Shandra agrees.

Ralph looks comfortable propped in the bed so I sit and talk with Shandra and Maisey at the table outside his door. It is social chit chat about all sorts of things, especially about food and cooking. I feel slightly restless – a need to do something rather than just sit here. But the unit is quiet . . . I must focus on silencing myself and dwelling. After about 20 minutes, Shandra excuses herself to do something and I can focus the conversation with Maisey more towards herself. She is one of 16 children, her mother first had twins when she was 16 and had Maisey when she was 46, thirty years of constant childbirth. Maisey is the youngest at 66. Just 6 children remain alive, the eldest being 86.

They have a large house near Luton . . . Maisey says she will stay there after Ralph dies even though it's so big, I think out of loyalty to Ralph. His presence will be in the house, and also because of her network of friends. Another part of her would like a more peaceful place to live away from the traffic.

Soon, I too give my excuses, it is hard to just sit for an hour. My body is tuned for more direct action at this time of the morning.

Later I help Shandra freshen Ralph. She asks me to hold him as we roll him so she can do a rectal examination. She has a sense that he is constipated which might further compromise his breathing. It will help him at home if we tackle any such problems now. But his rectum is empty. He has sores over his body and an elbow pressure wound drains copious fluid into a collection bag.

He struggles to stand and use a bottle. Indeed he is a large man . . . now we feel he should remain in bed so as not to compromise his breathing and provoke the SVC obstruction – we become more conservative, but does it really matter? Ralph agrees standing is now difficult although using a urinal in bed is not something he contemplates positively. A catheter is offered in view of him going home, but he declines, for the moment.

We finish his wash and tidy the room. I note his emaciated and dried legs. The skin is rough and dry and must feel uncomfortable. Another large pressure sore dressing covers one heel. I offer to moisturise his legs. Maisey says he has used aqueous cream but I suggest my reflexology cream may be nicer. It is my 'stock' jar with patchouli and frankincense. As before, I note the way Maisey and Ralph respond positively to the smell and rationale for these oils. For about 10 minutes I massage his legs and feet, moving my hands towards the heart, helping the sluggish circulation. Ralph is most appreciative.

Maisey sits close to Ralph . . . I sense Ralph's tears and then Maisey breaks away, tearful, and asks me to talk to him. She gestures through her tears and leaves the room. I know it's about the decision to go home. I sit with him, his lips tremble. He is caught in a dilemma: he does not want to be a burden to Maisey but he would like to be at home. He does not know what to do. We are silent and then he says he will stay. Just then Maisey comes back in, more composed. I inform her of Ralph's decision and immediately I know she is relieved because it takes an enormous pressure off her. She holds him, cradles him and says she will be here every minute with him. He needs this reassurance. I sense the fear rise in him and burst forth, his immense sense of losing Maisey, of being alone to die, fearing dying will be a lonely and frightening experience.

I observe them and feel such love. It is simply astonishing to be with people at such a moment. Maisey stands up and I sense the emotion flooding through her. I know it's right to offer a hug and she melts into my body and puts her arm around me . . . and for a moment or so I feel the tension ripple through her and then relax.

I inform Shandra that Ralph is staying, or at least he is staying for now. She goes to see him and Maisey as she must cease her discharge planning! I set up an aroma-stone with benzoin, lavender and frankincense. Ralph has a troublesome cough and I am mindful of using this approach with some success with Maxine [another patient]. I love the vanilla smell of benzoin. I talk through the benefits of the oils and they think the smell in the room will be beneficial for them all. As the warm smell percolates through the room I sense the spiritual dimension of the oils. Using the oils is also another sign to the family of our concern, that we are paying attention.

After a teaching session away from the unit, I return to say goodbye to the family. They are gathered like a tribe around the table, six of them. I am reminded of being with Elsie, Carol's mum with the family around the bed when I went to say goodbye. But today I feel I hover less on the periphery, that I dwell more within them even though I have not met four of the six people before. Perhaps I sense they know me because Maisey says, 'We have been talking about you' . . . (I guess in complimentary ways). I know she has been touched by my presence, just as she has touched the core of my being. Saying goodbye is never easy. Will I see them again? Will Ralph have died by Friday? I bless them with my love.

Reflection

This reflection was triggered by my interest in the idea of dwelling with a family as a family member approaches death. Consider the way I have addressed each of the MSR cues and the pattern they weave through the story. Is there a logical flow? I do not overtly use the model when I reflect because reflection has become so natural for me. Perhaps some of the cues are not addressed within the story. I can use the MSR as a list to check I have paid attention to all the cues.

Reflective cue	**Commentary**
What issues seem significant to pay attention to?	My uncertainty in responding to Ralph as Maisey rushed from the room distressed saying 'speak to him', framed within the bigger picture of 'dwelling with' this couple at this time.
How was I feeling and what made me feel that way?	Deep compassion; Anxiety: in responding appropriately and skilfully to ease their suffering that had burst out of its containment.
What was I trying to achieve?	To ease Ralph's and Maisey's suffering; to make them both feel more comfortable and less distressed in whatever way I could; to help them resolve their dilemma of where best for Ralph to die.
Did I respond effectively?	I think so – I am comfortable dwelling with patients and families as death gathers and using my massage and aromatherapy skills to create a sacred environment.
What were the consequences of my actions on the patient, others, and myself?	Ralph and the family were very appreciative of my actions. I felt I had achieved what I intended. I also know it was also a momentous time for Shandra being with this family, although I am uncertain how my actions affected her.
How were others feeling?	Full of emotion as Ralph slides towards death. Very positive towards me. I did wonder if I stepped on Shandra's toes. I asked her and she reassured me that

	I hadn't (I have been anxious about this before in my complementary therapist role).
What made them feel that way?	The immensity of the moment as death approaches.
What factors influenced the way I was feeling, thinking and responding?	Some fear of not responding well enough or messing it up (expectation from myself that I could respond effectively); not knowing the family; limited experience and skills and lack of confidence; doing what I felt was right – to ease suffering; stepping on Shandra's toes?
What knowledge did or might have informed me?	Certainly knowledge of different essential oils and their possibilities to help ease suffering – but being open to new possibilities with the oils. I know that dry skin is uncomfortable, I know massage is deeply relaxing. I was less certain about hugging Maisey as I did not know her well – but I was mindful of reading the signs well enough. I have been reflecting on my use of touch and reviewing the literature.
To what extent did I act for the best and in tune with my values?	I felt the tension between Ralph and Maisey and the way this tension created suffering. My action was to ease this suffering without undermining Ralph's autonomy.
How does this situation connect with previous experiences?	I had recently reflected on two other situations concerned with 'dwelling with' patients and families when death is certain and imminent. I have been developing a theory of 'dwelling with' and this experience contributed to my growing understanding. I was conscious of spending time with people in social chit chat and silence – overly concerned with my own comfort?
How might I respond differently given this situation again?	Such situations are very unpredictable – perhaps to be more comfortable with spending an hour with Maisey just chatting and steering the conversation more into Maisey's relationship with Ralph? But it is important not to delve too deep too quickly (is there theory to support that?).
What would be the consequences of alternative actions for the patient, others and myself?	Maisey and I would have 'dwelt better' – but only in theory – we were strangers first meeting under these circumstances – we needed to grope about to tune into each other. I felt that Maisey's head was elsewhere through most of the chit chat. I could have said no to Maisey's request or got Shandra to speak with Ralph but the moment would have been lost and I would have felt inadequate – does that matter? Yes. Responding was not about technique but being there.

How do I NOW feel about this experience?	Emotional but satisfied – it was a profound moment being with Ralph and Maisey.
Am I now more able to support myself and others better as a consequence? Am I more able to realise desirable practice? (using appropriate frameworks).	I would like to share this experience in supervision. Shandra was very supportive when we talked it through at the end of the shift. She more than I – I know she is also very close to this family. The experience enabled me to reflect deeper on my ability to 'dwell with families' as they face death. I am left wondering why I was restless talking so long with Maisey when it was so important for us to know each other and comforting for her not to be alone at this difficult crisis. My emotional turmoil revealed my lack of empathy and helped me become more mindful. My relationship with Shandra is strengthened.

Have I learnt from this experience?

The final MSR cue, 'Am I more able to realise desirable practice?', guides the practitioner to consider ways in which learning through reflection can be adequately framed. In earlier editions of the MSR, up to and including the tenth edition (Johns 1998c), I utilised Carper's fundamental ways of knowing (1978) as a valid way of framing learning (Box 1.2). Yet many practitioners struggled to interpret Carper's ways of knowing in meaningful ways because it was too abstract and didn't easily relate to the form of everyday practice. In response I advocate using the 'Framing perspectives' and the 'Being Available' templates as more accessible ways to frame learning (see Box 1.10).

In the MSR tenth edition, I had arranged the reflective cues to tune the practitioner into each of Carper's ways of knowing. I ceased this arrangement for the thirteenth edition (Johns 2002), simply because I no longer advocated Carper to frame learning through reflection. For this book I have decided to re-integrate Carper into the margins of the MSR.

As I will reveal through the book, much of theory can be designed as reflective maps to position and monitor the development of self in particular aspects of practice, for example the development of assertiveness and managing conflict (see Chapter 7). The templates I offer to frame learning through reflection are not exclusive, and you might prefer other templates.

Framing perspectives

A comprehensive approach to frame learning through reflection is offered by framing perspectives. These are a set of lenses that represent the breadth of learning necessary for becoming an effective practitioner (Box 1.10). Besides being constructed from research analysis (Johns 1998a), they offer a more congruent way to view learning than using Carper's patterns of knowing.

Box 1.10   Framing perspectives – learning perspectives within dialogue (Johns 2004)

Framing perspective	The practitioner asks – How has this experience enabled me to:
• Philosophical	confront and clarify my beliefs and values that constitute desirable practice?
• Role	clarify my role boundaries and authority within role, and my power relationships with others?
• Theoretical	link theory with practice in meaningful ways?
• Reality perspective	appreciate and shift those forces that constrain my realisation of desirable practice (embodiment, tradition and power)?
• Problem	focus problem identification and resolution within the experience?
• Temporal	draw patterns with past experiences whilst anticipating how I might respond with appropriate skilful and ethical action in future?
• Parallel process	make connections between learning processes within my supervision process and my clinical practice?
• Developmental	develop my expertise using valid and appropriate frameworks (for example, the Being Available template)?

Philosophical framing

Beliefs and values ripple below the surface of every shared experience. These can be teased onto the surface and held up for scrutiny in order to consider any contradiction between the practitioner's espoused vision of practice and the way she actually practises. Words like holistic can be explored for their meaning. Through philosophical framing the practitioner develops a more valid, robust and committed vision of practice.

Role framing

Each experience reflected on is framed by the practitioner's role. As such role framing challenges the practitioner to clarify her role responsibility and authority to act within the specific situation being reflected on. Responsibility and subsequent accountability are diverse (Box 1.11). Is there role ambiguity and conflict? If so, what is its nature? In sharpening her understanding of her role, the practitioner can develop a sense of autonomy and respond with more certainty and tackle issues of role conflict.

Theoretical framing

The basic assumption is that the effective practitioner is an informed practitioner, able to assess, critique and assimilate into practice as appropriate, relevant knowledge. In a world that values evidence-based practice then clearly such ability is vital. However, as with Belenky *et al.*'s separate knower,

Box 1.11 The diverse nature of practitioner responsibility and accountability

Accountable to	Rationale
The patient and family	To help them meet their health needs and support them through the medical response
Self	To act with integrity according to beliefs and values and to ensure self effectiveness
Society	To fulfil and enhance societal expectations of nursing
The organisation	To fulfil role responsibility
The profession	To justify actions within the guidelines of the UKCC code of conduct
Peers	To work in collaboration and mutually supportive ways to ensure patients and families receive congruent, consistent and effective care

all knowledge is viewed through a sceptical eye (Dewey 1933) – the reflective practitioner accepts nothing on face value. Knowledge merely informs, always needed to be interpreted for its relevance within the specific situation rather than applied as a prescription (Carper 1978). As Dewey notes:

> 'Reflective action entails active and persistent consideration of any belief or supposed form of knowledge in the light of the grounds that support it and the consequences to which it leads.' (cited in Tann 1993, p. 54)

Of course, this is the old chestnut of the theory–practice gap, as if these were two distinct types of knowing: 'knowing how' and 'knowing that'. Reflection synthesises these ways of knowing into *praxis* – informed and committed knowing within the unfolding moment; knowing that is always contextual and subjective. How could it be otherwise?

Reality perspective framing

I call this perspective the 'reality wall.' It is the point where practitioners struggle to take action because of those factors, either embodied within themselves or embedded within patterns of relating, that constrain them. The intention of reality perspective framing is to acknowledge that it is not easy to shift the reality wall, but that's okay – it is a real world and it's tough sometimes. However, we can understand the barrier of reality whilst helping the practitioner to become empowered to act in more congruent ways.

Just because we can understand something doesn't mean we can change it. But understanding it *is* the first step towards changing it. We learn to plot, become strategic, devise tactics. We are resolute, committed and patient.

Problem framing

Problem framing focuses the practitioner's attention to the way she has framed and resolved particular problems that are evident within the reflection. Once framed, the practitioner can see the problem for what it is and begin to consider ways of resolving it – to test in future practice. In this sense, reflection is very practical, and resembles an action-learning spiral of problem identification, understanding, resolution, subsequent action and reflection (Kemmis 1985).

Temporal framing

Reflection is never an isolated event but a moment of paying attention within the endless flow of experiences. This framing perspective guides the practitioner to consider how the present experience is informed by previous experiences. Are there patterns of behaviour evident? Do we keep falling into the same stream? Temporal framing facilitates the continuity of meaning between the present and past that Marris (1986) considers crucial in order to focus on the future in meaningful ways. If we are looking back at the past (with regret, resentment, disappointment, longing, fond memory) then we are not looking forward to new possibilities.

The other side of temporal framing is to anticipate the future – to be creative and imagine new ways of responding within situations. Over time, the practitioner can look back and reflexively plot a developmental journey through her experiences.

Parallel process framing

Parallel process framing perspective really only applies to situations where the practitioner has been guided. It invites the practitioner to consider the way the dynamics of guidance can inform her practice. It assumes the therapeutic relationship between the guide and the practitioner is a mirror for the therapeutic relationship between the practitioner and the patient or client. Box 1.12 shows this relationship.

The guide becomes a role model in the way she responds to the practitioner. As such the guide's responses, for example the guide's use of Heron's Six-category intervention analysis (Box 5.2), can be analysed, viewed and rehearsed in terms of the practitioner's practice.

Box 1.12   The guided reflection/clinical practice link

Guided reflection relationship ⟷	Clinical practice relationship
The guide works with the practitioner to help her to find meaning in her (work) experience, to make best decisions, and take best action to meet her developmental and practice needs.	The practitioner works with the patient to help her to find meaning in the (health–illness) experience, to make best decisions, and take best action to meet her health and life needs.

Box 1.13 Framing perspectives questions of Ralph and Maisey

- *Framing perspective*: How has my reflection about caring for Ralph and Maisey enabled me to . . .
- *Philosophical framing*: Is my vision of practice strengthened or developed?
- *Role framing*: Do I identify and resolve any role ambiguity or role conflict?
- *Theoretical framing*: Is my practice more informed?
- *Reality perspective framing*: Have I overcome constraints to practice more in tune with my vision?
- *Problem framing*: What problems have been resolved?
- *Temporal framing*: Have I drawn conclusions about responding more effectively?
- *Parallel process framing*: Are there patterns of learning between my experience and sharing it within supervision?
- *Developmental framing*: Am I more available to work with patients and relatives as a consequence of this reflection? (See also Box 2.6).

Developmental framing

How might I frame my realisation of desirable practice? The solution to this teasing question was to analyse the nature of desirable practice from over 500 experiences reflected on and shared by practitioners in guided reflection relationships. The result was the Being Available template (Johns 1998a). I explore this template in Chapter 2.

In Box 1.13 I use the framing perspectives to pose a number of questions to reflect on my learning from Ralph and Maisey's experience. I leave it to the reader to answer.

Writing a reflective journal

'What dark caves must you walk through? What do you fear? What are the things that make you hard and tighten your jaw? What memories still bite you? What situations or people do you avoid, postpone, run away from or aggressively blast through? These are your dark caves. Take the time to write these things down. Become intimate with your fears, for if you pretend they don't exist they are empowered, and then, they rule your life. Learn to walk through your fear. It is okay to be afraid and nervous and scared. You will not break. Each time you walk through your fear you become stronger and your fear becomes weaker. Each time you walk through your fear you learn more about yourself. What possibilities await you? Knowing the colours of your strengths, fears, challenges, and joy, what possibilities appear? Your dance can be danced with a variety of steps, a variety of expressions, a variety of emotion. Keep a journal of your strengths, fears, challenges and possibilities. Add to it when you can. Reflect on this often. Take the time to look over the results of the above discoveries. This is the mirror of your self. From this reflection, the final dance will appear.' (Blackwolf and Gina Jones 1996, pp. 52–3)

As a reflective practitioner I write reflections or stories of my practice in a journal. I wrote my reflection about caring for Maisey and Ralph the evening after the shift. I was tired but these thoughts and feelings were swimming in my head and I knew I wanted to write about them and to explore further the idea of 'dwelling with' the family as death becomes imminent. As always I doubted myself: in the intensity of the moment had I responded well enough? I felt I had moved into a new space within my practice that felt exhilarating but also uncertain.

Although I carry my reflective journal around with me in my briefcase, I usually write my reflections in the evening when I can dwell with my thoughts and consider the events of the past few days with less distraction than at work. I always reflect after each visit to the hospice or following a community visit. Even the most ordinary events have great significance for the mindful practitioner. Yet, interestingly, I rarely reflect on my educational work as a university lecturer, at least in a written format. Part of the reason for this is that I use my practice reflections as educational material and research activity. I like to teach the palliative care students 'around the camp-fire' where I share my own stories of palliative care to trigger stories in others and to role model the art of reflective writing.

I know that 'just take some time out to reflect' sounds like easy advice, but when our lives are addicted to being busy, it may be hard to focus one's thoughts within rather than be scattered outside. As Rinpoche (1992) says:

> 'We are fragmented into so many different parts. We don't know who we really are, or what aspects of ourselves we should identify with or believe in. So many contradictory voices, dictates, and feelings fight for control over our inner lives that we find ourselves scattered everywhere, in all directions, leaving nobody at home. Meditation (reflection) then helps to bring the mind home.' (p. 59)

Although Rinpoche was talking about meditation, reflection is a similar experience. If you consider that 'who I am' is the major therapeutic tool I use in my practice, then clearly I need to know myself well in order to use myself in the best therapeutic way. Reflection is about coming to know 'who I am', so I can refine and sharpen this tool for therapeutic work. As George Elliot wrote in *Daniel Deronda*, 'There is a great deal of unmapped country within us which would have to be taken into account in an explanation of our gusts and storms.' Reflection is mapping, charting the unknown self, to better recognise, understand and control these gusts and storms.

In his book *Awakenings*, Sacks (1976) says:

> 'In our study of our most complex sufferings and disorder of being, we are compelled to scrutinise the deepest, darkest, and most fearful parts of ourselves, the parts we strive to deny or not to see. The thoughts which are most difficult to grasp or express are those which awaken our strongest denials and our most profound intuitions.' (p. 15)

However, the deeper we go, the more defended we are likely to be, yet this is further reason why reflection may need to be guided to explore these depths within a trusting, caring relationship. It is our feelings that give access to the inner world, this is often a negative feeling or sense of discomfort about something that has happened during the day. So write a description of the feeling in your journal, in the middle of the page:

> I feel angry
>
> I am frustrated
>
> I am sad
>
> I feel so good

And then ask yourself some questions about the feeling – Why do I feel angry? Do I often feel angry in similar situations? Could I have not been angry? Etcetera.

Another approach is to simply write a story:

April 30
Today I felt angry at Jane, the junior nurse because I asked her to help a patient wash, but she ignored me and went to help someone else. I was puzzled why she did this. It made me feel angry but I could not challenge her . . . I just didn't want a fuss . . . but it made me angry . . . and I'm still angry at myself for letting her get away with it.

You might draw a line down the middle of the page and write the description in the left hand column and ask questions of the text in the right hand column. The questions flow naturally from the text yet are all grounded in the MSR cues:

Today I felt angry at Jane, the junior nurse because I asked her to help a patient wash, but she ignored me and went to help someone else. I was puzzled why she did this. It made me feel angry but I could not challenge her . . . I just didn't want a fuss . . . but it made me angry . . . and I'm still angry, at myself for letting her get away with it. I want to scream but it's bottled up inside me.	Why did Jane respond like that? How was she feeling? Does she normally respond like that? Was I sensitive enough in the way I asked her? Why am I so angry? How can I shift this anger? When I see her tomorrow, how will I feel? What do I need to do? Does transactional analysis help me understand the pattern of communication between us?

However, reflection does not need to be triggered by strong emotion, either negative or positive. As I have suggested, the most mundane experience can be a focus for reflection for the mindful practitioner. Reflection may be triggered by reading a publication or by interest in a specific aspect of care, as illustrated in my story of Ralph and Maisey.

Richardson (1994), in her review of 'the health diary' as a method for data collection, acknowledges that diaries can be structured or unstructured. The structured view focuses the research respondents to collect specific information about their life experience and illness management. The unstructured diary enables the respondents to focus on issues which they consider most significant. Structured diaries are easy and quick to write, thus making it more likely the diary is completed. This may be significant for people who are fatigued. However, some people may like to journal extensively in order to help find meaning in the illness and as a cathartic expression, for example the journaling of Moira Vass (see Chapter 5). Structured diaries are also easy to analyse whereas unstructured diaries require coding and interpretation. Both types require respondents to be able to read and write in the same language, thus excluding people from participation.

Therapeutic benefits of writing a reflective journal

The subtitle of Rachel Remen's (1996) book *Kitchen Table Wisdom* is 'Stories that heal', that in telling our stories, by reflecting on our experiences we can connect to something vital within us, something healing. In sharing our stories with others we realise we are connected to them and that we are not alone in the world. Connection is healing. Pennebaker and his various colleagues over many years have demonstrated the therapeutic benefit of journaling in well being, notably the benefit of connecting strong feelings to past traumatic events. Smyth *et al.* (1999) has developed this work to show the physical benefits of journaling on reducing symptoms in asthma and rheumatoid arthritis.

Smyth's (1998) review of the literature suggested that emotional expression has a salutary health effect, whereas emotional inhibition has a detrimental health effect. Emotional expression may take the form of writing or telling another person your story. Smyth cites Pennebaker *et al.*'s (1997) claim that:

> 'Written emotional expression leads to a transduction of the traumatic experience into a linguistic structure that promotes assimilation and understanding of the event, and reduces negative affect associated with thoughts of the event.' (p. 175)

Smyth's review highlighted that the ten review studies demonstrated significant superior health outcomes in health participants: psychological well being, physiological functioning, general functioning, reported health outcomes, but not for health behaviours. Smyth noted that these studies demonstrated that short-term distress was increased but is thought to be related to long-term improvement. Pennebaker *et al.* (1990) note:

> 'The present experiment, as well as others that we have conducted, found that writing about transition to college resulted in more negative moods and poorer psychological adjustment by the end of the first semester. Our experiment may have effectively stripped the normal defences away from the experimental subjects. With lowered defences, our subjects were forced to deal with many of their basic conflicts and fears about leaving home, changing roles, entering college.' (p. 536)

All indications from this study suggest that the power of confronting upsetting experiences reflects insight rather than cathartic processes. In follow-up questionnaires, for example, the overwhelming majority of the subjects spontaneously wrote that the value of the experimental condition derived from their achievment of a better understanding of their own thoughts, behaviours and moods. The stripping away of defence mechanisms means that practitioners and patients may need guidance to support them through the consequences of the writing experience (see Chapter 3).

Pennebaker *et al.* (1987) investigated whether it made a difference if the respondents told or 'confessed' their stories to another person rather than into a microphone. 48 respondents were randomly assigned to either talking to a microphone or to another person hidden from view (as in a confessional box). The only noticeable difference was that SCL (a response to inhibition) was higher for people when talking to another person, suggesting that talking to another person was inhibiting. The researchers state:

> 'The studies indicate that a personality dimension is related to the degree of disclosure. Those rated as high disclosers could be characterised as individuals who exhibited more negative effect and were more emotionally expressive than were low disclosers. Low disclosers tended to depersonalise their disclosures, even by their own admission.' (p. 530)

This is a pertinent observation in that journaling and self-disclosure will vary in its benefit. Indeed for some people who cope by non-disclosure, journaling or confession may be detrimental, at least in the short term. However, as Pennebaker (1989) noted:

> 'When given the opportunity, people readily divulge their deepest and darkest secrets. Even though people report they have lived with these thoughts and feelings virtually every day, most note that they have actively held back from telling others about these fundamental parts of themselves. . . . Over the past several years, my colleagues and I have learned that confronting traumatic experiences can have meaningful physiological and psychological benefits. Conversely, not confiding significant experiences is associated with increased disease rates, ruminations and other difficulties.' (p. 223)

An important dimension to coping with stressors concerns the degree to which people discuss or confront traumas after their occurrence. Jourard (1971) for example, argued that self-disclosure of upsetting experiences serves as a basic human motive. As such, people naturally discuss daily and significant experiences with others. When talking about a trauma with others can strengthen social bonds, provide coping information and emotional support, and hasten an understanding of the event, the inability to talk with others can be unhealthy (p. 213).

Smyth *et al.* (1999) shifted Pennebaker's focus on healthy college students to patients experiencing the specific chronic illness states of asthma and rheumatoid arthritis (RA). They sampled 112 patients with asthma or rheumatoid arthritis and assigned them in random controlled trial (RCT) groups to write either about the most stressful event of their lives or about neutral topics. Outcomes were evaluated at 2 weeks, 2 months and 4 months after writing. They reported that patients with mild to moderately severe asthma or rheumatoid arthritis who wrote about stressful life experiences had clinically relevant changes in health status at 4 months, compared with those in the control group. These gains were beyond those attributable to the standard medical care that all participants were receiving. For the asthma patients, the primary outcome measure was forced expiratory volume in one second (FEV_1). An improvement is measured as 15% improvement in functioning.

Evaluations of RA patients were made with a structured interview completed by the treating rheumatologist, rating diagnostic symptoms, global assessment of disease activity, symptom severity, distribution of pain, tenderness, swelling throughout the affected joints, presence and severity of deformities, assessment of daily living capacity, and general psychosocial functioning. This was based on a categorical scale (asymptomatic/mild/moderate/severe/very severe), and a shift in category gave on overall rating. There was 47% improvement in experimental groups, compared with 24% in control groups. Improvement was maintained in asthma patients whereas the change for RA patients was not evidenced until the 4-month period, suggesting that underlying physiological processes differ in different chronic processes.

The study by Smyth *et al.* indicates that writing about illness experience does reduce physical symptoms. Alexander (1998), in her role as writer-in-residence at a hospice noted:

> 'Writing is no solution to pain or illness. It cannot cure or heal physical damage but it can help a person to feel whole again, a human being with a story to tell.' (p. 178)

Alexander's role was to help others to express themselves in words. Whether words can heal is an interesting challenge and the focus for her present study.

Reflection as humanities

There are a number of poems scattered through this book that capture the poignancy and intimacy of the moment, expressing the self beyond a rational or cognitive level of knowing. Writing a poem is a release of tension, an expression of compassion, that honours self and other and the connection between you.

On the reflective practice course I direct at the University of Luton, my colleague Val Young does the *umbrella exercise*, asking students to write about themselves as an umbrella or as the wind. The results always astound the students. It is liberation from the bonds of rationality, a setting free in the world to be an artist, creative, imaginative, empathic, uncensored and caring. Often, after writing a poem, practitioners say that they do not know where their words have come from. Many are astonished that they can write poetry, as if it is some untapped, latent potential within us all. Yet in a technology-driven world, the latent artist may be buried under the demand for the rational, scientific, masculine perspective.

In one workshop I painted a reflection on my feelings after the death of Iris, a patient I had given reflexology to over two years. The painting was simply the six colours painted horizontally that represented each of the major chakras I balance as part of reflexology. In the middle of the painting I portrayed a gapping dark grey hole that represented the disruption of the energy fields with Iris's death and my sense of loss. Inside the hole I spread the shavings from sharpening the colour pencils, each shaving representing the fragments of Iris's life, the memories of being with her collected together. I wrote the poem *Shavings* to accompany the painting.

Shavings

I sense the black hole
Blown open inside
Its angst leaking out
Across the anguished soul

I sense the shavings of your life
Fragments of wholeness
Reflecting all the different colours
that flow within

like broken bits they float
about; unconnected
like bits of self
now lost

yet I see your colours bright
that surround the gloom
my hand connects you
to sense your beauty.

Christopher Johns

Richmond (1995) offers a Jungian perspective, that aesthetic expression taps the collective unconscious:

> 'a more profound layer than the personal unconscious and containing inherited patterns of behaviour revealed in the Universal symbolic images of phantasies, myths, dreams, or works of art.' (p. 218)

Perhaps that is where the words flow from, shaped into a beautiful creation. It is this sense of creativity that softens suffering and enables people to learn through reflection. As Parker (2002) writes:

> 'Art and aesthetic expression unite us and contribute to our wholeness. They are essential means of communication and move us all toward increased well being.' (p. 104)

Undoubtedly, caring is a form of aesthetic expression (Wainwright 2000) that both reflects and nurtures caring. Art opens up a creative possibility that moves beyond, although the practitioner may need a guiding hand to move beyond barriers that portray art form as soft and flakey.

One risk of introducing models of reflection is to structure writing to stifle the spontaneous flow of words. It is easy to get locked into the technology of reflection, 'how to do it', simply because we live in a technological world that demands explanatory models. Poetry is like taking a short cut to the unconscious, by-passing the cognitive realm. As such, aesthetic expression balances the more cognitive approaches to reflection, a more holistic approach that draws on and uses all the senses and tap the deep pool of tacit knowing (Polanyi 1958).

A number of studies have used art and poetry to help practitioners find meaning in their experiences of being with suffering patients (Begley 1996; Brodersen 2001; Eifried *et al.* 2000; Parker 2002; Vaught-Alexander 1994). Of course this is no surprise, because it is the essence of art therapy (Mayo 1996; Tyler 1998). These studies reflect the way humanities can open a space where practitioners can dwell with their own vulnerability within a safe space, where expressions of vulnerability can be expressed in whatever form and learnt from. As McNiff (1992, cited by Picard *et al.* (1999)) eloquently puts it, '*Whenever illness is associated with a loss of soul, the arts emerge spontaneously as remedies.*' Put another way, whenever activity is related to the soul, the arts emerge spontaneously as soul food.

Wagner (1999) interviewed 18 nurses for their reflections of family impact on the dying experience. She then reduced these experiences into a set of categories using fragments of the nurses' reflections to justify each category. In doing so, I felt she lost the meaning in these nurses' stories. However, Wagner then re-interpreted the nurses' words into poetry 'as a way of knowing subjectively and inter-subjectively the fullest meaning of the data' (p. 21). Her poetry reflects a deeper level of interpretation beyond cognition. In my mind it heals the story and makes it possible to connect with the experience because it is whole, it is felt rather than read.

Evaluating reflection

Reflective practice has been criticised for its lack of definition, modes of implementation and for its unproven benefit (Mackintosh 1998). Mackintosh singles out the Burford reflective model for criticism. She states:

> 'The benefits of reflection are largely unaddressed by the literature (*that is beyond unsubstantiated claims*), and instead the underlying assumption appears to be that reflection will improve nursing care or the nursing profession in some intangible way. This is demonstrated by Bailey (1995), who although describing the introduction of reflection into a critical area and claiming that an improvement in problem–solving skills occurred, gives no evidence that the quality of care was improved in any way. These failings can also be found in much of the literature describing the Burford reflection in nursing model (Johns 1996a, b) which attempts to integrate reflective practice into a clinically grounded nursing model through use of a series of 'cues'. Much of the published evidence regarding the model's impact on clinical practice appears to be based on personal anecdote, and again, evidence in support of its impact on patient care is of a mainly qualitative and descriptive nature.' (p. 556) [italics my inclusion]

Of course reflective accounts are subjective and singular. The accounts within the *Burford NDU model: Caring in Practice* (Johns 1994) were not cited in the above references. Yet in this book there are four collaborating accounts from Burford practitioners and accounts from four other nursing units besides Burford, accounts that testify to the impact of the Burford model on clinical practice. In other words, Mackintosh reviews the literature with her own partial eye, seeing or interpreting what she wants to read to support her prejudice against reflective accounts and qualitative methodologies. As Wilber (1998) highlights, different paradigms have their own rules for injunction as to what counts as the truth, and who better to know their own truth than the practitioner? To dispute that truth would mean that every survey, interview and psychometric test is flawed, tainted with the 'suspicion of authenticity', and perhaps more so because the truth is obscured behind an objective illusion. As I explore in Chapter 3, the role of the guide is to help the practitioner see herself more objectively and to challenge the basis for perceptions and assumptions.

The limitations of reflection as a mode of learning have been highlighted by, amongst others, Platzer *et al.* (2000). Platzer *et al.* noted that students may be resistant to revealing self, a point also highlighted by Cotton (2001) that reflection becomes a type of surveillance, assessment and control. Yet education has always been a socialisation process. Where teachers use reflection from a teacher-centred perspective, then it may be resisted. Platzer *et al.* further note that embodied ways of learning and organisational culture impose tremendous barriers to reflecting on and learning from experience. Without doubt there are barriers, but the barriers are a focus for learning and shifting, both within self and within the organisational culture. Real education isn't necessarily easy. Students may prefer to be fed what they need to know but is that an adequate preparation for developing critical thinkers? The MSR has been tested and found to be beneficial in enabling students to develop self-awareness and caring potential (Novelestsky-Rosenthal & Solomon 2001).

Burton (2000) has noted:

> 'It will be argued that reflective theory and practice has not yet been adequately tested and there is a pressing need for evidence to demonstrate irrefutably the effectiveness of reflection on nursing practice, particularly with respect to patient outcomes.' (p. 1009)

Burton challenges why the UKCC and ENB insist that nurses at all levels of experience reflect, when the evidence to support its benefits is unsubstantial. Perhaps she should ask, why do people think in the first place and read research findings? Yet Burton's words, again like those of Mackintosh, reveal the way people who inhabit a behavioural paradigm view reflection. They impose their own rules of injunction without appreciating the nature of reflection.

Reflection is *not* primarily a technology to produce better patient outcomes

Reflection is essentially about personal growth, and its impact on personal growth can only be known through the stories people tell. As narratives can exquisitely illuminate, the impact on patient care shines through yet not in any reductionist sense. For example see the research narratives published in Johns (2002).

Chapter 2

Constructing a Reflective Framework for Clinical Practice

In this chapter I reveal a reflective framework for clinical practice to guide practitioners to be reflective within their everyday practice. In the first edition of this book I described this framework as a reflective model for nursing. However, this terminology is no longer appropriate for two reasons. First, the usage of models of nursing has no contemporary value and second, the framework is appropriate to guide all health care practitioners.

Vision for practice

The vision for practice should be strong (Senge 1990) yet flexible. A vision for practice must always be a dynamic structure, always open to scrutiny and development. Until now I have used the expression *a philosophy for practice* but now prefer the term *vision* because it is more descriptive of seeing a way forward and avoids the difficulty people have with the word 'philosophy'.

A vision is a statement of desirable practice made up of the beliefs and values that practitioners have about nursing that gives meaning and direction to everyday practice. So ask yourself, Why do I go to work? What are my values? What am I trying to achieve as a nurse or health care practitioner? Are my values appropriate? How do my/our values fit within external agendas for health care services?

Taking nursing as an example, vision is a fuzzy idea because nurses (in the UK) have tended to view themselves in terms of what they do rather than in terms of what they believe. It is a functional, as opposed to a philosophical, understanding of self.

Functional perspective   ◄────────►   Philosophical perspective

Defining practice in terms
of what practitioners do

Defining practice in terms of
practitioners' beliefs and values

Nursing as functional gained prominence during the 1960s with the rise of technology and the medical model. Within the medical model, the ill person is reduced to the status of a patient with a set of symptoms that require investigation, diagnosis and subsequent treatment. Little significance is attributed to emotional, psychological, spiritual and social aspects of being ill or causes of illness. The nursing response is primarily to support the medical task. I am sure many readers will remember being told not to sit on the bed and talk to the patient – there is *work* to be done! The implication is that talking to patients is not work. Within this culture nurses suspended their own (caring) beliefs as relatively unimportant to the medical task. Even today, caring has been increasingly subordinated to unqualified staff as nurses continue to embrace medical technology work, despite the emergence of a holistic ideology.

As nurses have endeavoured to define nursing and construct nursing models, nursing as caring has become a sub-culture furtively taking place alongside the 'real work' of supporting the medical model. Whilst it is imperative to assume that all health care practitioners value caring, when the head is locked into the medical sphere and the medical sphere is most valued within organisations then practitioners may lose sight of the caring ideal and fail to realise caring. I know many readers will have experienced this state of affairs when visiting family or friends, or experienced heath care for themselves.

It is important to bring this conflict to the surface because only then can nurses take action to resolve the contradiction to realise caring as a lived reality rather than as some nice ideal. Yet in a world where the health agenda is dominated by productivity and a culture of 'more for less', times are hard for caring. Practitioners may switch off their caring simply because it is too painful to witness suffering and the failure to ease it. Indeed, as Halldórsdóttir (1996) suggests, suffering is caused by the *lack* of caring. Although most practice areas comply with the idea of writing a philosophy, these philosophies do not seem to profoundly influence practice. They are often written in vague rhetoric, often by the practice leader some years ago, and are found pinned on office walls covered by layers of organisational memos or, worse, buried away in a policy file. The rhetoric is often grounded in caring clichés such as 'we believe in holistic care' that has no meaning for practitioners and is clearly contradicted by even the most casual observation. It is one thing to say 'I believe in holism'; it is another thing to realise that as a lived reality. As I suggested in Chapter 1 there are many forces that constrain nurses from acting out their values. Of course, the failure to realise our values is felt deeply and frustrating, eating away at our integrity. Perhaps under such circumstances it is better to have no *real* values or at least to rationalise ideas as holism good but unrealistic.

To reiterate, at the core of a reflective framework for clinical practice is a *valid* vision. Where groups of practitioners work together it is self-evident that they need to share a common belief system in order to ensure a consistent and congruent approach towards patients and families. A written statement becomes a public statement that others – patients, clients, families, other health care workers, and society – can relate to. It sets up the possibility for dialogue and collaboration.

The process of writing a shared vision creates an opportunity for practitioners to discuss the meaning of their practice, nurturing a dynamic practice environment in which beliefs are constantly challenged and clarified for their meaning within practice. For example, words like *holistic* have become pervasive, but what exactly does *holistic* mean in practice? How does a holistic practitioner go about her work and relate to others? A vision or philosophy is the bedrock of practice, a springboard to guide all aspects of clinical practice and practice development.

As Senge (1990) so vividly states:

> 'When people truly share a vision they are connected, bound together by a common aspiration. Visions are exhilarating . . . they create the "spark," the excitement that lifts an organisation out of the mundane.' (pp. 206–8)

In writing a vision, practitioners reconnect themselves to their caring beliefs and values, beginning the process of empowerment that is central to realising the vision as a lived reality. As such, constructing a vision must always be a bottom-up approach to change that enables practitioners to grasp their own destiny rather than have it imposed on them. In doing so, practitioners become active creators of their own practice and take responsibility for realising their beliefs in practice.

Constructing a valid philosophy

In 1989, I challenged staff at Burford Community Hospital to reflect on the meaning of nursing within the hospital. First, I asked them to tell me about the hospital's philosophy. They struggled to respond to articulate this. At that time, the hospital philosophy was 'imported', based on the philosophy of the Loeb Center in New York (Alfano 1971; Hall 1964). Hall's work was a vision of nursing as the primary therapy in its own right, alongside a complementary and supportive role to medicine. In 1982, when Pearson (1983) introduced this philosophy, it made sense in terms of his vision to establish nursing beds. Pearson had departed Burford some three years previously to my appointment. Yet the philosophy remained, untouched, no longer relevant despite being a potent exemplar of a vision for therapeutic nursing. From the nurses' responses, it was apparent that the Loeb Center vision had faded. Practitioners who remained from that era vaguely remembered bits of it.

I realised that an 'imported' philosophy had imposed some sort of reality on practitioners, but had denied the expression of their own. In response I facilitated the construction of a vision that would both reflect the individual's beliefs and be a collaborative statement to give meaning and direction to our collective practice. I asked Burford practitioners to write statements of what they believed nursing at Burford should be on large sheets of paper pinned to the wall. Over the next three months more and more statements were added to the sheets. I then word-processed the statements and gave each practitioner a copy. We then explored these statements during two staff meetings, resulting in a composite statement. This was eventually agreed and became the hospital philosophy. The second edition (Box 2.1) was written six years after I had left Burford, reflecting the development of my own understanding of holistic practice and the fact that visions must always be dynamic, evolving in light of reflection of its value to adequately represent the nature of clinical practice.

Box 2.1   Burford Community Hospital Philosophy for Practice

We believe that care is centred in the needs of the patient. The nurse works with the patient as a person, from a basis of concern and mutual understanding, where the patient's experience and need for control in their life is acknowledged. In this way trust is developed between patient and nurse. The person is seen and responded to as a unitary human being, which includes all the person's social and cultural world.

Effective care is the first priority of this hospital. Caring is holistic, and intended to enable the person towards recovery and growth of health through rehabilitation, respite care, loss, dying. The hospital is integral with the community and responds to and promotes the community's needs, whether in the hospital where this is necessary, or in the person's own home. Assessment is carried out with sensitivity in a non-intrusive manner grounded in understanding the meaning of the event for the person. Through the hospital's status as a nursing development unit, we accept a responsibility to continually strive to improve our caring. By appropriate monitoring and sharing, we contribute to the development of the societal value of other nurses, health care workers, and nursing.

Our caring is enhanced when we mutually respect and care for each other within our respective roles. This means being free to share our feelings openly but appropriately, acknowledging that as persons, we are stressed and have differences of opinion at times. This is the basis of the therapeutic team that is essential to reciprocate and support our caring to patients.

Explicit assumptions

Based on the tradition that nursing models are underpinned by a set of explicit assumptions I deduced the following assumptions about the *Burford model: Caring in Practice* (Johns 2000):

- Caring in practice is grounded in a valid philosophy for practice underpinned by the unifying concept of human caring (Roach 1992; Watson 1988).
- All persons are seen and responded to as unitary human beings (Rogers 1986).
- The intent of nursing is to enable the other to realise recovery and growth as expanding consciousness (Newman 1994) through appropriate caring–healing responses.
- The nurse works with the other through a continuing advocacy dialogue (Gadow 1980) mirrored by an internal dialogue with self (reflection-within-the-moment).
- Caring in practice is made manifest, known and developed through reflection-on-experience.
- Realisation of caring in practice is determined by the extent to which the practitioner is available to work with the other (Johns 1996a).
- Growth is a mutual process of realisation.
- Caring in practice is a responsive and reflexive form in the context of the environment in which it is practised.

On reflection, it is startling to see the level of abstraction between this set of assumptions and the written philosophy (Box 2.1) created in 1997. I was

Box 2.2 Revised vision for clinical practice

We believe that caring is grounded in the core therapeutic of easing suffering and enabling the growth of the other through his/her health–illness experience whether toward recovery or death. The practitioner is mindful of intent and is available to work with the person and the person's family in relationship, on the basis of empathic connection, compassion and mutual understanding, where the person's life pattern and health needs are appreciated and effectively responded to.

Caring is seamless across health care settings and responds to and promotes both the local community's and society's expectations of effective service. In this respect, we accept a responsibility to develop a leaning organisation that continually strives to anticipate and develop practice to ensure its efficacy and quality. By appropriate monitoring and sharing, we contribute to the development of the societal value of nursing and health care generally.

Our caring is enhanced when I work in relationship with our (multi) professional colleagues on the basis of mutual respect and care for each other within our respective roles. This means being free to share our feelings openly but appropriately, acknowledging that as persons, we are stressed and have differences of opinion at times. This is the basis of the therapeutic team that is essential to reciprocate and support our caring to patients.

obviously intent on trying to ground the philosophy in current and contemporary theories of nursing alongside my own emerging ideas of reflection and caring theory. The lack of connection between the philosophy statement and the explicit assumptions is reflected in the fact that I rarely used these assumptions in public representations of the Burford model.

The third edition

Writing the second edition of this book has given me the opportunity to reflect on how I would now articulate a vision for clinical practice at Burford. The answer is shown in Box 2.2.

Revised assumptions

As the reader can discern, the essence of the old Burford philosophy for practice (Box 2.1) remains intact within the revised vision for practice (Box 2.2). However, based on the revised version I now make the following assumptions:

- Caring in practice is grounded in a valid vision for practice.
- The practitioner is mindful of easing suffering and nurturing growth as she goes about her practice moment to moment.
- The core therapeutic of nursing practice is the practitioner *being available* – a working relationship focused to enable the other to find meaning in their health–illness experience, to make the best decisions and help take appropriate action to ease suffering and meet their life needs.
- Growth is a mutual process of realisation.

- Practitioners accept responsibility for working toward creating the learning organisation (Senge 1990).
- Caring in practice is a responsive and reflexive form in context with the environment in which it is practised.

I shall consider each of these assumptions in turn.

Caring in practice is grounded in a valid vision for practice

What makes a vision valid? Retrospectively, I reflected on the original Burford philosophy for practice to consider what factors would need to be addressed to ensure its validity as a representation of caring practice, resulting in the development of the *four cornerstones*.

The four cornerstones

The vision must articulate in enough detail what is necessary to fulfil its function to give meaning and direction to practice. To ensure a philosophy is *valid* I have suggested that a vision for practice has four cornerstones that need to be addressed within the vision statement: the nature of caring, the context of practice, the internal environment of practice and social viability (see Box 2.3).

Box 2.3   Four cornerstones for a valid philosophy for practice (Johns 1994)

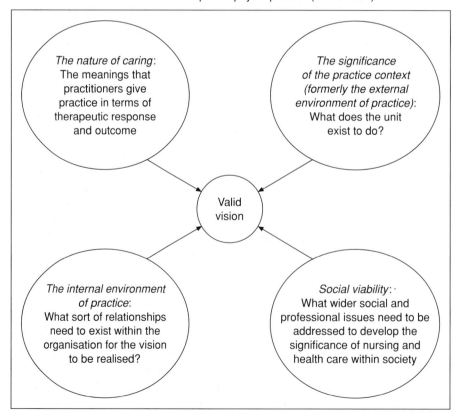

The context of Burford's practice was a community hospital. We felt strongly that the hospital was an extension of the community it served and provided in-patient services for those members of the local community who needed medical care but not admission to the local general hospital 20 miles away in Oxford. The hospital also took local people following major illness or surgery for rehabilitation, respite care and people with terminal illness. Caring is influenced by specialised knowledge that responds to particular needs: consider what is effective terminal care, effective rehabilitation, effective medical nursing and effective respite care? In addition the hospital provided minor surgery, minor accident and emergency, day care and out-patients. Clearly, to respond appropriately to such diverse needs the nurses needed to take an active and leading role in determining and realising the level of required expertise.

The *internal environment of practice* is reflected in the vision with its emphasis on the therapeutic team based on collaboration, mutual respect and care. The nature of the therapeutic team is explored in depth in Chapter 7.

Social viability

Social viability draws the practitioner's attention to three criteria (Johnson 1974):

- *Social congruence*: Do nursing decisions and actions which are based on the philosophy fulfil social expectations or might society be helped to develop such expectations?
- *Social significance*: Do nursing decisions and action based on the philosophy lead to outcomes for patients that make an important difference to their lives and well being?
- *Social utility*: Is the conceptual system of the model sufficiently well developed to provide a clear direction for nursing practice, education and research?

These questions challenge practitioners to look beyond the immediate context of the practice setting towards the wider social and professional communities. The questions demand that practitioners pay attention and incorporate both societal and professional ideology into their vision. In other words, the vision cannot be idiosyncratic. It is a public statement that challenges society to 'see' nursing differently, as making a significant contribution to the lives of its members and more generally to the health care of the community. This is an important point considering that so many people in society view nursing as a subordinate role to medicine, and nurses as the ubiquitous 'doctor's handmaiden'. Make no mistake, the general practitioners would have been happy to patronise nursing. Nursing's insistence to pursue its own philosophy resulted in much conflict, yet within the collaborative mind-set it was usually resolved to mutual satisfaction and, most importantly, in the health care interests of the local community.

To re-orientate society to value nursing requires positive action, yet such positive action is also required to ensure that society's 'new perception' of nursing is constantly reinforced by nurses living out the philosophy through their everyday dialogue and actions. To know whether nursing does make a difference to patients and to health generally within society requires programmes of development, evaluation and research that *adequately* demonstrate social viability.

The nature of caring

The reader can pull from the Burford vision its key caring concepts: the ideas of being mindful, easing suffering, nurturing the growth of the other, being available, connected and empathic relationship, compassion and appreciating pattern. These concepts are integral to the idea of wholeness or holism, that people cannot be reduced into parts or systems without reducing their humanness.

Without doubt, despite the best efforts of nursing theorists, an adequate definition of caring remains elusive. Caring is a subjective experience. It cannot be known objectively, reduced into types or attributes or a cluster of concepts. Such effort reflects a conceptual need to know the thing in itself, in order to teach, research and ultimately control it (Morse 1991). Caring can only be experienced within the unfolding moment as a moment between the practitioner and other. In other words it is ontological, a way of being. Shunryu Suzuki (2002) helps put this into perspective:

> 'Hashimoto Roshi, a famous Zen master who passed away in 1965, said that the way we [Japanese] cook is to prepare each ingredient separately. Rice is here and pickles are over there. But when you put them in your tummy, you don't know which is which. The soup, rice, pickles and everything get all mixed up. As long as rice, pickles and soup remain separate, they are not working. You are not being nourished. That is like your intellectual understanding or book knowledge – it remains separate from your actual life.' (p. 127)

However, this is not to say that caring philosophers or theorists cannot inform and challenge the practitioner to reflect on the meaning of caring. Jean Watson, in her transpersonal model of nursing (1988), states that the goal of nursing:

> 'is to help persons gain a higher degree of harmony within the mind, body, and soul which generates self-knowledge, self-reverence, self-healing and self-care processes while allowing increasing diversity. This goal is pursued through the human–human encounter caring process and caring transactions that respond to the subjective inner world of the person in such a way that the nurse helps individuals find meaning in their existence, disharmony, suffering and turmoil, and promote self-control, choice, and self-determination with the health–illness decisions.' (p. 49)

Watson's words focus on the individual nurse–patient relationship and perhaps needs to say something about the role of nursing within the wider community and in working collaborative ways with other health care workers. Yet, when I still read this now so many years after it was first published, I find there is resonance with the Burford philosophy. Interestingly, I took two

Burford primary nurses to listen to Watson speak in Oxford around 1990. They said she sounded just like me.

Savour Watson's words and sense the meaning. Can nursing be defined in this way? Would it suit all practice areas, health visiting, psychiatry or midwifery? Watson spirals nursing out of the realm or shadow of the medical model into a world of existential suffering where the uniqueness and mystery of what it means to be human is fundamental to healing and the fulfilment of human potential. Disease and illness are part of that pattern, although that part can so often create crisis for the person.

Watson's words are offered as a moment for reflection, as a challenge to widen the readers' vision of what caring might mean, not as a prescription of how the nurse should think about nursing. I know that such statements may seem far removed from the messy, everyday world of practice. Yet Watson (1988) does pay explicit attention to this messy world by noting the risks to caring both on an individual and societal level:

> 'Caring values of nurses and nursing have been submerged. Nursing and society are, therefore, in a critical situation today in sustaining human care ideals and a caring ideology in practice. The human care role is threatened by increasing medical techno-logy, bureaucratic–managerial institutional constraints in a nuclear age society. At the same time there has been a proliferation of curing and radical treatment cure techniques often without regard to costs.' (p. 33)

Watson's words emphasise the need to pay attention to 'social viability.' Practitioners may think that these 'political' issues are above them but unless they accept a responsibility for caring on a societal plane as well as within their everyday practice, then there is little chance for nursing to become more valued or assert any political clout to realise its therapeutic potential. The caring ideal as love may be scorned when we as nurses are so damaged or wounded that we cannot care or love. Watson says that it is this love that pro-vides the driving force to care. As I shall explore, it is this sense of concern or love that makes the practitioner more available to the other. Simply, without love for the other person, we cannot care because care is love. Without doubt, nurses, midwives, health visitors and all health care practitioners are aching to care. Such ache is like a flower that has not bloomed, like a sun lost behind a cloud; if caring is unfulfilled then it turns into acid to scar and burnout. Without doubt, patients and families need to be loved by nurses. They ache for this love and when they do not receive it they suffer. The sense of being uncared for is life depleting (Halldórsdóttir 1996) and increases, rather than eases, suffering.

The practitioner is mindful of easing suffering and nurturing growth as she goes about her practice moment to moment

This assumption focuses my interpretation of 'desirable practice' as easing suffering and nurturing the growth of the other through the health–illness experience and gives meaning to the idea of 'human caring.'

Easing suffering

Suffering manifests on the physical, emotional, psychological and spiritual planes. People suffer because they feel alone, isolated from themselves and from others. Hence, at the heart of easing suffering is connection – connection with self by listening to our own stories and connection with others who listen to our stories and say through words and actions that 'you are not alone.' Sometimes people need doctors to diagnose their suffering and prescribe treatment. Sometimes they need courage and support. Most often, people need a mixture of both. They always need someone available to guide them to ease suffering. Of course, the practitioner may also be suffering for whatever reason, and may need to know their own suffering so it does not interfere with seeing and responding to the other's suffering. To eradicate suffering is impossible, yet it can be eased by a compassionate and skilful response.

Nurturing growth

Whilst suffering is an expression of inner turmoil it does seem to offer an opportunity for growth, provided that people can face and respond to their suffering in a positive way. As such, caring is always the effort to enable the person to grow through their suffering towards a more harmonious state of being. Mayeroff (1971) states:

> 'To care for another person, in the most significant sense, is to help him grow and actualise himself.' (p. 1)

There is no mystery or mysticism to this idea. It does not need to be wrapped up in a web of scientific jargon or elaborate artistic strokes. It is fundamental to life itself and as such must be expressed in its exquisite simplicity. To actualise self is to fulfil one's human potential, whatever that might mean.

Newman (1994) has illuminated the way suffering creates the opportunity to stand back and take stock of self, especially when suffering becomes life-threatening. Then, one's taken for granted mortality is shaken, forcing self to contemplate life as impermanent. Forced out of our complacency we may question the very essence of our existence and the things that are really important to us. Newman expanded a view of health care beyond the narrow and reductionist focus of nursing models' focus on disease and health deficit. Yet disease does confront the sufferer with the taken for granted nature of health and much of life, prompting crisis; a breakdown where things no longer go smoothly, where things spiral out of control creating anxiety. The breakdown is experienced as a period of disorganisation and uncertainty. Old patterns of organisation no longer work. The person feels threatened on a deep existential level and is thrown into crisis. To overcome the crisis the person needs to learn new ways of organising self conducive with health. As Remen (1996) suggests:

> 'In the struggle to survive our wounds, we may adapt a strategy for living which gets us through. Life threatening illness may cause us to re-examine the very premises on which we have based our lives, perhaps freeing ourselves to live more fully for the first time.' (p. 156)

This can be very difficult, as the person is locked into ways of living that are not so easily changed. The practitioner's role is to help the person 'see himself' and to guide the person to reorganise their life pattern in ways that the crisis is resolved. This can be achieved by enabling the person to exchange energy with their environment, whereby the practitioner is a catalyst (Prigogine 1980, cited by Newman 1994) until the person can emerge from their crisis at a higher level of consciousness.

In the following exemplar I share my story of working with Tom one morning. I have used this story before in the context of giving meaning to being a reflective practitioner (Johns 1998c). The story has been constructed from my reflective journal I wrote following a shift one day at a community hospital. The story offers a point to reflect on the way Marie and myself responded to Tom to ease his suffering and nurture his growth.

REFLECTIVE EXEMPLAR 2.1 – TOM'S STORY

I went with Marie, a health care assistant (HCA) to wash Mr Sturch. I said, 'Hello Mr Sturch,' and explained who I was. He replied, 'Call me Tom.' I immediately sensed his need to be recognised and respected for who he was, together with his need for familiarity. We had been informed at the shift report of how miserable Tom was, being in hospital and being shut in a single room, because of the risk of cross-infection due to his diarrhoea. We were waiting for results of a bowel culture. If Tom's stools were clear he could be moved back into the main ward. As I was scheduled to work with Marie, I paid attention to who she was. She was in her fifties and very committed to caring. She loved it and would love to be a nurse. She was experiencing some strain in her personal life as her mother was very ill. She and her husband had moved here some years ago. Now she was having to travel every weekend, driving about three hours each way to care for her mother. I listened and was mindful of being available to her and helped her talk through her options, even though she had not met me before.

Marie's approach to Tom was familiar and caring, but task-focused. I immediately noticed the characteristic pattern of parent–child communication. Tom was like a little boy, upset but trying hard to be good. Marie was the mother, protective, kind, although her tolerance was limited to the extent that there was work to be done. I asked Tom how he felt this morning. He easily expressed his distress at being in hospital and shut up in this room. His tears were close to the surface. He felt lonely inside a side room and embarrassed that these poor girls had to clean him up. Marie kindly informed Tom that we were going to wash him. This was not negotiated with him. He needed considerable physical help as he had Parkinson's disease. His left hand in particular continued to tremor and his right side was weakened by a previous stroke.

We began to wash him as he lay on the bed, when he asked for the commode. I noted the impact of his Menière's disease, characterised by his nausea on standing. The symptom was poorly controlled. Ensuring he felt safe, we left him to use the commode. Afterwards, we helped complete his wash whilst sitting on the commode. I helped him stand whilst Marie washed his bottom. On seeing Tom like that I was struck by Mary Madrid's (1990) account about the nurse imagining who the patient is in terms of his past. Tom told me that he had been a staff sergeant in the army during the Second World War, working in recruitment training. I imagined him like that. How straight and proud he must have been, and now, what a different way to parade. And yet I could say that to him with humour, acknowledging his past while being empathic with this moment. I realised the significance of this approach in respecting people. Tom had been an engineer in microwaves, work that reflected his intelligence. I resisted a sense of pity at his current state. Instead I felt a wave of compassion towards him. I had learnt from previous experiences about acknowledging self-discomfort towards patients and families and confronting this through enabling the other to talk through their experience. In this way I converted my negative energy, pity, to positive energy, compassion. Stephen Levine (1986) helped me understand the tension between pity and compassion when he wrote:

> 'When you meet the pain of another with fear, it is often called pity. When you're motivated by pity, you're motivated by a dense self-interest. When you're motivated by pity, you're acting on the aversion you have to experiencing someone else's predicament. You want to alleviate their discomfort as a means to alleviating your own. Pity creates more fear and aversion. When love touches the pain of the other, it is called compassion. Compassion is just space. Whatever the other is experiencing, you have room for it in your heart. It becomes work on yourself – to let go, to stay open. To feel that being within you.' (p. 168)

After his wash, Tom cleaned his own teeth. He usually had an electric razor shave because the nurses felt clumsy with wet shaves. Tom liked a wet shave and I was able to do this little thing for him. I was reminded of the title of Martha MacLeod's (1994) paper *It's the little things that count: the hidden complexity of everyday clinical nursing practice*, and how this 'little thing' of shaving Tom made a difference in caring. I knew this informed Tom of my concern for him and, by paying him attention, my concern was fed and grew. I experienced a mutuality in his response. He began to care for me.

Although we had only just met, I had been involved with him in intimate physical care – washing him, being here while he was on the toilet, wiping his bottom, shaving him – and emotional presence. He easily disclosed other aspects of his life. He had been married for 59 years to 'wifie', his endearing term for his wife. Indeed, his diamond anniversary was in February. He became alive when talking about his wife and their life together. She visited in the afternoons. He desperately wanted to go home but he was anxious about the future. He was so dependent physically and even though they had a support package, he feared he would be too much of a burden for 'wifie'. I wondered if he would be happier with television, some music, or a paper? No, he just wanted 'wifie' and to go home. I was conscious of my need to 'fix it' for him, an almost overwhelming need to take his distress away from him. But of course, I was becoming anxious on his behalf, beginning to absorb his distress, which I recognised and could re-pattern to remain available to him.

He loved his shave. His happiness was for me to take a 'murray mint', his gift in return for my attention, my respect and kindness. In seeking to connect with me, he needed to give something back. By accepting, I could honour this need and he could honour himself. We began to tune into a reciprocal relationship, where I could respond with an appropriate level of involvement with Tom. In this way I synchronised our rhythms of relating with each other at this moment. Being in tune with him, I was most available to him.

I was mindful of the ways I paid attention to him in response to his feelings and needs, which had made him so happy this morning when he had been so miserable. Nurses are focused on the tasks of the morning and don't necessarily see him from his perspective. They may see him as a person but that's not their frame for responding. Marie noticed the difference in him this morning and passed this off as 'male company being good for him'. I was able to say when his doctor visited that Tom's stool was now semi-formed and to assert Tom's desire to move back into the main ward. This request was granted. I could also challenge the adequacy of the medical treatment for Tom's Menière's disease, to prompt a review of the medical response. The doctor welcomed my feedback. I felt good. I also had several 'murray mints' that morning.

Being mindful

In Tom's story I made a number or references to being mindful, mindful of who I am within the unfolding moment; mindful of the way I am thinking, feeling and responding within the moment; mindful of what I am trying to achieve, mindful of the impact of myself on the other and the other's impact on me. Yet Marie was not mindful of asking Tom what time he would like to bathe. Neither was she mindful of her impact on him. Like so much of care, it has become mundane and routinised. Such work has lost meaning. Paying attention to meaning is being mindful. Each human–human encounter is unique and, as such, essentially unpredictable. Each moment is an unfolding search for meaning and meaning will determine response. What time would Tom liked to have bathed? Probably, given the choice, he would say 'whatever time is convenient to you'. I know from previous experience that patients like Tom like to fit in with nursing patterns, they want to be co-operative, they do not want to be a burden despite their suffering. Perhaps they have learnt from previous experience it pays to fit in rather than be viewed as some difficult, dirty, demanding, old man. Perhaps Tom knows he will get more kindly attention if he does fit in.

Modes of being with another

Did Marie and I ease Tom's suffering or did we contribute to it? Halldórsdóttir constructed a typology of modes of being with another that ranged from

Box 2.4   Modes of being with another (Halldórsdóttir, 1996)

Modes of being with another	Description
Life-giving (biogenic)	A mode of being where one affirms the person-hood of the other by connecting with the true centre of the other in a life-giving way. It relieves the vulnerability of the other and makes the other stronger, enhances growth, and restores, reforms and potentiates learning and healing.
Life-sustaining (bioactive)	A mode of being where one acknowledges the person-hood of the other, supports, encourages and reassures the other. It gives security and comfort. It positively affects the life of the other.
Neutral (biopassive)	A mode of being where one does not affect the life in the other.
Life-restraining (biostatic)	A mode of being where one is insensitive or indifferent to the other and detached from the true centre of the other. It causes discouragement and develops uneasiness in the other. It negatively affects existing life in the other.
Life-destroying (biocidic)	A mode of being where one depersonalises the other, destroys life and increases the other's vulnerability. It causes distress and despair and hurts and deforms the other. It is transference of negative energy and darkness.

life-giving to life-destroying (Box 2.4). The typology offers a powerful reflective lens for the practitioner to consider her mode of being with another. The realisation that practitioners, through their attitudes and actions, can be uncaring and contribute to suffering, rather than ease, is a profound issue.

In my view Marie's mode of being with Tom was life-restraining, yet she would be horrified to view herself as such. Tom rationalised this approach as 'these poor girls' [having to look after someone like me]. Marie's response to Tom had become routinised and, as a consequence, her care of Tom had become depersonalised and focused around maintaining his physical needs. In contrast, my own mode of being was life-giving, connecting with him at the core of his own being and affirming his person-hood.

Patients and relatives need to feel cared for at a time of high anxiety. Studies by Reiman (1986), Mayer (1986), Larson (1987) and Halldórsdóttir (1996) are particularly significant in identifying the perceptions of both nurses and patients regarding caring and non-caring encounters. Halldórsdóttir worked with different groups of patients and women experiencing childbirth and cancer. Experiences of cancer were characterised by uncertainty, vulnerability, a sense of isolation, discomfort and redefinition. Because patients expect nurses to be caring, when they are not they often experience non-caring, characterised by disinterest, coldness and inhumanity, and this leads to a decreased sense of well being for the patient.

How was I feeling in this situation? I felt good as a result of my connection with Tom. I do not state my frustration with Marie and the unit generally. I did write in my reflective journal, 'why are we so blind to the patient's experience?' So how did I respond to my frustration? I did not share it with Marie although

I did write in Tom's notes highlighting the key issues in his care, notably his distress and fears. I also shared this verbally with the unit sister, having no confidence that the notes were an effective form of communication. I wrote in my journal:

> 'The nurse was receptive to my feedback, although again, I was sensitive not to overstep my welcome and be seen as some interfering academic. I thought to myself, we internalise self-regulation and yet how easy to marginalise self and become ineffective as a consequence. Another fine line to trip.' (Johns 1998c, pp. 21–2)

In these words the reader can sense that the factors that were influencing me were deeply embodied within me. I pick these issues up in Chapter 7. I hope I role-modelled a way of being with Tom that would influence Marie but I doubt I did influence her – she had already assumed that the difference in Tom was my male company, not because I had shown respect to him.

I have often used this story in my teaching to prompt discussion. The story evokes much passion, guilt and outrage. Yet the same nurses who express such strong emotion seem to be chained by their inappropriate models, seemingly unable to break free although they know there are more congruent ways of responding to clinical practice. Perhaps that is the guilt: knowing that they too slip unwittingly into routines that diminish person-hood and inadvertently cause suffering. They lead contradictory lives where the illusions of being a caring person barely paper over the cracks. In time, people who have contradictory lives become alienated from the self in the struggle to maintain the illusion. Jourard (1971) informs that people alienated from the self are unable to use themselves in any therapeutic way and hence are no longer able to care beyond a perfunctory response to the other as an object. Blindness is the refuge of those in despair, masking the truth.

Tom was in crisis yet the crisis presented an opportunity to search for and find meaning in his life. I could read Tom's crisis; it rippled across his being. I only needed to pay attention to who he was and read the signs that led to deeper underlying factors of which he and his family may be unaware. I was aware that Tom's needs (and his wife's needs) were not being met. The nurses' gaze was based on an 'activities of living perspective' (Roper *et al.* 1980) that obscured seeing Tom's crisis. He was seen as a collection of problems rather than as a whole, and yet his 'whole' screamed with suffering. I wrote in my reflective journal, 'why are we so blind?'

My effort was to guide Tom to learn from the crisis by helping him exchange his negative energy – despair, distress – for positive energy. I did this first by visualising myself as a space where he could exchange energy – a place where he could express and detach himself from his distress and despair – to look at it for what it is, to acknowledge, 'I am in distress and despair'. It was his pain, it belongs to no one else. So he had to own and accept it rather than try to hide from it. Second I helped Tom by understanding his story. To feel understood must be such a relief. I reinforced his humanness – that he was a worthwhile person with a positive future. This was not to give hope but to re-pattern the future as meaningful.

Finally, I attempted to reinforce his sense of self-determination and guide him to discover and take appropriate action to realise the possibilities. Tom has become dependent and may require more active help to realise his needs, yet I did so in negotiation and agreement with him rather than become parental and act in what I consider are his best interests. In doing so I am confronting and undermining his residual negative sense of self and reinforcing his positive energy for taking action.

Hopefully Tom will emerge through the crisis at a higher level of consciousness, having re-framed himself in ways so once again he feels in control of his life. His energy has been re-balanced. Once again life has meaning and he can be fulfilled. I became part of Tom's environmental field as he became part of mine. I can use my own energy as I do in body therapies, to channel and shift Tom's energy into a more positive pattern.

The core therapeutic of nursing practice is the practitioner being available – *a working-with relationship focused to enable the other to find meaning in their health–illness experience, to make best decisions and help take appropriate action to ease suffering and meet their life needs.*

In Tom's story I made reference to *being available* to him. Being available is not an abstract concept; it is always being available towards enabling the other in some way. In terms of my vision it is being available to ease Tom's suffering and help him to grow through his health–illness. It is being available to work with the person in order to enable him or her to find meaning in the health–illness experience, to make best decisions and to take appropriate action to meet their life needs. Gadow (1980) describes this as existential advocacy, contrasting it with a parental type of advocacy characterised by taking action in the other's best interests. Hence it is a *working with* rather than *doing for* relationship although, as I develop in Chapters 4 and 5, both are important types of relationships.

Six factors are significant in determining the extent the practitioner can be available (Box 2.5). These factors were explicated by analysing more than 500 experiences reflected on and shared within guided reflection relationships over a four year research period involving 15 practitioners in seven clinical practices (Johns 1998). The aim of the research was to understand the impact of guided reflection in enabling practitioners to realise desirable practice. The analysis resulted in the construction of the Being Available template as the core therapeutic of realising holistic practice. The analysis further enabled an understanding of the nature of effective guidance in enabling practitioners to become available. This work is developed in Chapter 3.

Read Tom's story again and consider each of the six factors that influence my being available to him. Does my vision shine brightly? Do I seem concerned or compassionate towards him? Does my compassion create possibility? How well do I know him? Do I grasp and interpret the situation well enough and respond skilfully? Could I have responded in other ways? Do I manage myself well enough within my relationship? Am I able to be available

Box 2.5   The Being Available template

The practitioner's ability to be available is influenced by:	Brief significance of each factor:
• The extent the practitioner has a strong vision of desirable practice	For my own practice this means being mindful of easing the other's suffering and nurturing their growth through the health–illness experience. Such vision gives meaning and direction to practice. It nurtures wisdom and focuses compassion.
• The extent the practitioner is concerned for the other	Concern for the other or compassion is caring energy. Concern creates possibility within the caring relationship – I pay attention to the other because they matter to me.
• The extent the practitioner knows the other	Knowing the other is empathic connection and appreciates the other in the pattern of their wholeness and the meanings they give to health. It is tuning in and flowing with the unfolding pattern of the person's experience.
• The extent the practitioner can grasp and interpret the clinical moment and respond with appropriate skilful action (the aesthetic response)	To be wise in the event (rather than after it) in making judgements and how best to respond within the situation. To be aware of my own limitations and take responsibility for ensuring I am skilful and to be confident in my intuition.
• The extent the practitioner knows and manages self within relationship	Being mindful of my own concerns so they do not interfere with seeing, responding and flowing with the other's concerns, and ensuring my energy is 100% available for caring work.
• The extent the practitioner can create and sustain an environment where being available is possible	Ensuring I work in collaborative ways with my colleagues towards our shared vision and can act to maximise available resources for caring.

considering the practice context? Do I work collaboratively with Marie? Do I surface and respond to conflict positively?

Each of the factors that determine the practitioner's ability to be available structure the next four chapters:

Chapter 4: Knowing the person and concern
Chapter 5: Responding to the person with appropriate and effective action
Chapter 6: Knowing and managing self within caring relationships
Chapter 7: Creating an environment where being available is possible

Growth is a mutual process of realisation

Being mindful, every experience is a learning opportunity for the practitioner's own growth besides the growth of the person receiving care. This is reflected in the fact that (holistic) caring relationships involve the therapeutic use of self within the human–human encounter. Reflecting on the efficacy of caring responses must always be a learning opportunity. This is exemplified through the text in my own and others' experiences.

Practitioners accept responsibility for and work toward creating the learning organisation (Senge 1990)

The learning organisation is concerned with establishing a work culture that is dedicated to creating the learning conditions whereby the organisational vision can be realised as a dynamic process. Learning becomes the norm in which every practitioner accepts a commitment and responsibility toward this common purpose. Senge (1990) identified five technologies that converge to innovate the learning organisation (see Chapter 10). These technologies are based on both individual and group reflective learning opportunities, such as clinical supervision as explored in Chapter 3, communication systems as in Chapter 8, and systems for monitoring quality as explored in Chapter 9. The key driving force of the learning organisation is the role of leadership, which is explored in Chapter 10.

Caring in practice is a responsive and reflexive form in context with the environment in which it is practised

This last assumption makes explicit what has been reflected in many of the other assumptions: the need to continuously gather relevant feedback to inform and nurture the development of practice. Being responsive is an open and proactive stance to both internal and external influences, whilst being reflexive is a dynamic learning approach that can adequately plot the emergence of new practices emerging from old practices.

A reflexive approach requires the development of systems that can sensitively monitor the quality of clinical practices, systems such as clinical audit and standards of care that are explored in Chapter 9. As with the learning organisation, these systems revolve around opportunities for both individual and group reflection.

From vision to reality

Whilst conceiving and writing a vision is a creative moment that gives practitioners a collective voice to articulate the meaning of their practice, how can such a vision become a lived reality? As Rawnsley (1990) challenges:

> 'Caring may be a desirable image for nursing, but is it meaningful? Is there congruence between the lived experience of nursing practice and the intellectual pursuit of caring as nursing's professional crest? When living the reality of their practice, nurses need ways through which they can connect the conceptual concerns of the discipline with the raw data of experience.' (p. 42)

Box 2.6   Structural view of a reflective framework for clinical practice

A culture that enhances clinical leadership	*A system for ensuring effective communication*	A culture of clearly defined role responsibility and collaborative teamwork
A system for operationalising the philosophy within each unfolding moment	**Vision of desirable practice**	*A system for ensuring staff are developed to use the model in effective ways*
A culture for creativity and positive risk management	*A system to ensure the model realises effective practice*	A culture that values holistic practice

My response was to construct a structural view of a reflective framework for clinical practice (Burford model – Box 2.6). The model consists of four reflective systems to facilitate practitioners to realise the vision as a lived reality against a cultural background that needs to exist to successfully accommodate a reflective model.

The four reflective systems

- a system for operationalising the vision within each unfolding moment
- a system for ensuring effective communication
- a system for ensuring staff are developed to use the model in effective ways
- a system to ensure the vision leads to effective outcomes

A system for operationalising the vision within each unfolding moment

How can a practitioner be guided to reflect on and respond within each clinical moment in tune with the hospital philosophy? It is proposed that a reflective model contains a series of cues to tune the practitioner into the caring concepts within the vision as a continuous process of grasping and interpreting the situation, envisaging the desired outcome, responding appropriately with effective action and reflecting on the consequences. This is essentially the aesthetic response (Carper 1978) I explored in Chapter 1.

A system for ensuring effective communication

How can practitioners who work in collaborative effort effectively communicate to ensure that patients and families receive consistent and congruent care? How do health care practitioners communicate in oral and written ways? Are these ways adequate or can more reflective ways offer a more satisfactory method? I shall address these question in Chapter 8.

A system for ensuring staff are developed to use the model in effective ways

How can the practitioner develop her ability to realise the vision as a lived reality? What skills are necessary? What attitude does she need? From Chapter 1, we might already state that the effective practitioner is a reflective practitioner who is committed and able to learn through everyday experience.

As I shall explore in Chapter 3, one developmental opportunity that is grounded in reflective practice is clinical supervision.

A system to ensure the vision leads to effective outcomes

How can practitioners get valid feedback that their practice leads to desirable outcomes for patients and families? In Chapter 10 I explore the way reflective techniques such as clinical audit and standards of care address this agenda from an organisational perspective, alongside the more individual process of clinical supervision.

Cultural accommodation

It is vital to acknowledge that the four systems are merely that – systems. Systems only work because of positive attitudes by practitioners to make them work. Hence systems need to be designed sensitively to ensure they work in ways congruent with caring processes and be open to review and change. Holistic practice is a reflection of deeply human–human encounters that seem a far cry from systems. Indeed, I sense from practitioners a deep distrust of systems, as if they represent a conspiracy against realising holistic practice.

There is a risk that innovative ideas that radically challenge usual ways of seeing and responding to the world will be rejected at worse or, at best, accommodated into practice in ways that fit with existing norms. Practitioners locked into normal ways may perceive the reflective practice as threatening and resist it in an effort to maintain the status quo, with which they are generally comfortable. When this happens, the ideal model is distorted and its impact minimised to the point that it makes no real difference (Latimer (1995) uses the example of the nursing process to illustrate this distortion). People may comply with the new idea if imposed from above but the result is a scratching of the surface. Perhaps a few missionaries embrace the ideal in relative isolation.

Hence, to accommodate reflective practice or indeed any radical change within practice, it is necessary to foster certain cultural conditions, as set out in the four corners of Box 2.6:

- a culture that values holistic caring
- a culture of collaboration teamwork
- a culture of creativity and positive risk management
- a culture that enhances clinical leadership

Understanding the way these cultural conditions support a culture of reflective practice acknowledges that managing change is a social process that will inevitably challenge deeply embedded social norms. These four cultural conditions always ripple just below the surface of all discussion and stories within the book. Sometimes the influence of these conditions is made explicit and sometimes it is understated, but it is always there for the discerning reader. A brief synopsis of each condition may be helpful.

A culture that values holistic caring

Reflective practice is symbiotic with a holistic approach to health care. As such, it will flourish in a culture that values holistic practice. Unfortunately (and here I might add, still unfortunately as the situation has not changed since the first edition was published) the prevailing culture of health care organisations does not seem to value caring beyond the rhetoric of 'patients first'. If this is true, then nurses and other health care practitioners must assert caring against a gradient of disinterest or resistance, where assertion threatens the status quo. To do so, the practitioner must become a political operator able to confront the organisation with the contradiction between its rhetoric of caring for patients and its reality of creating conditions where caring is not possible. Does nursing have an effective voice within the corridors of power? Ask yourself who your leaders are. Are they effective, or curtailed or have they sacrificed their caring ideals for those of the organisation itself? This is not easy work, if it is also true that nurses have been socialised to be a subordinate and powerless workforce (Buckenham & McGrath 1983) or to behave as an oppressed group (Roberts 1983).

A culture of collaboration teamwork

The essence of collaborative ways of working is for all practitioners to have a genuine appreciation and mutual respect of each other's role towards realising shared vision, whether I am a physiotherapist, nurse or a medical consultant. Further, each member of the team must take responsibility for their own performance within the team and supporting the collaborative ideal. This means confronting existing relational patterns that constrain collaborative work, most notably patterns that have emerged through hierarchical ways of relating that traditionally have fostered subordination.

As I shall explore in subsequent chapters, practitioners within the collaborative (or therapeutic) team must learn to dialogue and respond positively to conflict within the team, both of which require a high degree of self-awareness and assertiveness.

A culture of creativity and positive risk management

NHS Trusts are conscious of public image and litigation. Indeed, a cynical view might be that NHS Trusts are more concerned with public image than with patient care, although new public accountability bodies such as Commission for Health Improvement (CHI) really do seem to focus on patient care issues. As a consequence surface caring issues that have traditionally been shielded from view by other methods of accounting must be adequately addressed. However, nurses are in an unenviable firing line between management and the patient/family. Patients and families project their anxiety onto nurses. Management also projects its anxiety onto nurses to manage complaint. Nurses have internalised this anxiety by becoming consciously concerned with managing potential anxiety at risk of compromising caring ideals (Johns 1995b, 2002). Unfortunately this projection often results in nurses being blamed for situations and becoming the scapegoat. Inevitably, a blame climate leads nurses to become defensive and reactive and such a climate is not conducive to creative practice. Practitioners will sense a loss of control of their practice and feel powerless.

A culture that enhances clinical leadership

A collaborative or transformational style of leadership is required to guide shared vision, to nurture the collaborative team and generally resolve the cultural shifts necessary to effectively accommodate a reflective model for health care. Leadership is a very topical issue within health care. Government position papers emphasise the need for effective leadership at the clinical level and the pivotal role for nurses to manage change. Government sponsored programmes emerge such as the Leadership and Empowerment in the Organisation (LEO) programme to help foster leadership ability. The literature on leadership has a strong emphasis on transformational leadership; a style of leadership that is reflective and collaborative, with a strong investment in relationships and working with staff to realise shared vision. Again, this might be perceived as 'ideal' in a culture that might be regarded as essentially 'transactional' where leadership is perceived as driving a top-down agenda governed by outcomes rather than processes. In this approach there is considerable leadership anxiety to achieve outcomes, and, as a consequence, little investment in creating caring mutual relationships; indeed people are viewed essentially as a means to an end.

So at once we can see quite clearly a contradiction between normal NHS organisational culture and the transformational leadership to support a reflective and holistic model for practice. In Chapter 10, I explore a reflective approach to developing transformational leadership.

Reflect on your own culture. Do you work in a climate that fosters reflective practice? Do not despair if you are not optimistic. Remember the first step in becoming a reflective practitioner is to start from where you are and become open and curious about the way things are. As you explore the nature of contradiction then these cultural forces will emerge and can be understood for what they are, and a strategy can be planned to shift the conditions to better accommodate desirable practice.

Chapter 3

Clinical Supervision and Guided Reflection

And the stories begin

And the stories begin is part of the heading to Chapter 1 of Winnie the Pooh (Milne 1926). I use it because supervision is a space where practitioners, perhaps for the first time, can tell their stories. The essence of supervision is captured in the first few words of the chapter:

> 'Here is Edward Bear, coming downstairs now, bump, bump, bump, on the back of his head, behind Christopher Robin. It is, as far as he knows, the only way of coming downstairs, but sometimes he feels there really is another way, if only he could stop bumping for a moment and think of it. And then he feels that perhaps there isn't.' (Milne 1926, p. 1)

Milne might have been writing a text on clinical supervision such is his insight! Many nurses, like Edward Bear, are stuck in habitual and ritualised ways of responding to situations in which they feel powerless to change even though they know there are more caring–healing ways of responding. In busy lives that seem to be largely reactive to events it may be difficult to create the space (to stop bumping) to begin to think of better ways. In practices that seem to be governed by the interests of more powerful groups, as represented by Christopher Robin, it may be difficult to break free of established patterns of relating that represent the status quo.

The problem with thinking, is that it brings these issues into consciousness and creates a dilemma. How can we stop? How can we break free of the Christopher Robins? The words *'And then he feels that perhaps there isn't'* warn us of the need for practitioners to take action and break out of passivity or otherwise we are condemned to a life of suffering. Perhaps it is easier to conform and take pain killers for the sore head! Yet to do so will be to live an illusion where the contradictions between our beliefs and values and the way we practice are masked and defended from becoming invisible. The consequence is a gnawing away at our integrity as health care practitioners and ourselves as human beings.

Early days

I commenced working with practitioners using guided reflection in 1989 as part of a research project at Burford Hospital where I was both general manager and head of the nursing development unit. I was interested in exploring the use of guided reflection to enable me to fulfil my clinical leadership role to support and develop practitioners to become effective practitioners. This work extended over a four year period working with Burford practitioners and with practitioners in six other care settings. Dialogue from these sessions was recorded, making it possible for an analysis of the nature of effective practice and the dynamics of guided reflection (Johns 1998a).

Clinical supervision takes place as an adjunct to clinical practice characterised by a number of explicit aims, whilst guided reflection might be viewed as the developmental process that structures the clinical supervision space. Imagine clinical practice as a fast-moving river. In the busyness of the day, many practitioners feel they are being swept along in the current, reacting to events as they unfold about them. Now imagine an eddy within the fast-moving water that enables the practitioner to pause and observe what goes on in the fast-moving water. In this way, the practitioner may prepare herself to practice more effectively when she re-enters the current and not be so swept along. The eddy is still part of the dynamic harmony of events, it is not time out from the river itself. Yet the current is strong and the effort to find the eddy requires vision and resolve. The eddy must be seen as a desirable place. The current will not let you go too easily!

Clinical supervision

Clinical supervision has been defined as:

> 'a term used to describe a formal process of professional support and learning which enables individual practitioners to develop knowledge and competence, assume responsibility for their own practice and enhance consumer protection and safety of care in complex situations. It is central to the process of learning and to the expansion of the scope of practice and should be seen as a means of encouraging self-assessment and analytical and reflective skills.' (Vision for the future NHSME 1993, p. 3)

I have consistently used this definition because it reflects the fact that clinical supervision was promoted by the Department of Health in response to a perceived need for greater professional accountability or, put more sinisterly, surveillance to give the public confidence that nurses and health visitors' practice was being monitored. Midwives already have a form of mandatory supervision although the clinical supervision agenda by the Department of Health is a very different approach. The Department of Health approach was largely influenced by a psychotherapy and counselling model of supervision reflecting the backgrounds of the authors of a Government commissioned background paper (Faugier & Butterworth, undated).

The definition of clinical supervision suggests five key aims:

- to develop practitioner competence
- to sustain practitioner competence

- to safeguard standards of care
- to promote practitioner responsibility (for ensuring effective performance)
- to promote self-assessment (judgement of self performance)

On the surface these aims may seem contradictory. On one hand, we have an opportunity for practitioners to develop and sustain competence, but on the other hand a system that proposes surveillance to safeguard the public against standards of care. What are these standards? If they exist, then whose standards are they? Who will be making the judgement? If I thought that the main aim of a clinical supervisor was to judge my performance then I might be very careful about what I disclose, or reveal. Yet to see supervision as a learning opportunity I would need to feel safe to reveal any aspect of my practice. The contradiction is resolved, at least in my view, with the idea that supervision fosters the practitioner's responsibility to ensure and monitor her own performance against some idea of standard or competence.

Senge

A more dynamic and integrated perspective of the aims of clinical supervision are offered by the concept of the learning organisation (Senge 1990). Senge suggests that five component technologies converge to innovate the learning organisation, the realisation of which become the aims of supervision (see Box 10.1):

- to develop personal mastery
- to clarify and deepen our personal and collective visions of practice
- to scrutinise one's mental models and shift these towards realising effective practice
- to review and revise systems towards creating the optimum conditions for effective practice
- to develop dialogue expertise within supervision and practice situations to ensure effective practice
- to generate and sustain creative tension

These aims apply to all learning or developmental opportunities, not solely to clinical supervision and resonate strongly with the nature of reflection.

Models of supervision

Sloan & Watson (2001) distinguished between process and outcome models of supervision. They argue for a process model based on Heron's work (1975) and cite my own work as an example of such a model. Whilst I use Heron's work to guide practitioners to consider response options within situations, I have never explicitly framed supervision using Heron. I find a distinction between process and outcome spurious simply because I am mindful of both process and outcome.

Box 3.1   The intent–emphasis scale (Johns 2001a)

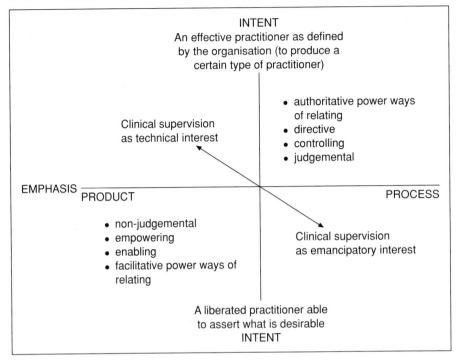

However, in my own research, I was able to make a distinction between those supervisors who are more outcome- or product-focused and those who are more process-focused depending on their intent and emphasis (Box 3.1) using Habermas's concepts of technical and emancipatory knowledge to draw a continuum between the different intent and emphasis of the supervisors (Johns 2001a).

In the research, I guided five managers and one practice development nurse to develop their supervisory skills whilst they supervised staff accountable to them. Three managed or developed discrete units, whilst the other three managed large district nursing practices. All the managers of discrete units were closely involved with everyday practice and held strong visions of what nursing should be like on their units. These managers were the most product-focused. The three district nurse managers who held vague visions of practice and were removed from everyday practice, were the most process-focused.

Given the small sample it is impossible to generalise, yet the distinction was strongly apparent.

The three managers of discrete units were more anxious about the perform-ance of the practitioners and, as a consequence, were generally more directive to guide practitioners to respond to practice in terms of their own ideals. They (unwittingly) saw supervision as a socialisation process to produce a certain type of practitioner. I say unwittingly because it was not their conscious intent.

Indeed, quite the contrary. However, they lived a contradiction that was very difficult to resolve. Listen to their words (Johns 1998a):

> *Pat*: 'it's obvious that the longer I've been here, the longer I know their patients and the more I question what is going on . . . and when I start challenging [in supervision], I sense the hairs on the back of their necks will start to rise and they become defensive.'

Linda had changed jobs but continued to supervise someone from her old practice:

> 'I can't monitor her effectiveness in practice. There is a missing link in supervision – if I was "on-site" manager I would be in a position to evaluate her development more clearly. How much is the contradiction in what I say effective – would it be more effective if I was there? Essentially I believe the supervisor should be the manager, otherwise there is or could be a large part of practice that may not be shared.'

Such understanding raises issues about who a guide might be and a cautionary note about being supervised by the practitioner's line manager. I say this despite the fact that I started supervising staff at Burford as line manager. I thought I had the practitioners' best interests at heart but on reflection I observed from patterns of dialogue that I focused practitioners to think, feel and respond from a holistic perspective. Clearly, genuinely sharing a vision is helpful.

Analysis of supervision dialogue (Johns 1998a; Johns & McCormack 1998) revealed a number of advantages and disadvantages with line management supervision (Box 3.2). Perhaps the most significant advantage is the development of collaborative relationships and the spill over of supervision dialogue into everyday practice. When this happens, reflection can be lived out in patterns of relating rather than be confined within the supervision bubble.

Supervisors will never perform well if they are anxious about the practitioner's performance. However, within bureaucratic systems such as the NHS, anxiety about outcomes and quality tends to be transmitted down through the system to unit leaders. Unit leaders know that they are held accountable for what takes place on their units rather than the individual practitioners. In an attempt to control this anxiety, unit leaders respond by using parental patterns. The effect is to impose conformity and stifle responsibility. This would be ironic as supervision has the specific aim of nurturing responsibility. The risk is that supervision is viewed in the old sense of the word 'supervision' to ensure a competent yet docile workforce (Foucault 1979).

The fact that practitioners did not reveal experiences that concerned me was startling. Was such the power of bureaucratic socialisation that they feared raising issues of potential conflict? My thoughts were confirmed by the fact that nowadays, all the supervision I give is from a non-line-management perspective, and that issues of conflict with management are frequently reflected upon.

Clearly, there are real advantages and disadvantages with line-management and even organisational supervision within a bureaucratic culture. Perhaps the bottom line is personal preference and whether the practitioner trusts her

Box 3.2   The relative potential advantages and disadvantages of line-management supervision (adapted from Johns & McCormack 1998)

	Advantages	**Disadvantages**
The supervisor knows the practitioner's practice	• Has a better understanding of issues the practitioner reveals • Opportunity for mutual reflection and supervisor growth	• Lack of vision to see other ways of doing things (tainted with the same brush as the practitioner)
Supervisor works with the practitioner	• Can tackle situations together • Spill over of supervision work into everyday practice	• Takes action of behalf of the practitioner
Pattern of management / leadership	• Work towards a collaborative relationship in practice as espoused within supervision • Opportunity to acknowledge and value practitioners	• Supervises as manages, reinforcing dependency and hierarchy • Manipulates agenda to suit own needs
Supervisor anxious about practitioner performance	• No advantage (should tackle such issues outside clinical supervision)	• Critical parent – overly critical and judgemental; need to 'fix it' syndrome • Nurturing parent – takes on board practitioner's distress ('hurt child')
Image of effective practitioner	• Work together to realise a shared vision of practice	• Moulding the practitioner or being remedial
Socialised within bureaucratic systems	• Fulfil clinical leadership role	• Practitioner may avoid sharing certain experiences, especially if grounded in conflict with the manager

manager? In Box 3.3 I set out the qualities of the ideal supervisor as identified by a training group at University College Hospitals, London that may help the would-be supervisee to choose a supervisor. However, I know organisations that impose patterns of supervision that deny the practitioner the option of choosing whether to enter supervision, who might be their supervisor, the mode of supervision (group or individual), and insist on auditing the outcomes by requiring notes to be made of each supervision session – all, in my view, against the ethos of supervision being a professional model of development.

It is patently obvious that if the practitioner senses any threat she will only reveal 'safe' experiences. If so, both the spirit and intent of supervision will be lost. It will be a sham, a game being played out that consumes time and fosters suspicion. It is the worse image of the 'confessional' (Gilbert 2000) – that the practitioner is expected to confess her 'sins' and will receive guidance and absolution. Under conditions of trust, the confession is an opportunity to reveal and learn through difficult experiences toward realising desirable practice.

Box 3.3　Qualities of a desirable clinical supervisor

• Strong sense of vision and purpose about supervision	• Concerned
• Listener	• Compassionate
• Challenger	• Experienced at reflection and supervision
• Non-judgemental	• Dynamic and powerful (not over me)
• I can trust	• Shares my clinical background
• Mutual respect	• Someone who doesn't know me
• Older and wiser	• Someone who I feel comfortable with
• Authentic/honest	• Someone who I'm attracted to
• Open/transparent	• Someone who I'm not dependent on
• Committed to the supervision relationship	• Someone who I'm not accountable to
	• Empathic

There is a real tension between supervision being promoted as a professional activity to benefit individual practitioners yet being implemented as an organisational quality tool – a tension played out along the continuum drawn in the intent–emphasis grid. If you are a supervisee, where do you place your supervisor? If you are a supervisor, where do you place yourself?

My own view is emancipatory, yet how realistic or ethical is it to promote emancipatory action within systems that clearly resist practitioner autonomy to act on new insights? Surely these insights could lead to the creation of conditions of practice where desirable practice can be realised. Is supervision at the level of emancipatory action no more than a furtive sub-culture of idealism? Do we end up playing in the safe shallow end, afraid of drowning if we step out of our depth where the obstacles of authority, tradition and embodiment await to snare us (Fay 1987)? Yet even in the shallow end, practitioners do become empowered to act on insights and shift practice for the better.

The need for guidance

For a number of reasons reflection needs to be guided to maximise its learning potential (summarised in Box 3.4).

To journal without guidance may be difficult and uncomfortable

Gray & Forsstrom (1991) note:

> 'The process of "journalling" may sound simple and easy to execute, but at times it was extremely difficult. Mostly the incidents recorded were identified because there was an affective component. This may be related to feelings of personal inadequacy to cope with the demands of the situation. Alone, it was emotionally painful to journal events that were largely self-critical.' (p. 360)

This is a significant warning to educators who simply expect students to reflect. Some practitioners may find writing helps them work through their feelings, but for others, writing about events, especially traumatic events, may lead to a

Box 3.4   Why reflection needs to be guided

- to journal without guidance may be difficult and uncomfortable
- to encourage and guide the practitioners to journal
- to listen to the practitioner's story
- to stoke the practitioner's felt conflict and support the practitioner to face up to anxiety rather than defend against it
- to reveal any self-distortion
- to see beyond themselves, to reveal possibilities for responding in new, more effective ways within similar situations
- to penetrate deeper, more critical levels of reflection to enhance the learning opportunity
- to plant and water seeds of doubt
- to co-construct meaning
- to nurture commitment and responsibility
- to challenge and support practitioners to act on new insights

sense of reliving the situation and distress because it confronts learnt ways of coping. As Cox *et al.* (1991) note:

'Reflection in isolation is difficult to sustain because of the difficulty in surfacing and transcending our own distorted self understandings, asking ourselves difficult, often self-exposing questions, facing difficult answers to such questions, and, perhaps most particularly, keeping our vision directed toward new possibilities for understanding and action.' (p. 285)

To encourage and guide practitioners to journal

Boud *et al.* (1985) observed how their model of reflection was something the student could do for themselves, but note that 'the learning process can be considerably accelerated by appropriate support' (p. 36). Yet many practitioners do struggle to keep a reflective journal (Johns 2002, p. 17). They are tired at the end of the day, they want to switch off, they don't see the value, they do not have the discipline, they don't find it meaningful, they reflect mentally, they work in a generally oral culture that eschews paperwork. I am sure you can add to the list!

Richardson (1994) cites Carp & Carp (1981), who observed that the quality of data from health diaries seemed closely related to the effect devoted by staff in encouraging diary keepers to maintain them. Keeping a journal makes reflection a daily activity and prepares the practitioner to share experiences within the guided reflection or clinical supervision relationship. If supervision takes place every four weeks, the practitioner who does not journal may only reflect every four weeks in preparation for the supervision session.

To listen to the practitioner's stories

Telling the story may be more significant than just writing it. Smith & Liehr (1999) note that when individuals tell their personal health story to one who truly listens, a change in perspective takes place. Citing Campbell (1988), they state:

> 'Self-discovery is embedded in story. Through story, persons search for clues or messages that potentate understanding and the experience of being alive described as a "resonance within one's innermost being and reality".' (p. 5)

Smith & Liehr (1999) demonstrated the therapeutic impact of enabling another person to tell their story in order to reduce blood pressure, suggesting that the therapeutic benefit of writing may be enhanced by sharing the stories with a person dedicated to listening and guiding learning through the particular experience. They give the example of a female attorney who experienced considerable stress in her work. In response to her story, the therapist (replace with guide) helped her to pay attention to her bodily responses, teaching her to breathe deeply and focus on calming images. Over the sessions she noted an increasing sense of calm as she came to take control of her life. Smith & Liehr describe truly listening as 'attentively embracing story as a process of connecting with self-in-relation to the person sharing their story through dialogue to create ease.' They note:

> 'As the disjointed story moments come together as a whole, there is simultaneous anchoring and flow through recognition of meaning, which empowers release from the confines of the old story. This is ease. It is calmness and vision even for a moment. It is a powerful moment creating possibilities for human development.' (p. 10)

Smith & Liehr did not ask their respondents to journal. However, as they note, the woman's story was disjointed, suggesting the difficulty many people may have in expressing their thoughts and feelings. Hence guidance may help to shape their reflection.

To stoke felt conflict and face up to anxiety rather than defend against it

Considering that reflection is most often triggered by negative feelings, the practitioner may naturally reflect to defend against anxiety rather than to face up to anxiety and learn through it. The role of the guide is to stoke the conflict of contradiction whilst supporting the practitioner to face up to anxiety, on the premise that the greater the felt conflict then the more likely the practitioner will do something about it. The key dynamic is the balance of high challenge – high support, whereby challenge is balanced with support to ensure any threat is contained.

I have already noted the significance of reflection as energy work – to convert negative energy into positive energy for taking action. The supervisor can guide the practitioner to visualise a space in which to place their feelings in order to look at them for what they are and focus on ways such feelings might be eased and converted into positive energy. In this way, the practitioner is unlikely to reabsorb the previous intensity of the negative feeling. When very strong emotions have been expressed or are apparent within the reflection,

I ask the practitioner to score the intensity of their feeling out of 10 and then again at the end of the session, when it is often much reduced. This gives feedback of the energy conversion.

To reveal any self-distortion

Reflection is always an interpretation of a situation, not the situation itself. So when practitioners reflect, they may unwittingly distort their experience of the situation for various reasons. It may be to defend themselves against some threat or anxiety, or simply because of habitual patterns of thinking about themselves. Clearly it is very difficult for practitioners to acknowledge their own distortions simply because of the difficulty to see beyond self in a rational way.

I do not think distortion is a phenomenon of memory although recall of an event obviously requires memory. Indeed, reflection has been viewed as a flawed process because of the limitations of human memory to accurately recall (Newell 1992). All stories are full of bias, contradictions and uniqueness (Remen 1996) and hence any firm grasp on reality is always tenuous. If people do distort their reality they do so for reasons that are, in themselves, a significant focus for reflection. As the practitioner becomes more mindful through reflection-on-experience, distortions become increasingly self-evident. The guide, especially if unattached to the situation being reflected on, takes a more objective view to help the practitioner see their flawed patterns of thinking and reveal distortion. Of course, the guide must be conscious of imposing their own patterns of interpretation, especially if they are attached to the situation, as can occur in line-management type supervision.

Because practitioners are generally 'normative', i.e. they take themselves and practice for granted, they may lack insight into current reality. Consider the story of Winnie the Pooh and the woozles from Chapter 3 of *Winnie the Pooh*: Piglet joins Winnie the Pooh as he was walking round the tree 'thinking of something else'. As they do, they become aware of their own tracks but misinterpret them, thinking that the tracks might belong to woozles. Christopher Robin is sitting up the tree watching and informs Pooh Bear what has been going on. Winnie the Pooh realises what he has been doing:

> ' "I have been Foolish and Deluded," said he, "and I am a Bear with NO Brain at All."
> "You're the Best Bear in All the World," said Christopher Robin soothingly.
> "Am I?" said Pooh hopefully. And then he brightened up suddenly. "Anyhow," he said, "it is nearly Luncheon Time." So he went home for it.'

In this story we can view Christopher Robin in a better light than bumping Edward Bear downstairs! Now he is a clinical supervisor with a helicopter view to help Pooh see things as they really are and to reassure him. He doesn't tell Pooh what to think or do, simply points out Pooh's flawed thinking. Often we get so caught up in things 'on the ground' that we miss the bigger picture, and lose track and panic. We feel stupid and beat ourselves up. We all get things wrong from time to time, so why make a big issue of it? Supervision helps put things into perspective and, after all, there are more important things . . . like luncheon!

To see beyond themselves, to reveal possibilities for responding in new, more effective ways within similar situations

Because practitioners get locked into themselves and practice in habitual ways, the practitioner may need challenging to think about things differently. The problem often lies with thinking patterns, our mental models that govern the way we feel, think and respond to situations. Lisa, a Macmillan support nurse in guided reflection with me, noted:

> 'I felt that being challenged is an essential element of supervision, providing that you feel comfortable in your environment and at ease with your supervisor. The challenge element encouraged me to think further than I had been and to deal with issues in a way I would not have considered before.' (unpublished supervision notes)

To plant and water seeds of doubt

I touched on the work of Margolis (1993) in Chapter 1; the idea that through reflection the practitioner plants seeds of doubt and possibility. Margolis considers that new ideas compete with existing ideas. The success of adopting new ideas depends on the robustness of existing ones and the force of argument available to support the new idea. The supervisor's role is to help plant these seeds of doubt in tune with desirable practice and to water them so the seeds grow and blossom, whilst weeding away old ideas that are no longer tenable.

Accepting the new idea is just the beginning, the ensuing congruent action cannot be guaranteed. As we have discussed, practitioners do not change their responses simply on a rational basis (Fay 1987). This point highlights the folly of imposing liberating structures such as supervision on people, in that practitioners, like nurses, who have been socialised to be powerless and subordinate, are unable to respond to liberating opportunities when they present themselves. The emphasis must be on the practitioner coming to find a new reality for themselves, rather than have this reality explained to them. For example, all shared experiences concerned with conflict have a fundamental power inequality at their root which manifests itself through different attitudes, beliefs and behaviours. This is not difficult to see or understand providing it is sought, and not just taken for granted as part of the 'natural' background of the experience. All understanding is cast against the practitioner's background while at the same time, the naturalness of social arrangements is challenged so that the practitioner and the guide become cognisant of both the restraints and the potential to change the situation so that the seeds of doubt will flourish and blossom. Through the continuity of clinical supervision or guided reflection sessions, new ideas can quickly be put into practice and subsequently reflected on. If the seeds don't take because the soil is stony, then the stone is chipped away slowly, until the moment when the new seed takes hold. This understanding reinforces the idea of change as a social process (Ottaway 1978), the need for patience, and emphasis on process not outcomes.

To penetrate deeper, more critical levels of reflection to enhance the learning opportunity

Powell (1989) in a small study with eight nurses on a post registered diploma course, used Mezirow's levels of reflectivity (Box 1.6), to demonstrate that every student, with one exception, did not naturally reflect at the level of critical consciousness. The one person who demonstrated some critical consciousness thinking was very experienced. The study doesn't outline the extent or quality of the guidance given. Although it is impossible to generalise from this study, it does suggest that critical consciousness thinking is outside the scope of most people's natural abilities, even with some guidance, but easier for people who can draw on experience. People have often challer.ged me, 'don't we all reflect?' That's probably very true but not at the depths Mezirow suggests are necessary for perspective transformation.

To co-construct meaning

The effort of reflection is to find meaning in experience and, on this basis, to contemplate new ways of being and responding. As the guide listens to the practitioner's experience she refrains from imposing meaning on the experience. Rather, she may tentatively suggest her own understandings after the practitioner has explored her own. This exploration is best done by picking up cues that seem significant and posing confronting questions rather than statements of fact. For example, using the Ralph and Maisey exemplar from Chapter 1:

'Maisey seemed very upset – why do you think that was?'
'What do you think she was thinking at that time?'
'Perhaps Maisey is torn between wanting Ralph at home and feeling she can't cope with him at home?'

Whilst this last question reflects the guide's interpretation of the situation, the guide is mindful not to impose it as a truism but simply to offer it as a possibility for exploration and mutual understanding, or what Gadamer (1975) describes as a fusion of horizons whereby the perspectives of both practitioner and guide are transcended in reaching new perspectives.

To nurture commitment and responsibility

The practitioner's commitment to practice may be blunted or that they fail to take responsibility for ensuring their own effectiveness. Given the significance of commitment and responsibility for clinical practice and reflection, the guide must first focus on helping the practitioner to re-kindle commitment before any real development can take place.

Karen, a practitioner, noted the flowering of her commitment to her practice and reflection:

'Sessions 1–6 were very much led by my supervisor, but in session 7 we had a sudden breakthrough and I took control. From then on I felt I was growing through supervision – I remember telling Chris I felt like a seedling in spring which has felt the sun and is now growing big and strong into a tree.' (Johns 1998a)

The growth of commitment to herself and to her practice was an emotional and revelationary experience for Karen. She noted how she increasingly looked forward to her sessions: 'I knew how much I benefited, but I also knew how much energy it took and I often felt drained afterwards' (Johns 1998a).

Initially Karen felt ambivalent toward supervision not just because of the effort of reflection, but because she felt threatened that her lack of competence would be exposed at the very time she was anxious to demonstrate that she was competent after qualifying with a nursing degree. At the time she needed most support she resisted it, which was an ironic twist.

In general, practitioners like Karen, once they had accepted responsibility for their learning, came to value supervision because it gave them positive feedback about the impact of their caring on the well being of patients and families and helped them resolve difficult situations and emotions.

To support practitioners to act on new insights

Effective guidance is the balance of high challenge and high support; high challenge as we have explored through each point why guidance is necessary, and high support to sustain the challenge, nurture commitment, infuse the practitioner with courage to take action to resolve contradiction and realise desirable work as a lived reality. Without adequate challenge the practitioner may rationalise the contradiction and decide to let matters lie, particularly where practitioners sense themselves as subordinate and powerless. They may fear disapproval and sanction. As Smyth (1987) notes:

'Most of us, unless we feel uncomfortable, shaken, or forced to look at ourselves, are unlikely to change. It is far easier to accept our current conditions and adopt the least line of resistance.' (p. 40)

Again the idea of stoking conflict arises. Guides who have the interests of the organisation at heart are unlikely to encourage the practitioner to 'rock the boat'. Hence organisational culture is such a significant background for the impact of clinical supervision for defining and enabling the realisation of desirable work. Lieberman (1989, cited by Day 1993) notes that:

'working in bureaucratic settings has taught everyone to be compliant, to be rule governed, not to ask questions, seek alternatives or deal with competing values.' (p. 88)

In response to Lieberman, Day (1993) asserts that reflection will bring the practitioner into tension with prevailing dominant organisational values, suggesting that reflection will struggle to make an impact unless the organisation is sympathetic to more collaborative ways of working. As I noted under the advantages of line-management supervision, supervision is potentially a way to move towards collaborative ways of working.

The participants in Kieffer's (1984) study of empowerment of grass root community leaders in the USA referred with great emotional intensity to the importance of the external enabler to support their struggle against more powerful others who were motivated to maintain the status quo. The practitioner connects with her guide or supervisor as a representative of the wider community; the gatekeeper and guide to this new world. In order to do this, the guide must connect with the practitioner in terms of her existing reality and, simultaneously in terms of a potential new reality. Fay (1987) puts it like this:

> 'Coming to a radically new self-conception is hardly ever a process that occurs simply by reading some theoretical work; rather it requires an environment of trust and support in which one's own preconceptions and feelings can be properly made conscious to oneself, in which one can think through one's experiences in terms of a radically new vocabulary which expresses a fundamentally different conceptualisation of the world in which one can see the particular and concrete ways that one unwittingly collaborates in producing one's own misery and in which one can gain emotional strength to accept and act on one's new insights.' (pp. 265–6)

These are powerful words that set the scene for effective clinical supervision. Clearly the attitudes of both the practitioner and the supervisor are important. Yet I meet few practitioners who are happy with 'their lot'. It is a tough world working within the NHS and practitioners are tired and frustrated. I get this message time and time again through the stories practitioners share with me on courses I teach or in clinical supervision. My hat is tipped toward the emancipatory intent, not because I am an 'agent provocateur' but because I value caring and sense its vulnerability in the prevailing organisational culture. I do not like to see nurses suffer because of lack of caring. Yet I must be careful because reflection can hurtle people against walls that are unyielding. Reflection can be painful. Hence the need for commitment, that my practice matters to me, to sustain the challenge and live through the pain.

Carl Rogers (1969) noted how people were ambivalent to learn because any significant learning involves a certain amount of pain, either pain connected with learning itself or giving up previous learning. He notes that the first type of ambivalence is illustrated by the small child who is learning to walk. He stumbles, he falls, he hurts himself. It is a painful process. Yet the satisfaction of developing his potential far outweighs the bumps and bruises. Or in the immortal words of CS Lewis spoken by Anthony Hopkins in the film *Shadowlands*:

> 'I've just come up against a bit of experience. Experience is a brutal teacher but by God you learn . . . you learn.'

But you learn more with support and challenge from an appropriate guide. So practitioners, choose your guides with care and take control of the supervision agenda – it is *your* practice!

Reflection may create a sense of crisis of confidence and even identity as one's 'old ways' are challenged. The practitioner is caught between defending self from this anxiety and opening self to new possibilities. However, in exploring new, more congruent ways, the practitioner may experience a crisis of isolation or separateness (Isaacs 1993) whereby group norms and ways of relating must shift. This may overflow into personal lives as practitioners find their voices and speak out. Isaacs notes:

> 'Such loosening of rigid thought patterns frees energy that now permits new levels of intelligence and creativity.' (p. 38)

The voice of freedom is a powerful cry and may be resisted by those affected by the practitioner's new ways of thinking, feeling and responding to situations. Through dialogue the practitioner can emerge transformed into a new dawn, ever mindful. We need to choose our guides carefully.

The nature of the supervisory relationship

As a formal relationship, clinical supervision needs to be contracted.

Contracting

> 'If supervision is to become and remain a co-operative experience which allows for real, rather than token, accountability, a clear, even tough, working agreement needs to be negotiated. The agreement needs to provide sufficient safety and clarity for the student/worker to know where she stands; and it needs sufficient teeth for the supervisor to feel free and responsible for making the challenges.' (Proctor 1988, cited by Hawkins & Shohet 1989, p. 29)

In establishing a clinical supervision relationship, both parties need to be clear about the intent of supervision. For example, it is not about the self per se but the self in context of her practice. In other words, a distinction needs to be made between what is construed as clinical supervision work and therapy. To some extent the two issues can overlap. For example, a practitioner in exploring her feelings about the death of a patient, also explores her feelings about her mother's death. Perhaps, in responding to her anger towards her manager, the practitioner notes that 'he acts like my father'. The supervisor or guide will point out the association and transference, but should keep the dialogue focused on the practice event. Practitioners do not generally want to be therapised and those that do are often playing a 'needy' game.

Contracting is negotiating a working agreement between the practitioner and the proposed supervisor. Remember, supervision is always the practitioner's developmental space, it is not an organisational space, even though the organisation may create this space. As such, the practitioner must have the right to choose their own supervisor, although there are always resource limits. Choice may be limited for multiple organisational issues and some compromise may need to be negotiated, yet always within the spirit of supervision. The supervisor and practitioner must always agree their positive intention to work together within a set of mutual expectations and responsibilities. Such issues include maintaining confidentiality (especially in relation to reporting of unsafe practice), writing and storing notes, termination and pattern of meetings.

Mode of supervision

There are advantages of both individual and group supervision. In groups, although practitioners have less 'air' time, they can relate to the experiences shared by other members of the group. This may benefit less vocal or reticent practitioners who feel threatened by individual supervision. Many practitioners say they learn more by listening and relating to others' experiences than they do by sharing their own. In groups there are more diverse views and more support for practitioners, especially if others do relate to their experiences. However, people can feel more vulnerable sharing their experiences in groups. As such groups may take longer to gel and create a safe environment, moving through forming norms. Groups should be limited to no more than 6 people. Groups are also vulnerable to irregular attendance which makes group norming more difficult. Practitioners within the group who work together may feel very vulnerable about sharing experiences that criticise other group members, constructing social norms within the group to ensure maximum comfort. The group guide will need to be experienced with group dynamics to counter game playing. Perhaps groups under these conditions need a more concrete focus, for example clinical audit.

Perhaps a mixture of both individual and group supervision might be ideal. Despite the forming difficulties of work based group supervision, I do think that they foster collaborative teamwork, shared vision, team learning, mutual support, role responsibility and quality – all advantages over individual supervision.

Supervision process – the nine step model

The process of clinical supervision can be summarised and viewed as a linear model through nine steps (Box 3.5). Each of the nine steps is essential to achieve effective supervision. 'Pick up' is commencing a session by picking up issues from the previous session. This is best done when some notes have been taken that identify specific actions to be taken before the next session.

Listening and the art of dialogue

The key to guidance is to listen. Only when the supervisor *really* listens can she hear what is being said or not being said. Clarifying – checking out that the guide has heard correctly and determining the significance of what is being shared – and listening are key elements of *dialogue* between the practitioner and the guide that seeks to resolve contradiction towards realising desirable practice as a lived reality. Isaacs (1993) summarises dialogue as:

> 'a discipline of collective thinking and inquiry, a process for transforming the quality of conversation and, in particular, the thinking that lies beneath it. The central purpose is to establish a field of genuine meeting and inquiry [which Isaacs describes as a container but I prefer the word clearing] – a setting in which people can allow a free

Box 3.5   Supervision process – the nine step model

(1)	Preparation	Creating the best possible environment for successful supervision.
(2)	Pick up	Ensuring continuity of supervision from session to session.
(3)	Listening	Listening with intent to draw out significance from the supervisee's story.
(4)	Clarifying	Ensuring you have heard correctly from the supervisee's perspective, guiding the supervisee to draw out significant issues, and picking up and feeding back cues.
(5)	Understanding	Enabling the supervisee to gain insights into why he/she feels, thinks and responds as they do within situations.
(6)	Options	Enabling the supervisee to see and explore other, perhaps more appropriate, ways to respond in future situations and their consequences.
(7)	Taking action	Guiding the supervisee to draw conclusions as to how they might like to respond in a future, similar situation.
(8)	Empowering	Infusing/empowering the supervisee with courage to act on their insights.
(9)	Wrap up	Ensuring the supervisee has summarised the session and feels okay (complete notes).

flow of meaning and vigorous exploration of the collective background of their thought, their personal predispositions, the nature of their shared attention, and the rigid features of their individual and collective assumptions.' (p. 25)

Dialogue is not a natural way of communicating. It must be learnt. The onus is on the guide to coach the practitioner to dialogue, which of course, assumes that the guide can dialogue herself. The guide actively creates a clearing to dwell in dialogue with the practitioner. In listening to the practitioner's reflection, the guide suspends her own values and judgement in order to connect with the experience in terms of the practitioner's experience with the intent to co-create meaning with the practitioner (Bohm 1996). This is the same empathic connection that practitioners need to listen and connect with patients (see Chapter 4). It follows that the guide must also be mindful of their own mental models, manage themselves well within relationships and be non-judgemental.

Self-disclosure

The guide might disclose her own experience as a way of helping the practitioner to see an experience more clearly or to illuminate a particular way of responding. The emphasis is on the word appropriate. For example, my supervision of the team leaders at the hospice where I practice is based on mutual disclosure yet always with a purpose of using my experiences to move the supervisees and myself towards new insights. It's also how I get my clinical supervision!

Monitoring the supervision relationship

As with any developmental process or innovation, it is important to monitor its impact. Supervision relationships should be periodically monitored, for example every six months, so the practitioner and supervisor can see if development is taking place and the supervision is working well. In tune with a reflective perspective, review is a dynamic continuous process of reflection–action–reflection. I always encourage practitioners to keep a record of each supervision session, although many are reluctant. They seem to have a natural reticence to writing and resist any formal record for which they might ultimately be held to account.

The record has four headings (Box 3.6):

- pick up issues from last session
- summarise aspects of practice shared within the session
- summarise significant issues that have emerged from discussion
- summarise actions that the practitioner and supervisor will either consider or take action on before next session

Writing notes reinforces the issues that have emerged during the session and provides continuity between sessions. The practitioner experiences a further level of reflection on reading the notes and pays attention to issues that might otherwise have been defended against within an oral mode. If a session lasts for one hour, as is typical, I suggest spending the last five summarising the

Box 3.6   Record of supervision

Clinical supervision Record of Session

Session ....   Date.............................

Pick up issues from last session

Summarise aspects of practice shared within the session

Summarise significant issues that have emerged from discussion

Summarise actions that the practitioner and supervisor will either consider or take before next session

session and ensuring the MSR cue 'How do you now feel?' is adequately dealt with, to focus on converting negative energy into positive energy and mopping up any residual feelings.

The notes, as a whole, provide the data for the practitioner to look back and review their reflexive development through the series of unfolding sessions. The practitioner can evaluate the supervision process for its efficacy in facilitating practitioner development using the Supervision Evaluation Questionnaire (SEQ) (see Appendix 1). The effectiveness of the supervision process should never be taken for granted and be constantly scrutinised. Evaluation is itself a significant developmental exercise for the practitioner to analyse the supervision process and to give critical feedback.

Parallel process

I want to end this chapter by returning to the idea of parallel process framing (see Box 1.10), to emphasise that clinical supervision is fundamentally a caring and healing relationship that parallels the clinical relationship, as set out in Chapters 4–7. If practitioners are expected to care then the systems that organise, develop and support practitioners must themselves be caring. Anything less is a contradiction. Clinical supervision *is* caring, a place of deep compassion and wisdom, of empathic connection and critical thinking, of authenticity and intimacy. Clinical supervision must have the primary focus for liberating practitioners to unleash their caring and realise their caring destiny.

I wrote the poem 'River of tears' following an emotional clinical supervision session with a ward sister. She was distressed about events and cried throughout the session. I was a container for her tears and metaphorically held her as she moved through the dark void to emerge into a light of possibility. As she said, it paralleled the way she often held her patients and families at times of distress.

The river of tears

This space between us
A river of tears
Where your tears flow,
The flow of pain
Hurt to the quick.

This river of tears
Where once your passion flowed
And where your passion will
    flow again
When the storm has passed
And the sun shines again.

And when I gaze across at you
I feel the touch of my concern
My gaze as an eagle's wing
That gently touches
the blue mood of despair.

The dark woman has broken
I feel her tears flow
Into the dark river that flows between
No words spoken
A clear winter's day within shadow.

I feel the swarm of bees about me
And the song of the bee about me
The dark woman stung
My words a balm
To loosen the binds that bound

Tears like dewdrops
Sweep across the soft lids
Eyes glisten as the smile breaks
    through
Her anguished cry stops
In the soft dawn of hope.

Within each tear spilt
I sensed your hopes and fears
Your sense of being betrayed
The machine says 'tilt'
No longer can you play.

Nerve shredded along the raw edge
Cut to the quick
You recoil hurt and vulnerable
Frailty exposed along the ledge
Take my hand.

I meet you in this space
Where we can move beyond
With energy renewed for the task
The past already a blur
We have learnt from.

And on another day
and in another place
We can look back
And bathe in this river of tears
Where the demons drowned.

Revised from the original published in the first edition

Chapter 4

Knowing the Person

What does it mean to know a person from the perspective of enabling that person to understand and respond to their own health needs? A number of points should be considered:

- that the focus of health care is health not illness, although illness most often brings people into the domain of health care
- that understanding is the basis for responding, yet it must be an understanding based on the person's perspective to balance the health care practitioner's own perspective
- that people have complex and unique human needs that are not stereotypical despite the best efforts of science, and which cannot be reduced or viewed in isolation from the whole, at least not without diminishing the person's humanness.

As Hall (1964) notes:

'It is impossible to nurse any more of a person than that person allows us to see. If we permit him to utilise our freely offered closeness, he will not only let us see more of him, but he will allow himself to see "more of him", so that he may, with excellent professional nursing, emerge as a "whole person".' (p. 152)

In other words, knowing a person emerges from the practitioner opening up a caring space where the person can reveal themselves, not only to the practitioner, but to him or herself. If the practitioner only glimpses who a person is or views them through a diagnostic lens then the basis for care is partial and unsatisfactory. This process is usually referred to as assessment – gathering the necessary information in order to reveal, anticipate, understand and respond to the person's health needs. Information comes from various sources: medical investigations, observations, taking a history, and listening to the stories from a person and their family. Asssessment is an ongoing process of grasping, interpreting and evaluating the situation as an unfolding process although it is often 'done' on admission, a significant process in the transition from person to patient. For many people, admission is a time of considerable anxiety where disclosure of self may be masked (Hughes *et al.* 1986), and that information may be limited or distorted.

Pattern appreciation

I prefer the term 'pattern appreciation' (Cowling 2000) to represent the complex interplay of the signs to which I need to pay attention in order to know the other person; reading the person's life pattern as a complex whole, a pattern continually shifting moment to moment along the person's health–illness journey. This is achieved by reading the signs on the person's surface, for example pain, anxiety, high blood pressure, sadness in the eyes, and pursuing these signs into the deeper self as appropriate. Pattern is always shifting in light of unfolding events. To appreciate pattern the practitioner must tune into the other person to find their wavelength. Only when the practitioner is in tune with the person can they understand and respond appropriately to the person's unfolding needs. Newman (1994) notes:

> 'The new paradigm of health, essential to nursing, embraces a unitary pattern of changing relationships. It is developmental. The task is not to try to change another person's pattern but to recognise it as information that depicts the whole and relate to it as it unfolds.' (p. 13)

Of course sometimes this can be difficult when the person is confused or not conscious. From a medical model perspective, assessment is centred around the illness or disease process. Nursing models such as Roper *et al.* (1980) have extended the medical model to include the impact of the illness on activities of living, the intention being to return the person to normal levels of activity. The Roper *et al.* model is typical of many models that emerged from the USA between 1960 and 1990 as representations of nursing, a rich period for the development of nursing theory. These models were based on systems theory, the idea that the whole is made up of a number of discrete parts, for example Roper *et al.* identified ten activities of living. However, such models are inherently reductionist, breaking the person into bits, with the consequent risk of losing sight of the whole. They also tended to be prescriptive in responding to the patient's problems. Later models from the USA were more holistic-based, understanding and responding to the person in their wholeness, for example the work of Parse (1987), and Rogers (1986). Yet in my view these theorists also prescribed a set of values with which nurses were expected to conform. The problem with all models of nursing is that they tend to impose a reality that limits practitioners' imagination, creativity and reflection. These models have rigid assessment criteria based on systems theory that 'encourage' the practitioner to fit the patient to the model, rather than using the model creatively to see the person, and to see the person as a set of parts in isolation from the whole. This is a far cry from holism. Yet, nurses in the UK, despite espousing holistic values, still persist in using such models despite their obvious contradiction. This state of affairs was evident when I prompted a review of the use of the Roper *et al.* model of nursing at Burford hospital in light of the hospital's newly developed philosophy of practice. A strong sense of its inadequacy emerged that reflected many of the points I have mentioned.

Practitioners viewed assessment as a task they did on the patient's admission in contrast with viewing assessment as a continual process that had real meaning and practicality. Practitioners thought the Roper *et al.* model was inadequate because it forced them to fit patients to the model's assessment framework, reducing the person to boxes that had to be filled in, often in a superficial way. The constant failure to adequately complete the boxes on sexuality and dying acknowledged the difficulty in seeing these as activities as part of everyday functional living. Sexuality reflects who people are. It is synonymous with the person's identity. Even responding to sexuality in terms of the 'sexual act' could not be addressed because of its social taboo. It is difficult to talk to a stranger about their sex life. It is even more difficult when such issues may be irrelevant to the health care experience. In other words, assessment using formal methods can be insensitive and intrusive. Being assessed was also felt to be a ritual of de-personalisation, of transition from person to patient. The problem with assessment schedules is that they demand to be completed, especially when audit systems are linked to completion. Hence when an activity of living box is not completed on a form, it indicates the practitioner has not assessed adequately. The effort is to complete the assessment sheet rather than to know the person.

Undoubtedly, the functional approach to nursing has encouraged practitioners to perceive models of nursing from a utility value, often taking or modifying bits from models, but breaking up the integrity of the model. For example, *self-care* may have an attractive appeal because it suggests that a target for nursing care is to enable people to regain their independence and return to their level of functioning before the illness event. Yet on a philosophical level, self-care must mean self-determination, being able to take control of one's life in a positive frame of mind. If this is true, then the focus of self-care on functional issues would be misplaced because the functional would always need to be viewed within the meanings the illness or disease had for the person. The focus on functional self-care may lead practitioners to fail to see the person and their distress at a crisis point in their lives. Self-care at a functional level is a deficit model rather than a growth model, with its emphasis to return the person to a normal level of activity. The patient becomes a series of deficits that need fixing rather than a person whose illness pattern is understood within the whole pattern of their life.

The Roper *et al.* model is easily understood from a functional perspective because it seems to represent what nurses already do. Hence adopting the model requires minimal accommodation. Neither is it written in an obscure intellectual language that characterises so many American models of nursing. Pearson (1983), in justifying the use of the Roper *et al.* model at Burford, noted the way the model:

> 'speaks to nurses in a language which is familiar and related to nursing in this country and hence its greatest advantage then is its ability to convey meaning to clinical nurses.' (p. 53)

Whilst practitioner's identification is the model's advantage it is also its weakness because, if it fits in with what nurses already do then its impact on changing practice will be very limited. Pearson seems to imply that models *should* convey meaning to nurses but this goes against the grain that the nurse must first find meaning for herself and then collectively with her colleagues. Only then are practitioners in a position to consider the value of external prescriptions of nursing to inform their practice. But if practitioners have developed their own vision or philosophy for nursing, why would they want to use someone else's? The outcome of the review was to sweep away the Roper *et al.* model, as an inadequate representation of the hospital's new vision for practice (Boxes 2.2 & 2.3), and to construct a reflective model to tune practitioners into the Burford vision within each unfolding moment.

The Burford NDU model: caring in practice

The reflective model consists of a sequential series of nine cues (Box 4.1) that offer the practitioner a reflective framework to facilitate the practitioner to probe and appreciate aspects of the person's life-pattern. The cues are internalised as a 'natural' way to see and respond to the person as a continuous process of pattern appreciation throughout the care journey. By natural I mean they become part of the practitioner's mind-set rather than pay conscious attention to them. So, if I am admitted into your unit, you 'naturally' reflect on, 'who is this person?' 'What meaning does this health event have for him?' etcetera. Your intention is to tune into and connect with me within a holistic attitude.

Let's be clear that the cues are *not* a series of boxes to fill in as with the Roper *et al.* model. I emphasise this point because the practitioner who has embodied a reductionist systems approach may well use the model in this way. As Sutherland (1994) noted:

> 'Although at first I did find myself going back to the Roper *et al.*'s headings to make sure that I had not missed anything, omitting what was physically important, I did not need to do this for very long.' (p. 68)

Sutherland further noted the impact of the reflective cues in changing her mind-set:

Box 4.1   Burford NDU Reflective model: Caring in Practice reflective cues

---

Core question: What information do I need to be able to nurse this person?

Cue questions:

- Who is this person?
- What meaning does this illness/health event have for the person?
- How is this person feeling?
- How has this event affected their usual life patterns and roles?
- How do I feel about this person?
- How can I help this person?
- What is important for this person to make their stay within the health care setting comfortable?
- What support does this person have in life?
- How does this person view the future for themselves and others?

'Because the emphasis is centred on feelings and the total picture of that person's situation rather than on their ongoing physical needs, it forced me to move away from a need to find things out, fill things in and get things done as soon as possible in an orderly fashion. It forced me to start listening to what patients themselves were saying was important to them and then to plan care with them from this basis. It gradually became a welcome release for me.' (p. 68)

There is something astonishing in Sutherland's words about the way she felt the Burford cues *forced* her to listen to patients. I think it is true, as she suggests, that the 'old model' became the task, hence the effort was to complete it rather than really listen to what the patient or family were saying.

The Burford cues are a radical reconceptualisation of practice because the emphasis was person-centred and pulled nursing out from under the medical model influence. It is not doing the same thing differently. As Sutherland suggests, the key is listening and connecting, and *then* working with the person toward meeting their health–illness needs. Consider these points in terms of your own assessment approach? Do you really listen to your patients or clients?

Explication of the Burford NDU model reflective cues

Who is this person?

Ask yourself, 'Who is this person?' This cue prompts the practitioner's primary focus on the 'whole' and unique person; i.e. that person in the context of his or her family, social and cultural world. In other words, the person is not seen in isolation and it brings the family into the focus of care. From a holistic perspective, the person's family is naturally included within the concept of 'the person' and within the caring focus. The cue encourages the practitioner to see the person in terms of their humanness and counters any tendency to see the person primarily in terms of symptoms and diagnosis, as significant as these things are. Of course, humanness is a reciprocal thing. If the practitioner sees the other's humanness she is more likely to see and respond from her own.

What meaning does this health–illness event have for the person?

This cue prompts the practitioner to endeavour to understand the meaning the person and family gives to their health–illness experience. The dialogue between the person and practitioner establishes the caring relationship based on mutual understanding, where the person's right to be involved in the health care process is honoured and actively facilitated. Ask yourself, 'Whose life is it?' When the practitioner views the other person at a distance and makes her own interpretations and responds to the other based on the assumptions drawn, then the risk of misunderstanding is great. Clearly the meanings the person has about their experience will be influenced by any 'diagnosis' but that is part of the whole, not the whole in itself as with the medical model that reduces the person to the 'diagnosis' or 'differential diagnosis' when the disease pattern is unclear. For some practitioners such as midwives and health visitors, the focus for connection is a normal event such as having a child or child development. Yet even in these normal living activities, the hand of medicalisation stretches to create a potential world of dis-ease.

How is this person feeling?

This cue prompts the practitioner to pay attention to the person's affective state, acknowledging that the person is suffering and may be anxious about a whole host of things. In paying attention to this cue, the practitioner responds to ease suffering and deal with any anxiety, helping the person to feel calm.

How has this event affected their usual life patterns and roles?

This cue prompts the practitioner to appreciate the person's lifestyle pattern. The practitioner guides the person or meaningful others to review their life-style, reading the pattern for deeper underlying factors that may have influenced the current situation. Often serious illness can prompt a radical reassessment of lifestyle and what values people consider significant within their lives. It focuses caring as both a health promotion and illness prevention activity. In terms of this cue, the practitioner may utilise a check list to consider aspects of lifestyle, rather like the Roper *et al.* activities of living, or any other reductionist scheme. If you were to construct a checklist what would it include? Obvious issues include work, leisure, daily living and religious act-ivities. Related to this are issues which affect these activities, such as mobility, fatigue, sleep, nutrition, pain or mood, and social factors such as support, attitudes and finance.

How do I feel about this person?

This cue prompts the practitioner to pay attention to their own feelings, thoughts, concerns and prejudices that may influence the way she sees, responds or reacts to the person, especially if the person arouses strong feelings in the practi-tioner due to the person's suffering, or their manner or behaviour. As such, the cue acknowledges the 'who of the practitioner' and the uniqueness of the human–human encounter with all its mystery and vulnerability.

How can I help this person?

This cue prompts the practitioner to pause and consider the information gained, to feed back understanding and begin to plan with the person (as they are able) and other health care practitioners, the best ways to respond to meet the person's health–illness needs. Another way to view this cue is to consider the first five cues as creating a clearing where the practitioner and person(s) can dialogue and negotiate care, both short-term in view of presenting issues, and longer term through anticipating future need.

What is important for this person to make their stay within the health care setting comfortable?

This cue prompts the practitioner to acknowledge that admission into hospital, hospice, care home, district nursing service, or having a baby is a major disruption and potentially uncomfortable. The cue guides the practitioner to focus on the person's comfort and control especially those 'little things' that make a significant difference to the person's comfort and perception of being cared for (Macleod 1994).

What support does this person have in life?

This cue prompts the practitioner to guide the person or family to explore what support resources exist within the person's life. It orientates the practitioner toward the person's wider social and cultural world, and toward the possibilities of mobilising and developing resources to support the person's future. As with the previous cue, this cue is vital to focus care towards successful exit of the care relationship or transition of care across health care boundaries.

How does this person view the future for themselves and others?

This cue prompts the practitioner to guide the person to gaze into an uncertain future. Used sensitively, this cue opens a space where fears and hopes can surface and be explored. Such dialogue may raise many difficult issues and feelings, such as the possibility of dying, disability or losing one's home.

Empathy

Imagine I am admitted to your practice unit. As you see me for the first time, what do you think? Do you think illness or person? Perhaps if my vital signs are compromised you will think in terms of saving my life, and only then if I survive might you pause to see me as a person. If you are truly a holistic practitioner then no matter what my medical condition you will always strive to see me first as a person and connect with me in terms of the meanings I give to my experience. This ability is called empathy. Empathy is the practitioner's ability to connect with what the other is experiencing (Belenky *et al.* 1986).

Empathy is differentiated from sympathy (Morse *et al.* 1992), sympathy being an emotional response to the experience of the other as a result of absorbing the other's suffering to some extent. In contrast empathy is an objective view – a dispassionate glance yet motivated by deep concern for the other. My understanding of the nature of empathy was initially constructed

Box 4.2   A model for empathy

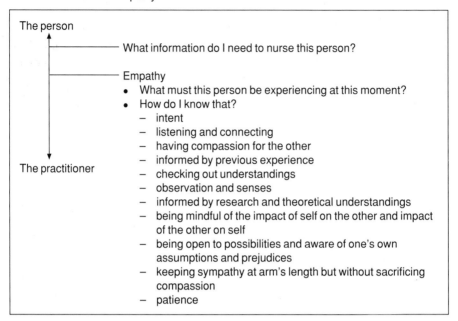

The person

What information do I need to nurse this person?

Empathy
- What must this person be experiencing at this moment?
- How do I know that?
  - intent
  - listening and connecting
  - having compassion for the other
  - informed by previous experience
  - checking out understandings
  - observation and senses
  - informed by research and theoretical understandings
  - being mindful of the impact of self on the other and impact of the other on self
  - being open to possibilities and aware of one's own assumptions and prejudices
  - keeping sympathy at arm's length but without sacrificing compassion
  - patience

The practitioner

with Helen Hardy whilst supervising her undergraduate dissertation at the University of Luton (Johns & Hardy 1998) resulting in the 'empathy model' (Box 4.2). Most of the issues listed in this box have been discussed within the cue descriptors above.

Compassion

Perhaps the most significant influence in being empathic, as with caring, is the practitioner's compassion or concern for the other person. Roach (1992) describes compassion as:

> 'A way of living born out of an awareness of one's relationship to all living creatures; engendering a response of participation in the experience of another; a sensitivity to the pain and brokenness of the other; a quality of presence which allows one to share with and make room for the other.' (p. 58)

I can only connect with you if I am interested in you; that you matter to me. This cannot be taken for granted. Compassion can sometimes be like a wilting flower if not watered. The patient might resist your approach, and have no desire to connect with you, and you may react negatively to such rejection, hence the need to be mindful. I have already discussed the significance of intuition and listening carefully, picking up and following the signs, and checking out interpretations with the person. Understanding the experience of the other is always intuitive – yet intuition is informed by past experience and knowledge.

Compassion is one of the key factors that determine the practitioner's availability to the person (see Box 2.6). Yet it is also a nebulous concept, difficult to grasp and certainly difficult to talk about and teach. Yet it is at the heart of caring and, perhaps as Roach suggests, it *is* caring. In Tom's story I quoted Levine (1986) who distinguishes compassion from pity. Pity is feeling uncomfortable with what the other person is experiencing and draws out the sympathetic response.

Levine equates compassion with love, a word that I suspect is difficult for practitioners to relate with. O'Donohue (1997) also uses the word 'love':

> 'When love awakens in your life, in the night of your heart, it is like the dawn breaking within you. When before there was anonymity, now there is intimacy; where before there was fear, now there is courage; where before in your life there was awkwardness, now there is a rhythm of grace and gracefulness; where before you were jagged, now you are elegant and in rhythm with yourself. When love awakens in your life, it is like a rebirth, a new beginning.' (p. 26)

These are such powerful words for every health care practitioner to reflect on. Do we who purport to care have a responsibility to develop our compassion if compassion is a vital ingredient of caring? Do we fail our patients and ourselves if we lack compassion? As a Buddhist I work daily on nurturing my compassionate self through meditative practice. I hope my compassion resonates through Tom's story and other stories in this book, illuminating the significance of compassion within caring. Empathy is a way of being, not a technique to know and apply. It is caring itself.

Patience

'Patience is a virtue' and in the mad rush to get things done it can easily be lost. Patience is tuning into, listening to and flowing at the person's own pace. Yet how hard it is to really listen if our mind is full of other stuff, if our heads are turned in other directions. To be empathic practitioners need to juggle a space in their minds to give the person undivided attention.

The colours of hope

I wrote the poem 'The colours of hope' after listening to a friend's extraordinary story of her journey through breast cancer. When she read the poem she cried, and said it was exactly how she felt. How did I know? Indeed, how did I know except by tuning into her story and tuning into my deeper sense of knowing that comes through experience of working with women with breast cancer and flows from my compassion. What does this poem say to you? Can you sense the woman's suffering and hope? Does it adequately capture the essence of empathy?

The colours of hope

In this place at this time
My mind with colours rhyme
As reflections of who I am
In this dark place of solitude.

A dark place . . . I think of black
Seeing only a black hole
That darkens the window of my soul
So I cannot see out and touch
My awaiting fate;
I strive to touch myself before too late
In my vain efforts to cope;
Black – a prison for hope.

Or is it grey?
Like these cold hospital walls
Where the paint flakes and falls;
Like me, my former glory gone;
Grey – like the woman's face across the way,
Like clouds on a gloomy day
That leaves no space for the blue,
No room for hope to shine through.

So I turn to blue . . .
The colour of my nurse's eyes
Whose nonchalance belies
Her concern for me;
I reach up to touch her face;
Not just another unfortunate case;
Blue – I sense the warmth of azure seas
And open my windows to its soft breeze.

I move to red . . .
My nurse's lipstick makes me dread
My own self-image fixed inside my head
Of some mutilated being;
Afraid that others might stare,
Despite my camouflage I feel so bare;
I grieve my lost breast; shapeless
No longer soft to my lover's caress.

And green. . . .
To thoughts of fields of long grass
On summer days long past
With children for whom I weep
In the loss of their dear mother;
Can I give them hope of just another

Christmas Day
Where joy can rule and hope makes play?

Lighter now I turn to yellow
Seeing the primroses, dried, pressed inside
Favourite pages of books I cried
Over in younger more romantic days.
Yellow – the sun's warm rays
Open my soul's window for me to gaze
Across the landscape of my mourning
To watch hope's dawning.

White – the bright light dazzles
Is this God meeting me so soon?
Is hope already past the moon
On this journey into the unknown?
I am transformed and grow through this ordeal
To know that I am real;
I sense my nurse's hand on me
And know not the hand of pity.

Eyes open to her warm touch,
a gaze upwards reveals her tender smile;
My children from the photo watch my trial
and test my hope in the colours of their dress;
Caring, being cared for in turn
I find peace in my nurse's concern
To face me;
Hope inside me breaks free
As tears clean the window of my soul.

REFLECTIVE EXEMPLAR 4.1 – STEPHEN

Consider my ability to empathise with the experience of Stephen and Stephen's sister. How well did I get to know these people? Stephen is a patient at the hospice.

Further along the corridor I knock and pausing for a moment, enter Stephen's room. We have not met before. He's buried beneath the bed covers so I decide not to intrude. I am informed that Stephen is a 49 year old African–Caribbean man, who was transferred from the local general hospital with cancer of the stomach and liver metastases. The cancer is newly diagnosed. His notes display his anger at his GP for not taking his stomach complaints seriously. Since admission he has been withdrawn, cocooned in his bed, shocked by the way his life is being torn from him.

Shortly afterwards, I return to find him on the floor on his knees. I guess rightly that he was attempting to reach the toilet. He is in pain but accepts my offer to help him get there. Just lots of wind. The effort exhausts him so I fetch him a wheelchair. I help him back to bed and fetch his breakfast but he has no appetite. He clutches his stomach complaining of pains. Dr Brown is around and sees him. He prescribes octreotide for his vomiting. Paracetamol settles his stomach pains, a reminder to think up the pain ladder[1].

I mention to Kerry, a staff nurse, that I found Stephen on his knees. She surprises me by asking, in her fairly jokey way, if he was praying. I'm not sure if this was a flippant remark, but he is a member of the Adventist church. A book lies on his bed locker; the title is *Preparing to Meet Jesus*; an ominous title under the circumstances.

He certainly is not well today . . . a real struggle for him with his pain. His legs and penis are greatly swollen because of the intestinal compression. He says he is drowsy . . . that he hasn't slept, but that he wants to be alert, and is anxious that his tablets will make him drowsy. He is fighting to be awake. I sense his fear, that he is frightened of dying. I pick up his book *Preparing to Meet Jesus* and ask if he has a strong faith. He affirms but I can see that conversation of such nature is not possible at least until his physical distress is adequately dealt with. Everything is kept in perspective. We have to help him deal with his pain and vomiting, but I wonder if some of his pain is a deeper psychological pain, what Kearney (1996) describes as 'soul pain.' I feel clumsy looking after him, struggling to find his wavelength but nevertheless, I hang in there.

Later I meet his sister, her two daughters and grandson who is just three months old but was two months premature. He stares at me and gives me a big smile. I stand on the threshold of this family. The family notice this and invite me to enter into their world. I make them coffee, chatting about things on a social level. In the background Stephen is restless and groaning – he projects himself into the foreground and the sister recoils. It is hard for them to sit here, listening to his suffering . . . but not being able to communicate with him or ease his suffering. I acknowledge this. She says, 'I feel helpless . . . I don't know what to do.'

I can't say what she can or cannot do. I also have a sense of helplessness. However, we have broken the ice, we have acknowledged her struggle to stay with her brother. Acknowledging the struggle makes it easier to bear. I simply dwell in the silence between us and communicate my presence to her . . . my being there is a distraction for her to face up to Stephen's overt distress. She is silent because she does not know what to say. Yet she diverts her attention because she is suffering. I suggest she can give Stephen silent attention, just being here and communicating love. Saunders (1996) says:

> 'Sometimes there will be no answers to give to those in apparently desperate situations, and we find ourselves with nothing to offer but silent attention . . . a feeling of helplessness may urge us to withdraw or escape into a zealous hyperactivity which can well exacerbate the patient's suffering.' (p. 13)

---

[1] The pain ladder (WHO) is a common-sense approach to pain assessment and management whereby the practitioner progress up three rungs in responding to the patient's pain: no opioids, weak opioids, strong opioids (+ adjuncts as necessary)

Being Available

Using the Being Available template (Box 2.5), consider the extent I knew Stephen and the way I managed myself within this relationship.

The first point of reflection is to consider how well I knew Stephen and was able to tune into and flow with his wavelength. I struggled with this, but why? Stephen was closed, defensive, angry, rejecting my desire to develop a relationship on my immediate terms. Indeed, I was a target to project his silent anger into. As it was I absorbed his struggle and had difficulty finding his wavelength. I think I was anxious to move Stephen into a more comfortable place for both of us to dwell because where he was was a tough place to be. He was suffering mental, physical and possibly spiritual torment. Or was he? Did I make this assumption?

How would I feel if the roles were reversed? How would I want myself to respond to me? Kant's moral imperative (Seedhouse 1988) is always a good tester. Firstly, I would want me to understand where I was coming from. I am whirling around uncontrollably in a whirlpool of intense feelings – much more than anger although the doctor's words ring in my ears. I feel there is no escape from this death sentence despite my weak denial, 'this can't be happening to me.' There is little room for bargaining, at least at this moment. Any threads of hope dangle out of reach. I am only 49 years old and this news has been swift and devastating. I feel abandoned by everyone, especially by my God. Indeed, my religion torments rather than comforts me because I cannot accept death's menacing shadow. I feel submerged by waves of depression; my emotions are haywire. Kübler-Ross's stages of dying (1969) merge and swirl about me in dark patterns. I plead, 'Please stay with me on this rollercoaster. I don't mean to reject you but it is hard for me to accept you just now. Am I dying?'

To imagine or empathise with Stephen I need to suspend how I imagine I would actually respond within this situation. Yet how would I respond? Would I be accepting or would I too have to run the gauntlet of denial, anger, bargaining and depression? Would my Buddhist belief of impermanence prepare me well enough to face death with equanimity or would I crumple in the utter oblivion of death's inevitability? How do you, the reader, imagine you would respond?

A salutary lesson, yet one that is central to wavelength theory and managing self within relationship (Johns 1996a). To tune into and flow with the patient the practitioner must be aware of and manage their resistance to the patient; requiring an almost unconditional acceptance to whatever the patient is experiencing without *imposing* expectations of how the patient should respond. Of course, human suffering knows no limits and consequently this can be extremely difficult work. This is the compassion litmus test. I am reminded of words by Thomas Moore (1992):

> 'Day by day we live emotions and themes that have deep roots, but our reflections on these experiences tend to be superficial . . . not only are our reflections often insufficient to account for intense feelings, but we may have been living from a place that is too rational and dispassionate. Rainer Maria Rilke advises the young poet

to "go deep into yourself and see how deep the place is from which your life flows". We could all take note of this advice, go deep into ourselves and discover how deep is the source of our everyday lives.' (p. 235)

To know Stephen in this moment I needed to go deep within me, to tune into him on a more intuitive level, perhaps on the level of the soul. How do we know things?

Wavelength theory

Perhaps the most significant skill the practitioner has is her ability to tune into and connect with the person – to literally get on his *wavelength* in order to flow with him as his experience unfolds. I have tried to capture this flowing between the person and practitioner in graphic form:

Patient's wavelength

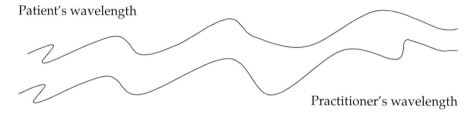

Practitioner's wavelength

When people like Stephen and Stephen's sister experience crisis in their lives, their wave patterns are likely to become chaotic; descents to ever greater depths as suffering and despair take hold zigzagged with moments of hope and salvation. By flowing with them I could be most available to them.

Tuning into wavelength is only the beginning. The practitioner must then flow with the other's wavelength as it unfolds. Newman (1999) describes this as synchronicity, a rhythm of relating in a paradigm of wholeness. This movement along the wavelength can be viewed as a dance (Johns 2001b; Younger 1995), each step a caring movement sometimes led by the practitioner and at other times led by the other as appropriate.

When practitioners lose sight of the person, they expect the person to fit into their wavelength of the 'good patient', a straight line that diminishes the human experience. The patient (diminished person) tries to 'fit in' to be accepted and cared for. Failure to fit in often leads to censure, as characterised by the image of the 'unpopular patient'.

Patient's wavelength

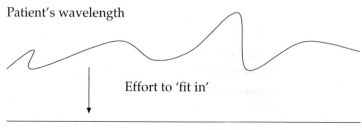

Effort to 'fit in'

Practitioner's wavelength

Blackwolf & Gina Jones (1996) capture the sense of wavelength for people in their portrayal of an eagle:

> 'Look up and see Eagle ride the invisible. Up and down, coasting, then back up and down again. With deliberate intent, she manoeuvres her wings in order to catch the next current, rising to a new height. Levelling and riding a straight course, she gains new sights. Then, accepting the inevitable downward drift, she surrenders to each experience. Invisibly changing and unpredictable, the air currents carry Eagle to the places she must go. Eagle understands the dance of life and accepts the downward as naturally as she accepts the upward.' (p. 185)

As my experience with Stephen illustrates, it is not necessarily easy to tune into the other's wavelength or to flow with the other on the pitch and roll of their journey. It may feel like surfing! To stay on the other's wavelength the practitioner must be mindful of the pitch and roll and manage any resistance they may have toward the patient. As Munley (1986) suggests:

> 'The hospice approach to terminal care is based on the premise that something more can always be done to give support to families and to keep dying patients as comfortable as possible. In concrete terms this "something more" means being responsive to physical, psychological, social, and spiritual pain. Responsiveness to pain [or suffering] in all its aspects requires great sensitivity on the part of caregivers and a willingness to take on the perspective of the person who is suffering. Entering into the world of the other leads staff to drop professional defences and opens them up to an experience of inner stress.' (p. 345)

I explore the issue managing self within relationship, resistance and stress in Chapter 6. However I would balance Munley's words by suggesting that *entering into the world of the other* also opens the practitioner to the intense satisfaction that caring brings which neutralises the stress that caring might create.

REFLECTIVE EXEMPLAR 4.2 – TONY'S STORY

Consider my effort to know Tony, a patient I met one morning on an early shift at the hospice.

> I went to help Tony get up for lunch. He is 53 and has a primary lung cancer with liver metastases. He is in the hospice for respite care. He has been here just four days and he wants to go home. In his words 'Not that it's unpleasant in here but . . .' Unspoken words but I sensed he didn't like the reminder of his forthcoming death that the hospice seemed to represent. Neither did he like being a patient. He had always been a very independent man and now he rebelled against the disease that was sucking away his energy and his life.
>
> There were cards on the wall made by his granddaughter. He became animated when talking about her and I could sense that she was very special to him, adding to his sadness and restlessness. Things that make us happy also make us sad. As Benner & Wrubel (1989) note, the things we care about are the things that make us vulnerable, because they matter to us. Caring

and vulnerability – two sides of the same coin. This is the same for me: in opening myself to being vulnerable, I also seek ways in which I can manage my vulnerability yet without diminishing my concern for the other.

As I gazed at Tony, I sensed that his life was in crisis, that he sought meaning in this cruel twist of fate that threatened his relationship with his granddaughter. I sensed his irritation with me. Did he want me to go? If so, should I accept his dismissal or assert my authority to be his helper whether he liked it or not? To be a good patient, he should conform to my authority, but what a potential for anarchy if we accepted that all patients had the right to choose which nurses cared for them. So I rejected his unspoken dismissal, which I rationalised as an expression of his suffering, his existential angst which he projected into me. I hung around him, communicating my availability to help him if he wished it. I had been told that he struggled to co-ordinate himself. He needed but didn't want my help. I picked up his ambivalence and felt uncomfortable, not wanting to irritate him further but recognising his need for help. I was trying hard to open and maintain a positive space in which we could work together even as I struggled to tune into his wavelength. Perhaps he wanted Susan [another nurse], whom he knew and felt comfortable with? Yet, being a good patient, he couldn't tell me that . . . at least not in words.

Tony got himself into the shower. I held him steady as he moved in and out of the shower. There was no resistance. Eventually he dressed. I helped with his socks and shoes. This had taken about an hour. His pain was well controlled but now I wonder: 'why are nurses so focused on pain?' Perhaps we understand, feel comfortable with, feel more useful with such concrete issues as symptom management than with responding meaningfully to his sense of irritation and search for meaning.

We talked about schooling, my two children, and his granddaughter. We talked about his work: he had been a plumber; he knew he was not going back to work any more and accepted that. All the while, he remained superficially accepting of my presence although I continually sensed his irritation rippling over him. I was tempted to let him know that I sensed this, to confront him: 'was I bothering him?' Such confrontation might prick the tension I felt, yet it might also embarrass him. I would be acting for my benefit rather than his. I never felt comfortable with him but then why should I? And why shouldn't he be irritated?

I decided to pick up the underlying reason for his irritation: being in the hospice when he wanted to be at home. I acknowledged this need, feeding back my empathy, understanding and acceptance of his predicament. However, the fact was he had no choice about going home because his daughter was away for the week. He seemed to relax more when he discovered I was an academic, as if he could accept my being here more easily, rather than being a new nurse he had never met before and the need to go through it all again – the effort of making a relationship. In my experience some patients like to tell their story over and over, and others prefer their own solitude. Tony was one of the latter, yet he was intrigued by my academic role at the hospice. This was an important understanding: he needed to know me, frame who I was, to put me into context in order to accept my presence more than simply as a 'visiting nurse'. Even though that was true – I was a 'visiting nurse' – it was a conservative truth. Why should he be pestered by an inquisitive visiting nurse when he was contemplating his own death and the loss of his relationship with his granddaughter? For whose benefit was the pestering? Did I pretend I was helping him? Does the need to be useful or, even worse, the need to fix his problems for him, become a mentality that threatens to reduce Tony to the status of some curious object? I know I didn't feel like that, but perhaps Tony felt that way.

We went to lunch in the communal dining room. Everybody else had gone. I joined him for lunch, and stayed with him until he had finished. There is something normalising about having a chat outside the immediate care environment and having a meal with someone. He had been a keen cyclist which gave us something concrete and interesting to chat about. By the time we had finished I felt as if I had tuned into his wavelength and sensed his ease.

On reflection, it had been an uncomfortable 90 minutes where I struggled to manage my ambivalent feelings towards this man, just as he struggled to manage his ambivalent feelings towards me. In this experience I can sense the way feelings are reciprocated. It highlighted for me the fundamental need to know people in order to respond appropriately to them on a level that is meaningful. This required a deep concern that Tony matters to me, a concern that was threatened by his barely concealed hostility and my ability to manage my feelings of rejection so as not to poison the possibilities. It also required a mutuality – it takes two to tango and dance well. Whilst Tony resisted me, no therapeutic relationship was possible. We got there but it took an immense effort. Should I have bothered? Perhaps I should have said to Susan, 'this man needs you,' and walked away. Did I hang in there because of my own need not to fail? This is a profound question because I, nurses, need to recognise that I, we, are not omnipotent and cannot impose our idea of relationships or help everyone all of the time. The very nature of suffering, dying and human relationship must always make nurse–patient relationships precarious. In getting to know someone who is dying and suffering loss we must trip along a fine edge of raw emotion.

Whilst I could have connected superficially with him by helping him wash, dress, escorting him to lunch, administering and monitoring his pain medication and other symptom relief, this was not the level of help he really needed. On a deeper level he was in spiritual crisis. I could read that, but that was my difficulty. I could not respond easily to the superficial caring issues outside that deeper context. Hence helping him wash and dress became difficult once I had looked into his eyes and touched his suffering. He also knew that, and perhaps resisted me because he needed to protect himself from this intruding stranger. Perhaps he would have preferred my superficial attention. As it was I did feel intrusive, as if my caring ethic had trapped me. Although he eventually accommodated me, I felt as if I had pushed his limits and challenged his control of the situation. The lyrics from the Doors comes to mind: *'break on through to the other side.'*

Later I shared this experience with Susan. She affirmed my feelings, acknowledging Tony's struggle in facing his death. She also acknowledged my difficulty in tuning into him, but felt I shouldn't worry unduly about that. Tony was 'difficult' and, *ipso facto*, my experience was normal, the flattening of sensitivity in order to cope with the stresses of the day. Susan's concern for me was genuine, but I was struck (again) that it is the patient who has the problem rather than the nurse being unskilful.

Writing has helped me through some issues that I had been conscious of within the moment but which are now clearer. Now I feel positive toward Tony. My compassion for him has been fed and grown. I feel no sense of pity toward him despite his impending loss. Indeed, I look forward to picking up my relationship with him although it is unlikely we will meet again.

Reflection

Perceive the way the Burford cues (Box 4.1) ripple through my story in my effort to know Tony. They are all present to a greater or lesser extent. At the time, I did not explore the support he had in life except to note that his stay in the hospice was for his daughter's holiday. I did not know his daughter. As with Stephen, it was not easy to tune into Tony, and yet, why should it be easy? His wavelength was turbulent, buffeted by raging storms. No wonder I wanted to shelter. And yet perhaps it is at such moments of resistance that Tony needs someone to stay with him, as if he has contradictory and competing needs.

In terms of what meanings Tony gave to his illness, his anguish at anticipating the loss of his relationship with his four year old granddaughter was most profound. It seemed to hang like a dark cloud over him. In terms of helping him, I could not lift the gloom. There are no off-the-shelf remedies to apply. He felt in despair and I unwittingly absorbed some of that despair, which was reflected in my discomfort.

REFLECTIVE EXEMPLAR 4.3 – HELEN AND KIM

In this exemplar consider the way Helen uses the Burford model cues and establishes a dialogue with Kim. Helen is a Clinical Nurse Specialist (CNS) for nutrition. The dialogue between Helen and myself has been edited from clinical supervision.

Helen: "Using the Burford model has confronted me with the fact that people have real feelings. It has provoked a chain of thinking, 'Why do I go to visit these patients? What am I trying to achieve?' I got an unpleasant feeling of not offering them anything except maybe to increase their safety . . . I am actively making this effort to see them as people . . . to see them differently from how I have been seeing them."

CJ: "Does this lead to increased satisfaction?"

Helen: "Yes! . . . although it makes it tougher. It has challenged my 'task' approach . . . now I probably see fewer patients in a day. That in itself is frustrating but I am more satisfied with what I do."

CJ: "A key aspect of your work is managing time and priorities?"

Helen: "It's the crux of the CNS role. I don't want to 'police' others' work but that's what has happened! At least the danger of it, if that hasn't totally happened. It may also be a problem of being part-time – I don't work enough hours or maybe it's a problem about the way I work, the 'beat the clock' thing. The reflective cues – 'How is this person feeling?' and 'How do I feel about this person?' – keep popping into my head. I had a situation with a patient, Kim, it changed the whole way the experience went. She is 26 with Crohn's disease. She has a nasty fistula pouring fluid. She is on total parenteral nutrition (TPN). I visited her on the ward. Her dressing had been done. The 'Hickman line' should have been fixed in . . . she had sat on it and it pulled out. The doctor said he would sort another one out but she had said 'no!' I went in. I knew she would not get better without a new line. My intention was to be forceful just like the doctors. And then I stopped myself. I asked myself, 'why am I acting like this?' I noted my feelings – that I was anxious she was not safe without the TPN. I asked her how she was feeling. She was reacting against having TPN forced on her. She has been like this for two years now. Her life has been turned upside down with no feeling of control – her only control was to say 'no!' I confronted her with this, 'Is this how you are feeling?' She said, 'yes! That's exactly how I am feeling. I am not having it!' I sat and talked it through with her. In the end we negotiated a compromise; that she could go home for the weekend to spend it with her children without the line and return on Monday to have the line resited. We agreed!"

CJ: "You saw the person instead of the problem?"

Helen: "It was wonderful. I went home beaming! Since then I have had other situations with doctors rushing her. For example, her Hb was 6.7 and she needed a blood transfusion. She told them to 'push off' saying, 'I'm a honorary Jehovah's Witness.' But give her time and she will mull it over. Eventually she said she was happy with this. When they put the second line in the intention was to put two units of blood through it before the TPN. I said to the consultant on the ward round, 'No, that line is for the TPN.' I confronted him. He agreed with me. But two to three weeks later the doctors tried to give her another transfusion through the 'Cuff Cath.' She said to them, 'No you're not, Helen said no.' The doctor went to the consultant who again agreed with me that they were not doing that. I had told Kim why it was important, that it contaminated the line with the risk of CVP sepsis."

Commentary

It was a shocking realisation for Helen that patients are real people, illustrating how easy it is to lose sight of this within the medical model, even for very caring people such as Helen. Helen knew that her therapeutic response was to be available to Kim, to help her find meaning in her health–illness experience and to find a way of having some control over her life. It was as if Kim needed to reclaim her own body that had been taken away from her by the medical system that was trying to fix her body but not paying attention to who she was – the classic mind–body split. In repositioning herself, Helen became a space in which Kim could reflect her feelings and claim her body. Helen's role was no longer to fix Kim's body but to work with Kim to help her regain a sense of wholeness.

Clearly Kim's suffering was more than physical yet no one had been listening to her existential angst. Helen could not take away Kim's angst but she could be a secure place where Kim could work out her thoughts and feelings and decide how best to respond to her treatment options. In doing so Helen shifted her ethical position from beneficence – knowing what's best for Kim – to patient autonomy – respecting Kim's rights to make decisions about her health care and creating the conditions where her autonomy could be exercised. Seedhouse (1988) considers that autonomy is the highest ethical position, although some authors consider that we have gone too far down this road (Woodward 1998) to the extent of jeopardising professional autonomy necessary to preserve the professional's own moral integrity. Helen takes the existential advocacy role to guide Kim to make her best decision (Gadow 1980). In doing so she helps Kim to identify and reflect on her options and their consequences, and where necessary confront Kim if she feels that Kim's decisions are ultimately not in Kim's own best interests. So Helen sits with Kim and enters this dialogue.

Part of the existential advocacy role is to help Kim feel empowered and take control of her illness trajectory, reflected in the way she is able to successfully challenge the doctors' potentially unsafe practice. Making decisions on behalf of another person is termed paternalism. Paternalism can be viewed on a therapeutic continuum with existential advocacy

Existential advocacy	← →	Paternalism
Enabling the other to make decisions; take action for themselves		Making decisions or taking action; on behalf of the other

At times, patients may be bewildered, or need to be dependent on practitioners. Indeed, asking patients to make decisions may put undue pressure on them. The mindful practitioner is sensitive to these dynamics and responds accordingly. For paternalism to be therapeutic, i.e. in terms of the patient's best interests, Benjamin & Curtis (1986) claim three factors need to be satisfied:

Harm factor	Is the patient likely to come to some harm if the practitioner does not take action?
Autonomy factor	Is the patient unable to make the decision for himself?
Ratification factor	Would the patient at a later time ratify the practitioner's decision as being in his own interests?

These criteria offer a reflective lens to consider taking action on behalf of others. The dilemma that often faces practitioners is the individual's right to self-determination measured against the harm factor, balancing one ethical principle (patient autonomy) against another (malevolence). All practitioners live out the daily tension between what is therapeutic and what is safe. Perhaps practitioners err on the side of safety because of the blame culture prevalent in the NHS and the growth of consumer litigation. In my experience with Tony, I stayed with him whilst he showered because he might easily have slipped and hurt himself. Was that a paternal act and an infringement of his autonomy?

REFLECTIVE EXEMPLAR 4.4 – AGNES AND RITA

In clinical supervision, Leslie talked about bathing Agnes and Rita, and how bathing them created a space where they could talk and he could get to know them. Agnes was a respite care patient and had had a number of strokes in the past, leaving her very dependent and difficult to communicate with.

> *Leslie*: "I felt I got to know Agnes for the first time this morning since she arrived. I took her for a bath and she talked about her legs, the swelling and pain. We made frequent eye contact and she showed me she was enjoying the bath and was quite comfortable. She was crying out for Toby, her son and carer, when she first came in. Now she seems more relaxed. She smiled at me after the bath."
>
> *CJ*: "Giving you positive feedback?"
>
> *Leslie*: "Oh yes . . . When I looked at her legs and changed her dressings she made it clear that she was pleased with this attention. After her bath I was helping her comb her hair, showing her the mirror, she said, 'Go on, give me a kiss'."
>
> *CJ*: "And did you?"
>
> *Leslie*: "Yes. I think I had perceived the 'stereotype' of a dependent, confused patient when she came in and now I'm seeing her as a human being."
>
> *CJ*: "Your honesty is profound . . . you highlight the significance of knowing the person and yet how easy it is to see the 'patient', especially in negative terms. In terms of knowing Agnes, did you check her self-assessment?"
>
> *Leslie*: "No. I need to contact Toby and make an appointment to talk through her self-assessment."
>
> *CJ*: "Doing this would create the opportunity to establish a dialogue with Toby and assess his own carer needs; reflect on the philosophy of self-assessment in respite care . . ."

After we had explored the philosophy of respite care in the context of knowing Agnes and Toby, Leslie continued by talking about Rita:

> *Leslie*: "Rita also had a bath this morning. We talked about Burford and the surrounding countryside – the places we know. She talked about the places she had lived, where her husband had died, her dog. Lots of personal parts of her life."

CJ: "Did you ask what she was really trying to say?"

Leslie: "No I didn't. At times she just wanted to burst into tears. It was certainly grief she was expressing."

CJ: "Some people find it difficult to talk about their grief so they talk about all the things that surround their grief."

Leslie: "Ummm . . ."

CJ: "You didn't feel like going in there . . . would that have been the wrong time?"

Leslie: "I think so . . . Rita wanted an early bath to be ready for the chiropodist, so she was anxious about that as well, but we did talk about the good things in her life that she valued. This was useful to know with her case conference coming up for nursing home placement."

Commentary

What do these brief snippets of supervision dialogue reveal about knowing people? Leslie highlights the risk of knowing Agnes only as a 'stereotype', as if she was someone who had 'lost her mind' and had become merely a body to service. Yet, given the opportunity, Agnes emerged to surprise and delight Leslie, even indulge in mild flirtation. He brightened her day and as a consequence she brightened his. The Burford cue, 'Who is this person?' acknowledges the humanness of the person; challenging the pull to depersonalise and categorise people as types.

With Rita, helping her bathe opens a space where Rita can explore her life. Leslie dwells at her side as she talks through her life in response to her grief at losing her husband and now her home. Her grief lays thick on the surface of who she is at this moment in time. Leslie tuned into this wavelength. Other cues buzz as he also collects information for her forthcoming case conference: 'What support does she have in life?', 'How does she view the future for herself?'

In both situations Leslie was helping these women bathe. Yet does bathing these two woman justify Leslie's time and priority? He is their primary nurse but why not ask the care assistant on duty to do this apparently mundane task? From a holistic perspective there is no such thing as a task, let alone a mundane task. Bathing these women is part of the whole. The holistic practitioner responds on simultaneous multiple levels rather than as a set of linear tasks. Bathing patients is often viewed as menial and unskilled work for care assistants to do, yet sense the poignancy and intimacy within the caring moment. Bathing enabled him, certainly for the first time with Agnes, to know these women at some deeper level, where the emotional, psychological and spiritual dimensions of being surface – a moment where the profane meets the sacred (Wolf 1986). Perhaps bathing these women is the most important work for Leslie that morning, that is if they are not uncomfortable with being bathed by a man. Leslie needs to be sensitive to the gender issue because these women are vulnerable.

Pick up the advocacy role

Leslie noted that some of the night staff were negative towards Agnes when handling her. In clinical supervision we explored why his colleagues might feel this way. Leslie felt it was because they did not know her as he now did, that they only saw the difficult patient not the suffering person. Based on this understanding we explored how Leslie might respond to his colleagues by opening up a dialogue to communicate his understanding of their feelings but also to undermine their negative attitude; for example, asking his colleagues directly how they respond when Agnes called out 'Toby' all night long. Their negative attitude confronted Leslie with a significant therapeutic challenge: how to minimise the impact of these negative feelings on Agnes's care? Leslie knew he needed to protect Agnes from this abuse but how? He felt like a protective parent toward Agnes and an angry parent towards the night staff in response to their 'uncaring'. Using Halldórsdóttir's criteria (Box 2.4), he could see the night staff's response as 'life depleting'. We agreed he needed to involve the night staff more in appreciating Agnes's life pattern, acknowledging their input in knowing Agnes at night and to plan with them how best to meet Agnes's needs, especially during the night.

As it was, Leslie had labelled the night staff in negative terms just as they had labelled Agnes.

This experience illustrates the way prejudice clouds the practitioner's knowing lens and that knowing the person must be a collaborative knowing. I develop the idea of the 'difficult' person phenomenon and parental responses in Chapter 6, and the nature of the therapeutic team and managing conflict in Chapter 7.

The clinical supervision dialogue reveals my 'line manager' supervisor response – confronting Leslie with his effective performance yet hopefully in a way that is supportive. Issues like checking Agnes's self-assessment is crucial to her appropriate care and involving Toby in the caring process, issues picked up in Leslie's next supervision session dialogue:

Leslie: "I met with Toby, Agnes's son and main carer. It's interesting to follow up the conversation from our last session. The family asked to see me about lifting and the possibility for further respite care admissions.
CJ: "To teach them lifting?"
Leslie: "Yes and for updating the assessment for them to feel more supported."
CJ: "Do they belong to the carer support group?"
Leslie: " I'm not sure . . . until the case conference I hadn't appreciated her daughter's real feelings. She had broken down and talked to the social worker about her relationship with her mother. Carers always seem to have to put up a front that they are coping. They seem uncomfortable about expressing any struggle because they are uncertain how we will respond."
CJ: "Do you mean how we might judge them?"

Box 4.3   Nolan & Grant's (1989) identification of (unmet) carer need

---

- Need for information on a variety of topics from who's who to a more detailed account of illness, treatment and services available.
- Need for choice and some degree of control in packaging services to meet individual needs.
- Need for skills training in relation to nursing care, such as dealing with incontinence, lifting techniques.
- Need for nursing support on a number of levels:
    (1)   Being recognised and valued for their caring.
    (2)   Having someone to talk problems over with.
    (3)   Help with recognising and dealing with emotional issues of guilt, anger, sadness, hopelessness and helplessness.
    (4)   Some form of regular respite care from their role as carer.

Leslie: "Yes, yes . . . who else is there for her to open up to? There isn't a husband."

CJ: "Yes, it's important to develop your empathy with the carers who deal with such situations. Perhaps review respite care theory in the carer resource file? In particular note Nolan & Grant's research into carer burden and the inadequacy of professional response to carer need (Box 4.3). Then use this research to reflect on Agnes's son and daughter needs."

Nolan & Grant (1989) considered that lack of professional sensitivity may inadvertently increase carer stress and inhibit carers from seeking further professional help. Leslie could see that his approach to the carers had tended to be reactive: waiting and responding to their approach, rather than proactive: taking the initiative and approaching the carers first. I asked Leslie, 'If you were the carer, what approach would you prefer?'

Of course Leslie appreciated the proactive stance. I challenged him. 'Why?'

Leslie responded, 'Because it would tell me you cared whereas if I came to you I might doubt that. I may not even come to you because I don't want to admit I'm struggling and don't want to burden you or make you feel I am a nuisance, and jeopardise existing respite arrangements.'

Leslie laughed. The revelation was profound. Not letting him off the hook I confronted him with his role *vis à vis* the social worker role – does he hand over responsibility to the social worker to work with Rita's daughter? Role ambiguity can lead to conflict so clarifying role responsibility and role relationships is essential to enable professionals to work together effectively (role framing – see Box 1.10).

Self assessment

Agnes was a frequent admission for respite care to give her family a break from caring. At Burford two beds were set aside for respite care. Often these patients had varying degrees of dementia and were poor informants. The reason for admission was usually for respite care for the home carers although also an opportunity to review and improve the caring situation at home.

As such, the carers were often not around to give information to the care staff except on admission. In response, a self-assessment form was developed to enable carers to provide information about the patient and to reflect on their own carer needs. The self-assessment form is based on activities of living and the carer needs to inform us of the person's and carer's needs at point of admission so the carer can be reassured that we know how best to care and hence minimise the risk of disrupting normal patterns of caring. It enables the carer to be acknowledged and feel involved in the caring process. Carers may well feel guilty at neglecting their 'carer role' (Dawson 1987). It is often difficult for carers to accept help because any disruption to normal patterns can create more stress than it eases. By negotiating care based on the self-assessment, the carer feels they have not relinquished either their caring or responsibility. Hopefully, the carer can then enjoy her or his break in a more relaxed frame of mind.

In summary, self-assessment aims to enable the staff to:

- appreciate and honour the carer's principal caring role
- recognise the person's needs and lifestyle in detail
- ensure the immediate continuity of care between home and hospice with minimal disruption to normal lifestyle patterns (unless beneficial)
- appreciate the little things that are significant to make the person's stay in hospital most comfortable and enjoyable
- know and respond to the carer's needs.

The self-assessment form has 10 parts that focus on particular aspects of daily living:

(1) personal hygiene needs
(2) dressing needs
(3) eating and drinking needs
(4) toilet needs
(5) mobility needs
(6) sleep needs
(7) daily activity/communication needs
(8) psychological and emotional needs
(9) additional information
(10) carer needs

In Box 4.4 I illustrate Mrs Gilbert's self-assessment of her carer needs, part ten of the scale. Mrs Gilbert's husband was terminally ill with bowel cancer. Mrs Gilbert presented a 'brave face' but actually was at the end of her tether – an impression masked in her written responses. Her comments were fairly typical, reflecting a significant level of carer burden. Completing the form was very revealing for the carers – it confronted their stoicism – and was often the first time they admitted to themselves that caring was both a physical and emotional burden. This was difficult to accept because they felt a duty to care and saying it was hard was somehow indicating that they were failing in some

Box 4.4   Mrs Gilbert's self assessment of her carer needs

10.0	**Carer needs**	
10.1	How are you generally coping at home?	*Reasonably well but there is no let up. I am 77 years old.*
10.2	Do you have any particular problems or areas of concern with caring?	*No, only cleaning up accidents – not so bad lately.*
10.3	What support are you receiving? Is this adequate?	*I have a certain amount of help with cleaning – a nurse to bathe Jim weekly. I am hoping for help from Social Services to help him wash and dress – this is in the pipeline.*
10.4	Are you able to identify any further support that might be beneficial?	*Not as yet, must see how the above works out.*
10.5	How do you anticipate the future?	*With trepidation, but I take each day as it comes.*
10.6	When did you last get a break from caring?	*Never, since the illness started apart from some sitting service with the church to let me go shopping.*
10.7	Do you get a break from caring from other sources?	*No.*
10.8	How would you describe your mood?	*Generally I grin and bear it, but it's getting harder and I feel I am getting irritated with him sometimes – which only makes me feel guilty and more stressed. Bit of a vicious circle.*
10.9	Has it been necessary for you to care for others in the past?	*Only with my mother many years ago.*
	How was that for you?	*Difficult because of my own growing family's needs.*
10.10	How does caring affect your pattern of living?	*One tends to drop out of local events because caring is so time consuming and exhausting.*
10.11	Are you anxious about ....Jim....... coming into the hospice?	*Slightly apprehensive as he's a home bird but I know he will have every care possible.*
10.12	What is your greatest fear?	*I know it sounds selfish but being left on my own . . . I know Jim is going to die.*
10.13	How is your partner feeling?	*Behind his brave face he is petrified yet he won't talk about it to me . . . it makes me feel alone.*

way. Discussing their responses opened a space where they could be acknow-ledged for their caring role and to release pent-up feelings, enabling the practitioner to respond to Nolan & Grant's challenge to provide emotional support. The responses also revealed physical and social aspects of care that the caring team could help with to improve the home situation.

Therapeutic journaling for patients

In Chapter 1 I indicated that journaling was therapeutic. Consider any patients you work with who have been having a difficult time or have difficulty in expressing their feelings. Ask yourself, 'Would keeping a journal benefit them?' Of course they might be reluctant to share their writing with you, but I suggest that such writing is revealing and helps you know the person.

REFLECTIVE EXEMPLAR 4.5 – MOIRA VASS – LIVING WITH MOTOR NEURONE DISEASE

Moira wrote her story of living and dying with motor neurone disease because she wanted her carers to understand what she was experiencing. Writing gave her dying some purpose and enabled her to express her feelings of despair and anger that she struggled to say. Moira wrote:

> "I have motor neurone disease (MND). This is a disease that relentlessly destroys the nerves that enable us to control all our movements, while leaving the intellect and senses unaffected. There is no cure for this disease. I was told the cause was unknown and it was terminal. However, there is a ray of hope – the drug Rilutek. This is not a cure, but has been shown in trials to extend survival in people with MND. Its cost is somewhere between £1000 and £2000 per patient per year, yet it gives the patient time and some hope. It slows down the paralysing effect. My attitude to Rilutek is if it does not cure then why take it? It only prolongs the agony and postpones the inevitable. The paralysis goes on unabated and death is by strangulation, a form of choking due to the fact that the intercostal muscles are affected and you cannot breathe or cough. From day one I became slowly and deliberately useless and within six months I could no longer speak, eat, drink or walk unaided. Artificial ventilation via an endotracheal tube merely prolongs the suffering. Patients remain alert to the end and many need treatment to relieve their distress, as well as oxygen to assist breathing.
>
> **Living with feeding at home**
> MND affects the nerve endings and consequently affects the muscles in most of my body, but particularly all the muscles in my throat which means I cannot speak, eat, drink, or swallow. I was referred by my neurologist to a dietician as the time had come for me to be fed by tube. My reaction was disbelief, anger and a lot of tears. Then more tears.
>
> By the time I came to see the nutritionist consultant, I had calmed down and accepted the fact that this was my only option if I wanted to go on living. The tube is attached to the gastrostomy. My reaction was despair. How can I live with this? The first thing that crossed my mind was no more baked or roast potatoes. No more pre-dinner sherry, wine, all the joys of living. One of my favourite hobbies was cooking: adventurous cooking, dinner parties, BBQ with the family, like any normal person.

The first feed was only 200 ml at 50 ml per hour. The feed type was Nutrison and it was not a painful procedure. When the feed was finished this was followed by a 60 ml syringe of water to flush out the tube and give you extra fluid and thereafter a water flush every four hours, totalling 240 ml per day to prevent me from getting dehydrated – feed at night and water during the day.

However, it did little to calm my anger. I just wanted to stop the whole business and go to God. I could not see myself living with a Kangaroo pump and a plastic bag full of 1000 ml of Nutrison Energy Plus to be given overnight. The idea of the night feed was to enable me to be free during the day apart from the water flushes.

I laid awake for the first three nights in hospital, my anger only getting worse. Anger that felt like someone pouring boiling oil over my body. On the third night, I reached down and closed the roller clamp. I forgot about the bleep sound from the pump, which brought two nurses to the pump who duly restarted the feed. They sat with me for a while and we had a chat. I was finding it impossible to come to terms with my new way of life, but I decided to take a more positive look at my feelings and especially the word ANGER. It struck me the word 'anger' is almost a cocktail of emotions:

A   Aggressive, to myself and the staff – zero tolerance
N   Negative thinking
G   Grief, crying
E   Emotions out of control
R   Resentful – 'why me' syndrome

So I decided, for the sake of my family, my husband but especially my three grandchildren, to make an effort because they all thought the feeding pump was a great idea. I made up my mind to come to terms with tube feeding at home although the sight of the tube at my stomach brought back the anger.

On Saturday morning, 14 February 1998, I was found unconscious by Gordon, who was unable to rouse me. It was decided to admit me to the hospice. I have no recollection of the tragedy. I came round with my grand-daughter Kerry, aged 16, crying, telling me to squeeze her hand if I could hear what she said: 'Please wake up Nan, we love you'. Twenty four hours later, I was awake to the reality of my condition. My living will meant they could not feed me if I went unconscious. As a result they were anxious to start the feed but I said, 'No, no, leave me be'. By the fourth day I gave in and the Kangaroo pump and plastic bag with the 1000 ml of food was back. I was back to square one – I had to give in for the sake of my family.

Once I had come to terms with home feeding I found it extremely easy to live with and having the feed at night was more convenient. You are free during the day to do what you please and go where you like. It is very easy to take a water flush with you. It took about six weeks to establish a routine. I would set it up downstairs in the kitchen, sit back in my armchair and watch TV. The feed takes ten hours to go through. When I am in bed I make sure the tube is free and that I attach the tube from the pump by holding it in place with sellotape on my thigh – so far it has never woken me up. If you can still eat anything that is a bonus.

The hospice
Following my admission to the hospice as an inpatient in February, I received wonderful care, especially as I spent four days on 'hunger strike'. To me, this was the only way out – to stop all treatments, drugs and feed. The staff respected my wishes and while I was unconscious my living will (advanced directive) stated *no treatment*. When I regained consciousness I made the decision to continue cessation of all treatments. I found my family were devastated and my three grandchildren cried and pleaded with me. On day five, I came back to earth to the delight of everyone. The nursing care in the hospice was a special kind of nursing but I would rather have had my rights and my way.

On discharge I was invited back one day a week as a day-care patient. On the first day this caused me unbelievable distress. They collected me in a hospice ambulance; there was the driver, a nurse and myself. As my husband waved goodbye I started to cry, another step down the MND road to death. Suddenly my anger exploded and I lost control, crying excessively and choking. The nurse told the driver to pull over to the side of the road until I had calmed down sufficiently. On arrival at the hospice I was taken into the quiet room and there I remained for the rest of the day. With their special kind of care and continuous oxygen for 20 minutes, I calmed down enough and fell asleep again.

I have come to terms now with the hospice-type care for terminally ill patients. I am going into the hospice for a week of respite care – the last week of the world cup!

Care in the community
Learning to live with a progressive neurological condition, and in my case the advance has been rapid, has not been easy. Since my collapse in February on St. Valentine's Day, I am totally helpless and require 24-hour care. The equipment needed to assist in my care has built up gradually over a period of time. It takes one nurse to get me up in the morning, washed and dressed. I bring myself down on the chair lift. We found the easiest dress code for my needs consists of a silk top, slacks, knickers with pad, socks and sandals. What does break my heart is that I can no longer wear my size 12 outfits. Since the introduction of the tube feeding my waistline has increased to size 16. The position the night team leave me in bed has to be the right one for comfort as there I remain until morning. I can no longer move in bed or raise my head. I was provided with an air mattress to prevent pressure sores. My gratitude to the team. They always chat to me about nursing, clothes and fashion. I feel guilty that I need so much of their time. My particular hate was losing my independence, and in particular my personal hygiene. This added to my despair and anger.

It is at times like this when I wish we had voluntary euthanasia. The patient should certainly have a say when and where to die. Life with MND is like a living hell on earth. Your whole body is dead. All I am left with is sight, smell, taste, hearing and sensation. Family gatherings and Sunday dinners have never been the same. I can take no part in family laughter and discussion. I take no part in the kitchen or food shopping. Anywhere I go I must take the suction machine, my talking machine, a large bunch of tissues and a carer familiar with my management. Controlling the saliva which flows from my mouth is not only depressing but also embarrassing. I fold the tissue into one-inch widths, fourfold deep and roll the top end down into a narrow roll. I put about three rolls in the side of my mouth since I can no longer cough, but if I have an occasional sneeze this prevents me from biting my tongue and my lip which is very painful. If I sneeze again within 5–10 minutes I hit the same spot. The surgery lent me a nebuliser to help remove very thick mucus.

Through Social Services I have obtained a wheelchair. I cried my heart out when it first arrived. Life in a wheelchair is a very different world. You feel so vulnerable and at risk. As the disease progresses I find waking up in the morning a slow process. My friend, the practice nurse, suggested 10–20 minutes oxygen is supplied. Someone has to open my eyelids for me – usually Gordon. The only way I can sum up the sad journey is with a poem I have written. What more can I say!"

My living hell on earth

I walk alone
Along this path
Leaving life's hope,
Sorrow, love and pain
Standing at my gate.

I speak no more
I sing no more
I eat no more
IN MY LIVING HELL.

Sometimes I wish
I could swallow,
But there's always
Something at my throat.

I drink no more
I kiss no more
I smile no more
IN MY LIVING HELL.

I see and hear
My world go by,
But reach out
I can not do.

My smiles have gone
I have no joy
I walk no more
To join my crowd
IN MY LIVING HELL.

I'm wheeled along
In my wheelchair
To a sea of knees
And a lot of pushchairs!

Some smiles I get
Some yawns and cries
Thank God they're not
IN MY LIVING HELL.

I tried to find
The peaceful way
But the road is closed
And I must stay.

Animal rights have a say
They can die
When they say;
Please God why can't I?
IN MY LIVING HELL.

Reflection

Moira was keen to publish her journal. Louise, the day-care senior nurse discussed this with me and I agreed to meet with Moira and discuss possibilities. I wrote in my reflective journal:

"August 4th. I arrive ten minutes late. Moira is not there. Louise says she has been delayed because her catheter had blocked and will arrive in about 20 minutes. I am happy to sit with the group preparing for the day. Moira arrives. We move to a table. She is small and frail in her wheelchair. She has a piece of tissue coming out of her mouth that soaks up the excess secretions she can no longer control. She has her 'lite speaker' with her to communicate with me. I tell her who I am and clarify why we are meeting together – to consider her journal on living with motor neurone disease and ways it might be published. I had been strongly moved by her journal. I also felt strongly moved by Louise's experiences that she had shared in clinical supervision. As one of Moira's carers Louise had become deeply involved with Moira.

Using her 'lite writer' Moira tells me about her experience this morning with her catheter being removed. The district nurse has asked Louise to replace it. Moira says it was awful. I sensed this and ask if it was embarrassing. Moira grimaces. She said she could write so much more. I say she has written enough, that her message is powerful and will enable others to understand and learn. I pause and wonder what it must be like to suffer from MND.

I say to Moira that I understand she wants to publish whilst she is still alive. I ask her 'How long do you expect to live?' I feel my pulse quicken on asking this question yet Moira takes it in her stride. She says her GP refused to answer that question, but she expects to die soon. Of course, no one knows for certain but do we as practitioners avoid such difficult questions and conversations? Does Moira's despair and obsession with euthanasia encourage us into avoidance tactics?

I understood Moira's need to write as a testament that her life and death were not without meaning. She had been a health visitor and teacher. She said she loved nursing and wanted to give something if it would help others to understand. Keeping a journal was a therapeutic act for her. It was cathartic, enabling her to pour out her feelings and helping her make sense of her despair in the face of her relentless physical deterioration towards death.

The catheter was yet another marker along this trajectory. She had become incontinent and she is a proud woman. Another devastating blow as it took away what pride she had left. I asked her if there was anything that made her smile – the sun shining in the morning or a sparrow singing? In response she did smile . . . but she said she felt like the weather. It was raining hard outside. Indeed, she had shed many tears that morning. In her absence of words she drew the tear lines down her cheeks with her fingers. There was no way anybody could take away her despair. There was no way she could rationalise what was happening to her, yet focusing on something positive as her journal and the possibility to publish it did ameliorate her despair, as if the sun had come out for a moment. She was grateful to me. She joined her hands in thanks. I felt touched by this woman in this moment, privileged to sit with her and experience her dying. I was conscious that she, like other patients I had met and written about, were teaching me something profound along my own journey to realise myself as caring. When I left her, I sensed a lightness, a soft spring in my feet. Why was this? Perhaps I should have felt burdened with her despair. But no, the contrary. I had been lifted by the experience, as if I had been touched by an angel. I felt such a calmness and sense of humility. I felt that I was an angel, that I had given Moira some warmth and light within her living hell, as indeed Louise gave her. Moira nourished others, comforted and cared for those who would care for her. She did not want to be a burden but sensed the struggle her carers must feel caring for her. She had shared her story with her carers when perhaps they had not realised how she felt and had been insensitive to her plight. They were touched and it changed their caring towards her. It had opened their eyes to what Moira was feeling inside."

Moira died shortly afterwards.

Such journal accounts offer deep insights into the way people respond to terminal illness and face death. Her writing became her sanctuary, her space where she could scream out loud and communicate to others so they knew and could understand. That was so important to Moira. Perhaps she sensed it was only too easy to see the demanding, complaining, depressed and angry woman rather than the suffering woman who deeply loved her grandchildren. Her writing made it easier for her and her family to dwell together.

How might you encourage and guide a patient to write? Well, most people will struggle with the idea because it is not something they usually do. Writing about feelings demands an acceptance of those feelings that the person may prefer to bottle up and defend against. So, I might sit with the person and help them talk about their experience and then suggest writing about the experience, perhaps as a letter to someone they love and want them to understand. Perhaps start by writing down the strongest feeling epecially if they have been resisting it. As such, writing the word down is both cathartic and confronting. I would then suggest they write something positive about their life, either something happening now or from memory. The intention is to balance any negative thoughts or feelings with positive ones, to seek balance and harmony through writing. To help find a still place inside themselves where they can be reflective (bringing the mind home) I might suggest writing in the afternoon, play some music, or have some complementary treatment beforehand. When they feel more at ease, I suggest they explore the feeling of thoughts they have written: 'Why do I feel that way?' And of course, to be available to the person to help them talk through the things they have written. In doing so, offer them guidance, courage, compassion and let them know they are not alone.

Chapter 5

The Aesthetic Response

In Chapter 2 I set out the Being Available template as the core therapeutic of holistic practice. In Chapter 4 I explored the way the practitioner's ability to be available is influenced by the extent she is concerned for the other and the extent she knows the person. In this chapter I reveal the nature of the asethetic response as another factor that influences the practitioner's ability to be available. The aesthetic response is coined from Carper's (1978) fundamental patterns of knowing in nursing (see Box 1.2) described as the ability to grasp and interpret what is unfolding, envisaging what might be, and responding with appropriate and skilful action that includes evaluating the efficacy of the response.

Clinical judgement

The ability to grasp and interpret the clinical situation is the essence of clinical judgement. If the practitioner does not grasp and interpret particular situations accurately, then the basis for subsequent skilful action is flawed. As Carper (1978) indicated, there are various influences on the practitioner's judgement:

- who I am as a person, my concerns, prejudices, attitudes, stress levels, values, feelings at the time; forces that are likely to influence the practitioner's judgement
- current research and theory that might inform the practitioner's judgement
- a sense of what is ethically the right thing to do
- past experience that includes what worked well and what didn't work well in similar situations, what interventions the practitioner is skilled at and feels comfortable with using, what responses are permitted, and resources available
- the practitioner's vision of practice.

Ethical action

Ethical principles exist within any society to guide people to act for the best. They are also the hallmark of professional accountability: 'codes of conduct' written by professional bodies to reassure society that professionals practise according to a set of ethical values, and for which they can be held to account.

However, ethical principles are only guidelines, they do not prescribe how the practitioner should respond within the particular situation. It is a question of judgement, being mindful of and balancing the influence of different ethical principles. There is always tension between professional and patient autonomy and the rights of the individual set against finite resources.

REFLECTIVE EXEMPLAR 5.1 – JANET AND MICHELLE'S STORY

This reflection concerns Michelle's response to Mrs Denver, a woman admitted to the five-day surgical ward for a breast biopsy. Michelle is a staff nurse who has been qualified 12 months and Janet is the ward sister. The data was collected as a part of a project to monitor the impact of clinical supervision as a model for developing clinical leadership (Johns 2003). The ward staff had recently written a new vision for practice based on holism and implemented the Burford NDU model: caring in practice. As you read, imagine you work on this busy surgical ward that does a drug round at set times.

> *Michelle*: "She was a nurse, a pleasant lady. Next morning I was on an early shift doing the drugs. I asked her whether there was anything she needed. She said, 'No . . . oh I do feel weepy,' and then she burst into tears. I pulled the drug trolley over and pulled the curtains around her bed. She said her friends had been saying how scared they would be if it was them [having a breast biopsy] . . . she hadn't appreciated these feelings until now. She said, 'Oh my husband and my children!' It made me think – she's a nurse and she's so vulnerable. I don't know if I did any good."
>
> *Janet*: "Put yourself in her shoes . . . you spent half an hour with her. How would you have felt if a nurse did this for you? Nurses often underestimate the work they do with patients. Could you have done more?"
>
> *Michelle*: "I made a conscious decision to blow the pills, no-one will come to any harm. It made me feel so vulnerable. What do you say?"
>
> *Janet*: "Did you have to say anything? Nurses aren't very good at sitting and listening . . . It's okay giving out information and advice."
>
> *Michelle*: "The silence is difficult . . . it's keeping quiet I find the hardest. Did we give her the opportunity to chat? Did we keep away because she was a nurse? Are we frightened of being patronising? Should she be treated any differently?"
>
> *Janet*: "You are the patient's named nurse and therefore it was appropriate for you to spend time with her. Finding someone to take over the drug trolley or even finding the named nurse if you hadn't been the named nurse would have lost the spontaneous moment for this lady. Did you discuss this with other staff?"
>
> *Michelle*: "Yes. We are not as sensitive to these ladies with breast lumps as we could be. Would a counselling course help? I'm at a loss to know what to

say to them. Am I helping or hindering? It's such a sensitive issue. They look jolly and jovial outside but inside it's like a bombshell."

Janet: "Did you use touch?"

Michelle: "I put my hand on her arm when she apologised for crying. Not knowing her well enough stopped me from holding her hand."

Janet: "Could you have done anything differently?"

Michelle: "I could have been more available to her pre-operatively. I couldn't have made it better for her . . . change what was wrong."

Janet: "What would have happened if this had been a busier morning?"

Michelle: "I wouldn't have left her but I wouldn't have been so calm. I'd have been thinking more about other work that needed to be done: premeds, eye drops, and things . . . thinking I wish you'd hurry up. That's really wrong. How do we get over that?"

Janet: "I don't really know. Perhaps as practitioners we need to be more prepared to defend our actions."

Commentary

Finding an upset patient whilst doing the drug round is probably a common occurrence on hospital wards yet in this dialogue it takes on profound significance. Mrs Denver is no longer a task to do but a suffering human being, a vulnerable woman having undergone a breast biopsy and now awaiting her fate.

On reflection, Michelle could express her own vulnerability and lack of ability and confidence to respond, and see the way she avoided the situation until the moment Mrs Denver's suffering bubbled over and confronted Michelle. Michelle's caring instinct made her respond as best she could. It is a sobering thought to consider how many women suffer in silence and how many nurses are ill equipped to respond to suffering and as a consequence avoid it. How would you want a nurse to respond to you? Do you think Michelle responded for the best? How would you know that? I have used ethical mapping to consider this question (Box 5.1). Remember the ethical map trail has six stages:

(1)   frame the dilemma
(2)   consider the perspective of different people commencing with the nurse(s) own perspectives
(3)   consider which ethical principles apply in terms of the best (ethically correct) decision
(4)   consider what conflict exists between perspectives/values and how these might be resolved
(5)   consider who had the authority for making the decision/taking action
(6)   consider the power relationships/factors that determined the way the decision/action was actually taken

Michelle is first challenged to consider the perspectives of different players, whether directly or indirectly involved, commencing with her own and then Mrs Denver. She is encouraged to empathise with each perspective, which as

Box 5.1 Ethical mapping: Should Michelle stop the drug round or continue it?

Patient's/family's perspective Mrs Denver was visibly upset and needed care at that moment. Anything less would have added to her suffering, possibly a complaint from relatives? Stopping the round was the best action. Other patients may be watching and expect nurses to be caring yet also know they are busy, and may also expect Michelle to give them their drugs first.	*Who had authority to make the decision/act within the situation?* We do not know if Michelle was the 'nurse-in-charge' or patterns of ward authority. Janet's response suggests that Michelle did have authority to respond as she felt best.	*The doctor's perspective* Most likely to see Michelle's primary role to ensure all patients received medication on time.
If there is conflict of perspectives/values – how might these be resolved? Yes – Michelle experienced intrapersonal conflict (see Box 7.3) – uncertain in her own mind what's best. Options: Michelle could have spent less time with Mrs Denver, could have gone back to Mrs Denver afterwards, or got someone else to speak to her, or to take over the drug round.	*The situation/dilemma:* **Should Michelle stop the drug round or continue it?** Michelle was ethically right to respond to Mrs Denver. However, a better option may have been to acknowledge the suffering, finish the drugs and return when she was under less pressure. I think it was important that she responded and not another nurse 'sounds like a task to ask someone else as if nurses are simply interchangeable'.	*What ethical principles inform this situation?* Ethically, she was weighing up the needs of the individual against the needs of the whole. Would other patients have come to harm? Michelle felt they would not have done. Virtue: what should a caring nurse do? – supports Michelle's action.
The nurse[s]' perspective Michelle could not leave Mrs Denver suffering. Do all nurses share this caring ethic? Unlikely. Some nurses may be irritated that the drugs have been left – throw the ward into organisational chaos.	*Consider the power relationships/factors that determined the way the decision/action was actually taken.* There was no conflict between Michelle and other health professionals.	*The organisation's perspective* Most anxious to avoid complaint from patients not receiving their drugs on time or medical angst about 'irresponsible' nurse behaviour. Tasks are appealing because they reinforce the primary value of 'smooth running' of the organisation.

we explored in Chapter 4, requires understanding and suspending her own perspective about the situation in order to appreciate and accept the perspectives of others. This does not mean she has to agree with them. Seeing the different perspectives is rather like a helicopter view. Then she can consider what ethical principles inform the situation and whether any conflict exists between these principles and different perspectives. Only then can she consider the best way to resolve any conflict. Yet doing what's best may be constrained by tradition, authority and embodiment: tradition: always complete the drug round; authority: can I act as I feel appropriate?; embodiment: my body urges me to finish the drug round as usual.

As you can see I do not entirely agree that Michelle acted for the best, even though her response was most caring. She was 'mopping up a mess' that might have been lessened by being more caring beforehand. It really does highlight the need for connection and relationship. Michelle needed to be more mindful of the impact of breast biopsy on Mrs Denver and other similar patients. Michelle's comment, 'I could have been more available to her pre-operatively' is very insightful; consider the Burford cues (Box 4.1) – 'what meaning does this breast biopsy have for Mrs Denver?' and 'how is Mrs Denver feeling about this procedure?', 'what factors are important to make her stay in hospital comfortable'? and 'how do I feel about Mrs Denver?' – paying attention to the idea that Michelle might be avoiding Mrs Denver because she is a nurse.

As Janet said, 'Put yourself in her shoes.' What would you be thinking and feeling? Having a breast biopsy may be a minor surgical procedure, but what does it mean to the woman? Reflect on Mrs Denver's fears, 'Oh my husband and my children!', that reveal the threat of death. The literature indicates that this is a very distressing time (Woodward & Webb 2001). As Woodward & Webb note:

> 'The quality of life a woman experiences during the process of investigation and treatment for breast disorders is linked with the communication and support provided by others, and includes family members, friends and clinic personnel. Knopf (1994) recommends that nurses working with breast cancer can develop strategies to help patients clarify, interpret and process information: this needs to be extended to all breast disorders. Greater attention should be given to the emotional experiences of all women during the diagnostic phase of breast disease. As Northouse *et al.* (1995) comment, a breast biopsy is not a benign experience.'

There is a significant literature concerned with breast lumps that Michelle might explore to inform her practice, and which Janet might direct her to in responding to the MSR cue, 'What knowledge did or could have informed my practice?' If Michelle had been congnisant of this literature she might have been more sensitive to Mrs Denver's potential anxiety and emotional reaction. In other words Mrs Denver's suffering and distress *might* have been lessened by a more proactive response. Butterfield (1990) describes this as 'upstream thinking': responding to prevent people falling into the stream rather than having to rescue them once they have fallen in. Perhaps on a short stay surgical unit that specialises in breast biopsy such thinking should be second nature.

Yet practitioners get so locked into a reactive culture, it is difficult to see ahead. We may need prompts to draw our attention to things.

In choosing to spend time with Mrs Denver, Michelle chose not to spend time with other patients. The juggling of priorities is ethical action. The reflective practitioner is an ethical practitioner, mindful of competing priorities, and mindful that her values are not compromised. So Michelle might take Mrs Denver's hand and communicate her care and understanding. She might say, 'I can see you are upset.' She might say, 'I can't be with you at this moment,' but because she has invested in creating a caring relationship, Mrs Denver knows that Michelle cares about her and will return at an appropriate moment. Mrs Denver will feel and bathe in Michelle's care even in that brief moment, and her suffering will be eased.

In other words, if we reflect deeper on Michelle's experience we can see that the conditions for caring were problematic. Michelle must be able to justify her decision to stop the drug round, to confront others' perceptions of priorities when these are misplaced, and to resist any blame as a consequence.

The drug round reflects task approach nursing – that all patients receive medications at uniform times, helped by the routinisation of drug administration times into fixed patterns. The task is considered as an efficient way of ensuring work is delegated and completed. However, because the administration of drugs is routinised it may detract from seeing and responding to people's individual needs. Tasks break up the pattern of holistic care by fragmenting aspects of the whole and demanding conformity to the organisational pattern. It is as if the organisation sets the wavelength that patients must find and flow with or else be viewed as deviant and all the consequences that such labelling brings.

A counter approach would be that nurses tailor drug administration to their individual patients, an approach in my view that takes no longer and yet creates a caring moment (rather like Leslie bathing Rita and Agnes – see exemplar 4.4) for being with the patient, *especially* on busy surgical wards, when being with the patient may seem like a premium. Again this brings in the question of values. Unfortunately, the mindset of tasks is to get the task done, and interruption is often viewed as a nuisance. From this perspective, the drug round was itself the problem. The solution would be to scrap the drug round and ask nurses to administer drugs on an individual basis.

Reflect on the routines and tasks of your day and consider whom they benefit. Is the routinisation of work through tasks arranged in a hierarchy of importance? In my research (Johns 1989a) I identified a hierarchy of work priorities:

(1)   executing medical responses and physical care
(2)   complying with organisational demands, for example completing documentation
(3)   talking with patients (emotional, psychological and spiritual care)

When I fed back this interpretation to the staff they felt uncomfortable because it shattered the illusion that they practised holistic nursing. The contradiction was stark. The hierarchical task approach to work was so deeply embodied and embedded within tradition that it could not easily be shrugged off. Failure to comply to this hierarchy led to conflict amongst staff and with nurse managers whose interests were reflected in maintaining the hierarchy. The staff knew that the solution was to collapse the hierarchy into a new culture of professional responsibility and judgement based on the unit's holistic vision but could they actually achieve that? Even they doubted that possibility.

In a world of shrinking resources (although I wonder why when the world seems richer and richer), practitioners are at great risk of role overload that inevitably squeezes the caring aspect and heightens the dilemma of managing priorities. Betz & O'Connell (1987) describe role overload as being responsible for more tasks than an individual could perform within shift time. They note that role overload is greater when associated with perceived 'low-level' tasks and paperwork. As Leslie noted in his role as a primary nurse at Burford hospital, 'When I focus on patient care my stress goes down and when I focus on workload, interviews, case conferences, my stress goes up' (Johns 1998a). One response to shrinking resources is to break down the 'shift-bound' culture and move to a new culture of role responsibility. When practitioners felt valued, felt they had a choice about issues, and felt in control of their own time, they were less stressed and willing to use their own time to fulfil their perceived role responsibility. Otherwise they resisted and resented impositions on their own time (Johns 1998a). This understanding is significant in creating a culture of responsibility and support. The two must be in balance. However, such a culture is always open to abuse by unscrupulous organisations who do not value caring, and who see nursing as a prime target for resource savings.

Besides being ethical, action also needs to be skilful. In the following exemplars I want to draw attention to the use of touch as an example of skilful action in response to need.

REFLECTIVE EXEMPLAR 5.2 – ALISON & NINA'S STORY

Alison is a senior staff nurse who works in an Intensive Care Unit (ICU). In one group clinical supervision session she shared her feelings of uselessness and panic when accompanying a woman from ICU for a brain scan. The team was rushing her back to the ward. Alison noted that *all she could do* was stroke this woman's hair whilst in the lift. Nina, her supervisor and colleague challenged her to reflect on the significance of her actions. Alison felt she had stroked the women's hair intuitively, a reflection of her concern for this woman who was the same age as her, just 32. They returned to ICU where mechanical ventilation was commenced. The woman's oxygen saturation recovered and she eventually made a full recovery. Nina wrote:

"I could see that Alison had felt useless and helpless, that she felt she had no role in the lift. All she had managed to do was stroke Jane's hair. I felt it was important that she should be able to see that *being there* was her role.

Nursing is said to be one of the few medical–healing professions that carries out a major portion of its functions through touch. Alison was stroking Jane's hair as a means of reassurance, to imply a presence and to convey her sense of caring. Touch has the unique ability to communicate empathy without using words, words that Alison felt difficult and inappropriate to say in the confines of the lift. Additionally, it is suggested that when a patient is intensely stressed no other form of communication compares with the speed of response to the comforting effects of touch. In our notes of the supervision session we questioned whether touch could have an impact that would reduce anxiety and lead to improved blood pressure and oxygen saturation. The research could not prove this quantifiably in the ICU setting, but all the papers examined did indicate this probability.

Alison can feel reassured that her use of touch was appropriate at this time in Jane's life. When she was critically ill and unconscious, it was an attempt to communicate through one of the senses likely to be intact. When Alison instinctively reached out to touch Jane's hair, she gave her life support; as she attempted to calm her and ease her anxiety. She tried to ensure awareness of a caring presence and to communicate that Alison was *there for her*. Surely this was a most appropriate, fundamental, and worthy role in the circumstances."

Commentary

The clinical supervision group was a training group for clinical supervisors I facilitated. I was present when this experience was shared. It had a profound impact, not just on Alison sharing her experience but on all of us present. It was as if Alison had touched the holy grail of caring, of realising her caring self.

Perhaps, in her state of panic, Alison touched Jane to relieve her sense of helplessness. To touch is also to be touched by the other, a mutual benefit. Reflection enabled Alison to bring touch into her mind as a powerful response to the other's suffering and physiological crisis. Expert practitioners do not deliberately consider how they grasp and interpret the situation, what they are trying to achieve and how best to respond. They just do this intuitively. If a situation is beyond their scope they may be more deliberative (Schön's idea of reflection-in-action – see Chapter 1), or they respond instinctively as Alison did. Perhaps she knew, deep within herself, that touch giving with care is a powerful comforter. Yet, also deep within her, Alison is uncertain of the value of touch, *'all I could do'* as if she was not conscious of the value of touch or *being there* as a therapeutic response. Do we get so wrapped up in doing that we have lost the art of being?

Within the ICU with its banks of technology such simple truths of the power of touch may be obscured or even lost, yet recent research has shown that a five minute foot massage for patients in ICU can significantly reduce anxiety (Hayes & Cox 2000). The use of touch is fundamental to nursing practice and yet how mindful and skilled are nurses at using touch? Every practitioner should be mindful of touch as an expression of caring presence and relaxation, whether bathing, comforting, massaging or whatever.

The impact of touch was the focus for Jill's learning portfolio whilst undertaking the 'Expanding horizons of palliative care' module[1] at the University of Luton. Jill's narrative is a profound story of great beauty that raises significant issues for those who claim to care and offers a good example of reflective writing for academic purposes at post-registration undergraduate degree level.

REFLECTIVE EXEMPLAR 5.3 – JILL'S NARRATIVE

Jill writes:

"This narrative focuses on my experience with Sally who struggled to accept her horrific circumstances as life slipped away. Sally was diagnosed with acute lymphoblastic leukaemia two years ago. She underwent a bone marrow transplant, which completely cured her illness. Eighteen months later she developed cutaneous T-cell lymphoma caused by graft versus host disease. There has only been one other case like this reported in the world! Filled with astounded disbelief Sally is left to suffer the consequences of this devastating condition with the knowledge that no curative treatment is available. On admission to the hospice Sally is in the terminal phase of her illness.

Using selective literature I enhance and substantiate my intuitive awareness that many skills used in palliative care are not formally taught in nursing school but acquired during life experience and personal study. I aim to explore the depths and meaning of touch to gain insight into its therapeutic value. By reflecting on my thoughts, feelings, and reactions of the care I administer, I aim to reveal ways in which I can improve my nursing.

Sally – Evening reports continued
'Her skin is burnt all over, each movement causes pain creating many difficulties with her care. She is having trouble coming to terms with her condition.'

Leaving the office I wander along the corridor greeting patients and informing them that I will be here tonight. A penetrating nauseous vapour fills the air leading towards an open door. Standing at the doorway my eyes transfix onto the small wispy figure covered only by a thin linen sheet. Her face, peaceful in sleep, is disfigured by ferocious, sore red patches which connect and weave their way into every crease and feature of beauty. The main attack centres on her eyes producing a monstrous appearance of two cracked shivering starfish oozing from tentacles. Small mounds of decaying skin cling desperately all around her head reluctant to completely give up and let go. Goose pimples emerge on my arms; my body shudders coldly

---

[1] This module is part of the palliative care pathway. It was previously incorporated within the ENB 285 programme. The module is a level 3 (degree) module.

ending the momentary glance. On auto-pilot I continue to the next room. Disgust and horror overwhelm my mind as I smile at the clean-shaven, unblemished tanned face of the gentleman sitting comfortably reading. Conversation readily flows, we discuss the beautiful view from the window but my brain struggles to dismiss the suffering in the previous room.

Sally has called for assistance; she requests that I cream a very sensitive sore area on her back. As my hand approaches, an invisible layer of heat three inches from her body penetrates my skin. Like entering a hot oven I carefully make contact with her slippery flesh. The cream has dissolved into oil and trickled onto the sheets. With gentle circular movements my fingers attempted to coat the raw burning tissues of Sally's back lubricating the rippled surfaces. Feelings of sadness and hesitance are replaced by pleasurable sensations. The moist warmth infuses through the dryness of my hands creating suppleness and ease. In silence I continue covering any area of need, enjoying the experience of Sally's relaxation radiating through my fingertips. 'That's wonderful,' she whispers, 'You're not wearing gloves.' Startled I question, 'Should I be?' 'Well I'm not contagious but everyone wears them because it's so revolting.' Sally's reply is nonchalant. Checking for approval I ask, 'Would you prefer that I wear gloves?' With eyes closed Sally relaxes, smiles and mouths, 'No, no it's lovely.' Continuing our intimate interaction until the peacefulness of sleep encompasses Sally, I leave feeling enriched by this encounter.

Returning to the office, thoughts of gratitude swell my mind. How privileged I am to work in an environment that values and prioritises time with patients. Gone are the days when I was considered a time-waster! (De Hennezel 1997, p. 61).

As morning slowly emerges I draw back the curtains enabling Sally to witness the beauty of the sunrise over the lake. She smiles whilst beckoning me to her. Taking my arm she thanks me for last night. Our eyes meet as I reassure her that I also benefited by creaming my neglected hands. Sally rushes into conversation about her history and prognosis; as if frightened that I might leave her she holds my hand tight. With resentfulness she recounts her story, bewildered how or why she has to suffer such torment. Restrained by her grasp I can only listen, no words are available to explain or bring comfort. Normal responses of stroking the hair or hugging are inappropriate due to causing excruciating pain. Motionless I stand as the painful darts of information enter my heart and compassion is portrayed through facial expression and contact. Consumed into the depths of reality and truth I feel Sally's pain opening disturbing craters in my soul. My mind wanders to things I should put right and others that I want to achieve before I die (Autton 1996, p. 123). Slowly an awareness of death is expressed as De Hennezel (1997) has observed many times. Like panning for gold I sieve through each word. Trickling down the mountains of despair is a tiny but clear meandering stream of hope and desire. The simplicity of Sally's needs bring tears to my eyes. Lowering my hand a spontaneous kiss reaches her erupting cheek; fragments of her scabby skin adhere to my lips but I only feel love. Sally mouths a return gesture, smiling we squeeze hands and disengage. 'See you later', I whisper, leaving her space. Sally nods, closing her eyes.

On reflection, Sally's history in report left me dumb struck. What could I say to her that would make a difference, alleviate anguish, and help her find peace? As Autton (1996) agrees, 'In some circumstances words can be more of a hindrance than a help' (p. 121).

By using touch as the first form of communication, I relayed my feelings to Sally (Talton 1995). I had the intention of achieving connection with Sally through physical contact. Sympathy and empathy can be exchanged by touch as Edwards (1998) explains when using the quote from Wyshcogrod (1981 p. 801) 'fellow feelings that you and I are one.' I wanted Sally to know I cared, to break down the barriers of being strangers and facilitate her journey of acceptance. Estabrooks & Morse (1992) use the beautiful phrase 'bumping souls', which sums up what I wanted to achieve (Frederiksson 1999, p. 7). Sally and I 'tuned in' to each other through the caring touch as Fredriksson (1999) has noted. I find amazing peace inside me that so much can be gained without the use of words!

Touch has been categorised as task-oriented, caring and protective (Fredriksson 1999; Talton 1995). Task touch is the most commonly used by nurses and does not always have the intent to communicate in a positive manner. It can be defined by 'hurried, rough, jarred movements' relaying 'frustration, anger, or impatience' (Frederiksson p. 2). I find this very disturbing and not true in the hospice where I work. Because of the horrific condition of Sally's skin I was very wary of how I should commence the application of cream. Taking time to register Sally's reaction to my contact and constantly reassessing our intention, I was able to ensure that we understood each other (Davidhizar & Giger 1997). To make the mistake of hurting Sally would create fear of me administering treatment and in turn cause anxiety instead of ease (Davidhizar & Giger 1997).

The disgust I felt on first seeing Sally produced intense guilt. The T-cell lymphoma had totally consumed her skin into a revolting, stinking mess. On reflection, I suppose as a nurse it would have been normal to reach for gloves. However, I feel they create a barrier within the touching process preventing skin to skin contact. I wanted to communicate my acceptance of Sally despite her disfigured body. Autton (1996) describes how reassuring physical contact can be by transferring a healing massage (p. 123). If I had created a barrier within the touching process, by wearing gloves, would Sally have received my message? No, I would have intensified her feelings of self-repulsion and ugliness. Sadly, when I tried to discuss this with my colleagues, they dismissed the idea and requested that we should all wear aprons as well to protect our clothes! How useful tacit knowledge becomes with experience. I knew she wasn't infectious. I didn't even consider using gloves and that brought Sally such pleasure.

Transmissions of pain and touch have joint nerve pathways (Talton 1995). The gentle movements of my fingers on Sally's back initiated relaxation and eventually sleep. What better way, during the night, can there be of dealing with personal mental trauma? So often, as hospice nurses, we turn to sedatives to induce sleep but through experience I am learning that giving time to patients is much more effective and rewarding. This can be demonstrated clearly in the way that Sally acted in the morning.

To conclude, Davidhizar & Giger (1997) state that 'touch has been described as the most important of all the senses' (p. 203). However it does not follow that touch is used more often than sight, hearing, smell or taste, all of which I observe to be in almost constant function. Chang (2001) observes, 'touching is an integral part of human life' (p. 2). Within the nursing environment using touch is a normal, frequent method of administering care both physically and psychologically (Chang 2001). Nurses are also allowed to enter the private zones of the individual through intimate touch due to societal agreement (Hickman & Holmes 1994). Surprisingly, Estabrooks & Morse (1992) note, 'One of the most neglected areas of touch in nursing research is the investigation of the touching behaviours of nurses.' These authors suggest that nurses develop their own touching style through individual life experience and training. It is a comfort to know that touching can be a learned behaviour especially when observing those who appear to have a comfortable natural ability of its proper use (Estabrooks & Morse 1992). Unfortunately self-evaluation and reflection is not a spontaneous process and therefore, some nurses do not learn to express positive feelings through touch.

This research has heightened my awareness of the physical and therapeutic areas of touch. Consideration must always be given to ethnic background, personal history and social connotations to ensure that touch is appropriate and authentic (Talton 1995). Ochs (2001) suggests that we should always ask permission before touching patients or family. I find it more agreeable to continually assess the person's reactions (Talton 1995). The meaning of touch is personal and can only be translated by the recipient (Chang 2001). To assist my own interpretation of touch I indulged in a full body massage. This opened my eyes into further pleasure of body therapies that complement nursing such as reflexology and aromatherapy."

Commentary

In this passage we can experience the exquisite beauty and significance of caring. Indeed it is beautiful because it is so significant, because Jill's action makes such a difference to Sally's care. The words are caught on the breath. Sally feels cared for, it is the essence of palliative care perhaps more than anything. Jill also had a sense of disgust at Sally's blistered and festering skin yet saw the deeper beauty. Sally had learnt that her skin was disgusting for the nurses to treat. She had embodied that knowing. Hence she expected Jill to wear gloves whilst applying cream. Jill was ambivalent, part of her wanted to wear gloves because the skin was disgusting. But another deeper and more powerful part of her rejected the gloves because she knew tacitly that she was rejecting Sally and this engendered guilt. She could not easily live with herself if she chose to wear gloves.

As practitioners go about their practice they touch people in different ways. I shall assume that touch is a vital part of healing, not just physical touch but also the sense of touching someone in an emotional way. Turton (1989) says:

> 'To put our hand on someone's shoulder or take someone's arm are such apparently simple and commonplace acts that we can easily forget that touch is the most import-ant sense in human growth and development.' (p. 42)

Turton reminds practitioners to be mindful of their use of touch and its therapeutic impact. Arthur Frank (2002), who was being treated for cancer, describes his experience with a blood technician:

> 'As this technician went about her work I remarked how skilful she was compared to some other technicians. She then said something to me that had a direct reference to my complaint but also elevated the occasion to a wholly different plane. "Remember," she said slowly, "everyone who touches you affects your healing."
>
> That technician (amongst many) is the one who drew me into a relation of care, in the full sense of *remoralisation*. She recognised, and she found a way to express that recognition, that she was not just extracting blood as a part of a diagnostic procedure, but was also affecting a change in who I was as a result of touching me.' (p. 18)

Frank makes the point that caring 'is not a substance or thing . . . not merely the taking of blood but is possible only within "relations of caring" . . . not as a puzzle to be solved but as a mystery.' (p. 13). Frank asks what the technician meant by using the words 'touch' and 'healing'? The words capture the sense of caring: the mutual exchange as something in Frank touched the technician, that she was open to and could listen to his suffering. From this perspective, touch to be recognised as caring, is more than a technical thing. Indeed, being touched without a sense of being cared for, without a sense of intimacy is demoralising, the sense of being treated as an object. It is the antithesis of caring.

Frank says his experience with the technician was remoralising; she placed him firmly on his healing journey. In other words, the role of any care-giver is to remoralise the patient, to help him or her grow through the illness experience, to emerge as more whole having been cut to pieces by the cancer experience, even for patients who are dying, who feel torn apart. Touch is then healing.

REFLECTIVE EXEMPLAR 5.4 – KAREN, MAVIS AND JOY

In this exemplar, Karen reflects on the way she positions herself in relationship with Mavis, a woman admitted for respite care, and with Joy, her daughter. It is intriguing to observe the way Karen responds as the drama unfolds. It gives an impression that Karen expects the family to fit with her wavelength and yet over time Karen shifts as she comes to understands Mavis and Joy and moves to flow with them. Yet Mavis and Joy have different and potentially conflicting wavelengths, so Karen must find a way to move along both simultaneously.

The text is edited from supervision dialogue recorded between Karen and myself. I am Karen's line manager. Karen has been qualified for six months. We meet for approximately one hour every three weeks. In session 13 Karen first talked about her relationship with Mavis and Joy. Mavis is a woman who has regular respite care at the hospital. Joy is her daughter and main carer.

Supervision Session 13

Karen: "It's the first time I've seen Mavis as Joy describes her at home. For the last few months Joy has been saying how demanding she's been, that she doesn't want Joy to go out. Joy's saying she feels trapped, that it's affecting her marriage. I haven't seen that before when Mavis was here. I'm just observing how she is this time. She is much more demanding, for example, take off my tights, put that there, etcetera."

CJ: "What are your choices?"

Karen: "To go along with it?"

CJ: "Do you have other choices?"

Karen: "To challenge Mavis's behaviour; for example, to ask her to be more polite, to ask her why she is acting differently than before."

CJ: "What would be the consequences of 'going along with it'?"

Karen: "She would receive care similar to what she gets at home."

CJ: "Is that significant?"

Karen: "It is in terms of the respite care philosophy not to disrupt people's normal life styles . . . and yet we also view respite care as enabling the carers to care more effectively and give emotional and psychological support."

CJ: "Okay, so we may have a dilemma as to how best to respond. Does her daughter do everything for her at home?"

Karen: "Yes."

CJ: "But grudgingly?"

Karen: "Yes, I think it's getting that way."

CJ: "You're not sure?"

Karen: "I'm not sure 'grudgingly' is the right word. Joy is getting tired that's for sure."

CJ: "But Joy is complaining to you?"

Karen: "She's justifying it; what Mavis did for her when she was a little girl."

CJ: "Like repaying debts . . . caring from a sense of duty?"

Karen: "Yes, very much."

CJ: "Are you doing something you don't want to do by mirroring Joy's behaviour with her mother at home?"

Karen: "It's not something you want to do. I'm carrying on for Joy's sake."

CJ: "But you would like to change Mavis's behaviour to make Joy's life easier, therefore why carry on?"

Karen: "Because it's the only way to observe the full picture at the moment."

CJ: "Let's look at your option to challenge Mavis."

Karen: "If I challenged her she might act differently than she does at home."

CJ: "Are you thinking that you might succeed in changing her behaviour here, in hospital, but not at home."

Karen: "Yes . . . if I ask her to be polite in hospital when she's here, she . . . she would try desperately hard. Mavis is morally correct. It would upset her too much. She would look at me with wide-eyed wonder and disbelief."

CJ: "Would you be asking her to be polite for our benefit rather than hers?"

Karen: "It wouldn't be for me. It would be for Joy's sake."

CJ: "What might be the reasons for her acting differently? Could the reasons possibly be organic . . . dementia?"

Karen: "Umm . . . I'm not sure about that although it's important to put her behaviour into that perspective . . . it's definitely possible. I feel she is in a strop because Joy has gone on holiday. She didn't want Joy to leave her."

CJ: "This has been happening for two years now. Do you think she has become more dependent? Could you use your empathy and be cathartic to enable her to surface this anger, 'You seem angry that Joy has gone on holiday?'"

Karen: "Thinking about the cathartic and catalytic ways of responding, I don't think I often do that. That's why I probably chose the carry on as before strategy, because I have a fear of using these responses. I haven't used them before."

CJ: "You probably have but not in such a self-conscious or technical way . . . perhaps you are avoiding delving into Mavis's feelings because of fear – fear of the unknown? fear of upsetting Mavis? fear of cocking it up?"

Karen: "Yes, upsetting Mavis . . . being confrontational. Mavis has some environmental problems being here. There's a nosey woman in the same room and sharing a ward with a man as well . . . it can't be easy for her."

CJ: "Are you suggesting that Mavis may be angry with us for these reasons? Consider the Burford cue 'What factors are significant for making this person's stay in hospital comfortable?'"

Karen: "I haven't considered whether these factors could have made her discontented. . . ."

CJ: "Something else for you to consider. Do you feel you have a good relationship with Joy?"

Karen: "I feel she trusts me all of a sudden. I've always been open and friendly with her. I thought no more about it until I became her primary nurse. I don't know what else I need to do with her."

CJ: "That seems a significant insight. Why not think about inviting her for a chat when she returns from her holiday, ostensibly to feed back how Mavis has been in hospital? How does that feel? How do you now feel about Mavis?"

Karen: "I did think she was a very nice lady. Now, I'm beginning to think that she is more manipulative than I gave her credit for."

CJ: "Does that make you feel angry toward her?"

Karen: "Hesitant."

CJ: "It's important for you to understand how you feel about her . . . how she makes you feel because it may influence your responses to her."

Karen: "That may be why I was going to observe her."
CJ: "How do you feel about Joy?"
Karen: "I feel protective towards Joy, more protective for Joy than I do about Mavis."
CJ: "Are you at risk of being caught between two people?"
Karen: "Definitely . . . not knowing where my priorities lie."

Commentary

Karen's frustration with Mavis triggered her reflection. The dialogue reflects the depth of knowing necessary to know the whole family and to understand the conflicting and competing needs of both Joy and Mavis. Mavis was a private and 'proper' person being compromised by her deteriorating intellect. Hence sharing a room with a man or with an intrusive other woman may well have been distressing to her, compounding her despair at being left by her daughter. Karen's sympathy lay with Joy, an emotional reaction rather than a deep understanding of the family's dynamics. As a consequence Karen feels entangled in a web of Joy's concerns to the extent that she begins to re-evaluate Mavis as a 'nice' person. The dialogue reveals the way guidance helped Karen to view herself within the context of the situation and explore her use of therapeutic responses using the work of Heron's (1975) Six category intervention analysis.

Six category intervention analysis

Six category intervention analysis (Heron 1975) is a framework of six therapeutic responses that practitioners can use within practice (Box 5.2). In response to the particular situation, the practitioner chooses the most appropriate response and can move easily between the different responses. Karen noted that she felt unskilled at using confrontation, catharsis and catalytic responses, and how her lack of skill constrained her ability to develop the therapeutic relationship with Mavis and Joy. She was anxious to use confrontation and catharsis because she wanted to avoid making Mavis upset. She also doubted her ability to work with feelings including her own.

Box 5.2   Six category factor analysis (Heron 1975)

Authoritative type responses	Facilitative type responses
• *Giving information*: enabling the other to make a rational decision	• *Being cathartic*: enabling the other to express some emotion
• *Giving advice*: helping another see other, better ways of seeing and doing things	• *Being catalytic*: enabling the other to talk through an issue
• *Confrontation*: challenging the other's restrictive attitudes, beliefs or behaviour	• *Being supportive*: communicating a sense of 'being there' for the other

Some evidence exists suggesting that nurses avoid using confrontational, cathartic and catalytic responses, preferring to give information, give advice and be supportive (Burnard & Morrison 1991). These researchers noted that using confrontational, cathartic and catalytic responses involved 'an investment of self which may be emotionally draining for the practitioner'. Nurses, like Karen, felt they had not been prepared for this type of work, confirming James's (1989) conclusions from her research into the nature of 'emotional labour' that this type of work was not valued and therefore not taught, being a natural extension of women's work. James considered that emotional labour was highly skilled, as suggested in Karen's dialogue. Without doubt, working with patients and families is emotional work. To be an effective practitioner requires the ability and confidence to engage in emotional work, even if it is personally threatening. As we shall explore in Chapter 6, knowing and managing self within relationships in order to be available to the other is itself skilful.

I have analysed a pattern using Heron's responses:

- When an underlying emotion is sensed, use a cathartic response. 'Mavis, you seem angry at Joy.' Or 'Are you happy sharing a room with a male patient?' The intention is to release and surface the emotion so it can be dealt with. At this level practitioners may fear releasing the emotion because they do not know how to respond to it.
- The use of a catalytic response to help the person talk through the issues with the intention of helping them find meaning in their feelings, and by talking through it, to understand deeper underlying reasons for their feelings. In this way the patient is helped to release the negative energy and begin to convert it to positive energy for taking action.
- Confrontation can then be used to challenge, yet always within a supportive framework. Confrontation is always easier when a trusting relationship has been developed, because the patient knows you care for them. As Karen's experience indicates, confrontation is often equated with conflict, which Karen felt was the antithesis of caring. Yet confrontation does not need to make the other person uncomfortable. Karen and I explored and rehearsed Karen's use of these skills, so Karen might confront Mavis, 'You aren't helping yourself so much this time?' or, 'Perhaps Joy needs a holiday?' These fairly innocent questions are confrontational yet in an indirect and less threatening way than saying something like, 'You are being demanding.'

Session 14

In our next supervision session three weeks later, Karen picked up her work with Mavis and Joy:

Karen: "I was so grateful we had the supervision session on it. I must make an appointment to see Joy as soon as Mavis is coming into hospital again in two weeks time."

CJ: "You are on a late shift today. Why not ring Joy this evening?"

Karen: "Maybe [cringes] . . . I was hoping we could rehearse again how I am going to be with Joy."

CJ: "Okay, so you ring her . . . ?"

Karen: "I could ask her to come to the hospital although she will have to make an excuse to leave Mavis . . . or I could go and visit Joy although Mavis might say, 'What's Karen doing here?' It might be difficult to have a conversation with Mavis listening."

CJ: "What's the best option?"

Karen: "To ask Joy to come here."

CJ: "What will you say to her on the phone?"

Karen: "I could explain the doubts I had about Mavis when she was last in and how Mavis had different perceptions to Joy's."

CJ: "How do you think Joy might respond to this?"

Karen: "She's likely to panic, 'What's mum been saying!?' She'll ask herself, 'What does Karen want to say to me?' I would not like to panic her, but yet to get her to see how important it is that we carefully plan our response to Mavis in the future."

CJ: "Okay, let's rephrase this so you don't panic her."

Karen: "I could ask her is there is anything she would like to discuss about Mavis's forthcoming admission beforehand?"

CJ: "What if she says 'no'? Or if she says, 'What things do you want to discuss?' Or wants to discuss what you have in mind over the phone?"

Karen: "I'm stuck."

CJ: "Okay, you may need a more direct invitation to her, for example, 'I've just returned from my holiday and notice that Mavis is coming in, in two weeks time. Can you pop in and see me at the hospital to have a chat about how things have been at the moment and for me to give you feedback about how she was during her last stay.' How does that feel?"

Karen: "That feels okay . . . if I went to her home it would become too social."

CJ: "So, she's here at the hospital. What's your agenda?"

Karen: "I wouldn't start by going straight in . . . some chit chat first . . ."

CJ: "For example, your holidays?"

Karen: "Yes."

CJ: "Okay, start by relaxing the situation?"

Karen: "No doubt the conversation would flow more easily after that."

CJ: "Let's clarify your agenda – highlight how Mavis was during her last admission and how she is at home. Then what?"

Karen: "Find out what Joy would like to happen, using the [Burford] reflective cues: How does she view herself and others? Does she want Mavis to change or does she want my shoulder to lean upon? The cue 'What support does she have in life?' would also be useful to explore."

CJ: "In that last respect you might use a cathartic response, 'How is your husband feeling?' Or, if Joy expresses non-verbal distress, you might say, 'Joy I can see this is upsetting you.' The aim would be to surface feelings because it *is* an emotional issue and feelings influence the decisions we make. Would you be able to deal with Joy's tears?"

Karen: "Yes."

CJ: "It might be an opportune time to confront Joy with her reasons for keeping her mum at home."

Karen: "Yes . . . I need to determine what Joy really feels about keeping her mum at home, and then look at ways to support her to do that, if that's what she wants . . ."

CJ: "And not lose sight of Mavis in the process . . . it would be easy to see Mavis as a problem that needs solving."

Commentary

The dialogue reflects Karen's uncertainty with opening a space for Joy to explore her feelings about her mother and the future. It isn't simply a question of applying confrontation and cathartic techniques – they are simply that, techniques; it is more about using herself as a therapeutic tool, about her own feelings and fears; fears of mucking it up or not knowing how to take it forward, fear of losing control, fear of becoming entangled, fear of upsetting Joy and Mavis.

As her guide I metaphorically hold Karen's hand so she can confront and move beyond her fear.

Session 15

I met with Karen again three weeks later:

Karen: "I didn't see Joy before she brought Mavis in. I was surprised that there were no grumbles from Joy. I said to her, 'Can I talk to you a minute without your mother hearing?' Joy seemed very relaxed and talked about everything under the sun except her mum! After all our rehearsing I just had to ask her outright. I was ready for a shock/horror reaction as I had fore-casted but I got none of it. She said, 'Yes, fine, when?' I think I was more amazed by that, more than she had been by my asking her to come in. I was trying to think of the reasons why she didn't react with shock/horror. I thought she either trusts me or she saw it as an opportunity to have my whole attention or, she wanted to talk to me too. But I don't think it was that because I didn't detect relief in her voice. I was glad I'd asked her directly and hadn't pussy footed around trying to break it gently. I had been me!"

CJ: "You just highlight how unpredictable these things really are, that the best laid plans of mice and men don't necessarily materialise. But the point you raise about 'being yourself' is interesting."

Karen: "Yes . . . I feel quite a lot of that down here anyway. I'm very con-scious of north–south differences in nature because I have had such bad reactions in the past to my openness and directness. Then I think I try to con-form to how I think people are expecting me to behave down here. It seems as if people act for a long time until they feel they've really got to know you."

CJ: "That sounds as if it interferes with communication."

Karen: "Probably. I need to be on people's wavelengths to be therapeutic."

CJ: "Even if that means conforming and compromising who you are to achieve this?"

Karen: "That's what I have been doing."

CJ: "What you say is really interesting on two accounts. First, the impact of our personalities, 'who we are' on the way we view and respond to the world, and whether, 'who we are' is adequate or not to realise desirable and effective practice; and second, the way we may try and conform to some type of stereotype of 'who we should be', and in doing so, go against the grain of our personality and create a sense of inner turmoil and conflict. Jourard (1971) describes this state of being as self-alienation – that we risk losing connection with our real selves in striving to be something we are not, and that, in doing so, we are unable to use ourselves in a therapeutic way. I see that as a great value of supervision: to acknowledge this inner turmoil and work toward resolving it."

Karen: "Yeah – I feel that . . . that it's good to express this unease . . . quite a relief."

CJ: "Let's reflect on the way the first five Burford model cues [see Box 4.1] enable you to get on the person's wavelength."

Karen: "After using those cues I do feel I understand the person's wavelength but it doesn't mean I'm on it with them."

CJ: "That's a good point. The skill is to monitor the impact of yourself on others and manage any resistance either from yourself or from them in order to ride their wavelength."

Karen: "I've realised that I have been doing that more and more, being more direct and following things through."

CJ: "What's prompted that?"

Karen: "Thinking back to that meeting with Joy, she brought Wilf, her husband, along as well. That was fine. He was waffling on so much about something that I stopped him and said, 'I'm asking you all these questions because I am worried about your marriage'."

CJ: "What was the impact of that, did their mouths drop open?"

Karen: "Not at all. They said, 'Thank you very much for telling us that, thank you for getting us here.' I wrote down in my journal, 'direct questions get direct answers'."

CJ: "How did they respond?"

Karen: "Initially they were quiet and then they started telling me things like, 'Why don't you tell Karen about the allowances. Oh yes, we can trust Karen with things like that.' It was as though I had confirmed their hopes that I cared for them . . . honesty was the biggest thing."

CJ: "Maybe I would use the word 'authenticity'; in being your 'real self' you were able to communicate your care and concern for them. You seemed to cut across the game-playing and enable them to reveal their true selves and make a real connection. How did the conversation end?"

Karen: "I reaffirmed to them that if they needed to talk to someone about their relationship with Mavis, then they could talk to me, that I was here for them. They responded to that by saying, 'If there is anything we can do for you in the world, anything, then please tell us and if we can we will.' I definitely got across that I cared. They appreciated that. I wasn't sticking my nose in where it wasn't wanted."

CJ: "You beautifully illustrate the mutuality of caring . . . it is very powerful."

Karen: "I wanted to say it went totally different to what I expected and it was good that I had the meeting to find out what they were planning in the future. They will have Mavis living with them until one or the other's health deteriorates to the point they feel incapable of caring."

CJ: "It's easier for them knowing that you are with them now."

The dialogue reveals Karen's breakthrough in tuning into and getting onto the other's wavelength. Joy had given Karen clues before about the impact that caring for her mother was having on her marriage. Now Karen pays attention to this cue and takes this sign deeper and enables Joy and Wilf to release the deep angst within them. The bubble is burst, and they feel understood and cared for. They had been screaming out for someone to recognise them as people, as valid recipients of care. Karen did this although not in ways we had anticipated. Karen had reacted intuitively and skilfully within the moment because she was tuned in and went with her instincts.

To achieve this Karen had to find and accept her real self – a self she felt had become diminished. Through reflection she could reaffirm her real self, legitimising and valuing her own qualities of being open and honest, and yet be sensitive to the unfolding situation. Jourard (1971) noted:

'People learn to quash their real selves because they have learned to fear the consequences of authentic being and blind themselves to much of their real self; impairing their ability to empathise with patients and disclose themselves.' (p. 184)

As I said to Karen in the dialogue, Jourard believes that such action leads to self-alienation, thus jeopardising the nurse's own health and limiting her ability to use herself in a therapeutic way. In enabling the growth of self, the self needs to be honoured and valued. If we are unable to honour ourselves then we will be unable to honour those with whom we work – either our patients or our colleagues.

Session 20

It wasn't until session 20, four months later, that Karen picked up her work with Mavis and Joy.

Karen: "Mavis is now very confused and very sad. Joy says that Mavis is more confused and that she doesn't know what to do about it, how to keep Mavis occupied. Mavis is less able to do her knitting, even to watch TV."

CJ: "And making more demands on Joy as a result?"

Karen: "Joy feels she should be spending more time with Mavis whilst she is in here."

CJ: "Can you reassure Joy about that?"

Karen: "I said that we will try and stimulate Mavis more whilst she is in hospital and pass on any tips to Joy and Wilf for them to try out at home."

CJ: "Has anything emerged?"

Karen: "She can talk about the past with some understanding. Therefore old photographs, or videos would be useful."

CJ: "We have a book in the library on reminiscence [Coleman 1986] that might be a useful reference for you to explore."

Karen: "Joy would have to sit with her to accomplish that . . . She won't go to any clubs because she's deaf. Yet she will sit with Ethel [another patient] and have a conversation. I really think she plays Joy up at home, I really do. I'm toying with the idea of doing a home visit to clarify in my own mind if that is so."

CJ: "Even if she was, what could you do about it?"

Karen: "I'm not sure I could do anything except be more empathic."

CJ: "How do you feel about this situation?"

Karen: "Frustrated . . . I know I am absorbing some of Joy's anxiety, I know that, and I am trying hard not to, but it's difficult when you get involved with people like this . . . that's why it's so helpful to share it with you . . . not just to get ideas or check my own out, but to help me keep things in perspective."

CJ: "That's so honest of you. Okay, let's focus on other options. What about other workers, for example the Community Psychiatric Nurse (CPN) for the Elderly?"

Karen: "No. The only contact is the GP. They have a lot of trust in him."

CJ: "Have you thought about the CPN as a resource?"

Karen: "No, but that's a good idea. I haven't met her. This would be a good opportunity to do that."

CJ: "Do you know how to contact her? Her contact is in the resource file."

Karen: "Knowing the home situation would lead to a better appreciation of her life-pattern and give me insight into the way Joy and Mavis normally relate to each other and the help Joy gives Mavis. For example, if Joy was helping Mavis to dress at home and Mavis was managing that by herself here, we could help Joy to change her management for Mavis at home."

CJ: "Of course the dynamics are different at home – Mavis may be more dependent to get Joy to help her, and Joy may want to help her more than we might, because of her perceived dutiful daughter role. We've talked about this role and her guilt before. Again, the CPN may help you with a cognitive assessment of time/space/place/orientation, etcetera. However, you need to consider whether that's appropriate or just intrusive. You seem hesitant about a home visit."

Karen: "I feel claustrophobic about Joy and Wilf. I feel almost smothered by their love. I'm dodging them! It makes me reluctant to go and to feel even more closed in by them . . . stupid things like them calling me 'sweetheart'!"

CJ: "I recall your aversion to being called names of endearment by Elizabeth [another patient]. You can't accept that from Joy and Wilf? Use the transactional analysis framework to position yourself?"

Karen: "I have to be in a certain mood to accept it. I can see the TA pattern – parent–child with me resisting their loving parenting! I know I should be mindful enough not to go into child mode. I appreciate this 'up here' [in supervision], but it's different when I'm down there."

CJ: "It feels like a situation of entanglement – of losing the boundaries between yourself and them. You've become aware of this and now want to take a step back to untangle yourself and yet they want you to take a step forward."

Karen: "Yes, I'm trying to maintain a professional distance."

CJ: "I'm not sure about this idea of 'professional distance' – it sounds like a barrier to retreat behind because you cannot manage your resistance to them. This seems to be a repeating theme through your experiences – where to pitch your involvement with patients and families. Perhaps you want to take a step back because you don't know what's waiting for you?"

Karen: "In light of past experiences I guess I should have seen this coming . . . but it's like it creeps up and grabs you. I don't know what demands it's going to make on me, but I don't feel comfortable."

CJ: "Do you know the best ways to resolve this dilemma: on one hand knowing your responsibility to help them and on the other hand wanting to flee from them?"

Karen: "I know a solution – to do the home visit but to spell out the objectives to them, emphasising that the visit is not a social visit."

CJ: "In other words to set the boundaries for the visit and for your relationship with them?"

Karen: "Yes."

CJ: "I agree with your actions. It enables you to be positive rather than defensive. In doing so you don't need to resist them but accept their need to be affectionate to you . . . it gives you some control, and anxious people need to feel in control. Do you feel able to be open and honest with them as you were before?"

Karen: "Being in control – that's important. I can relate this to my earlier work with them . . . the way they make me like a 'big soft puppy.' I think I can deal with it now."

CJ: "Do they have children?"

Karen: "Joy has two children from a previous marriage . . . are you suggesting they might want to mother me?"

CJ: "It's a possibility."

Karen's involvement with Joy and Wilf takes a paradoxical turn. Having worked hard to connect with them, she now recoils from the unexpected consequences. Joy and Wilf wish to reciprocate Karen's care at an unacceptable level. Hence Karen resists this demand, feeling smothered by love and treated like a little girl with such endearments as 'sweetheart'. Yet Karen also feels guilty of her resistance. As a result she is entangled, trapped by her 'ethic of care' (Dickson 1982); caught in a dilemma of knowing how best to respond. She cannot reciprocate the level of involvement demanded by the family but

Box 5.3   Reciprocal and non-reciprocal patterns within transactional analysis

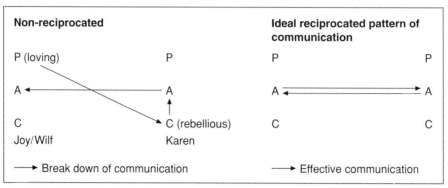

neither can she resist it openly because of her concern for the family. In response to her anxiety, Karen had flipped into rebellious child mode (see Box 5.3), fighting against 'her parents' who wished to impose a level of intimacy that was unacceptable and uncomfortable.

Transactional analysis

Transactional analysis offers a framework to reflect on patterns of communication between self and other. It is based on the theory that people communicate from one of three ego levels: parent (P), adult (A) and child (C). The child is essentially irresponsible, playful, demanding and can be either conforming or rebellious. The child grows into the adult, associated with the growth of responsibility and reason. The parent is associated with authority, and may be either a critical or protective parent. When people become anxious they tend to revert to 'script', an habitual ego level where they feel safe – usually the parent or child in order to manage their anxiety (Stewart & Joines 1987).

Effective communication, although not necessarily therapeutic communication, takes place from reciprocated ego state levels, for example parent–child, adult–adult. When communication is not reciprocated then lines become crossed and communication breaks down. Take Karen's experience with Joy and Wilf as an example. She resists being responded to as a child and demands being communicated with as an adult. However, as the dialogue reveals she did respond as a rebellious child. As a general rule adult–adult is the desirable pattern of communication based on mutual responsibility and being reasonable (see Box 5.3).

There may be times when a parent pattern of communication is therapeutic. For example, a patient may feel safer being dependent for a period of time. For the mindful practitioner, choosing a parent or child ego state to communicate is a matter of clinical judgement rather than an anxiety reaction. Being mindful, Karen will recognise and understand why Joy and Wilf are responding from a parental ego state. She can acknowledge that graciously whilst at the same time helping Joy and Wilf shift into adult mode. The key is for Karen not to become anxious. Perhaps inadvertently Karen does display child ego communication that she does not realise and which paradoxically encourages Joy and Wilf to be parental. As Karen says in the supervision dialogue, *I know I should be mindful enough not to go into child mode.* As with all responses, it is a matter of reading the signs and responding appropriately.

Session 21

Karen and I met again three weeks later.

> *Karen*: "Mavis has agreed to go into a residential home. I found out when she didn't turn up for respite care yesterday."
> *CJ*: "How do you feel about that?"
> *Karen*: "Very pleased for Joy and Wilf. The stress is removed from them. Mavis had been getting up three times during the night. They have a different stress now, whether they have made the right decision – is mum happy there? At least they have their home back again, plus Joy's own health problems have worsened. It will now be easier for her to cope with this."
> *CJ*: "How would you feel if Mavis wasn't happy at the home?"
> *Karen*: "I don't know . . . I may keep in touch with Joy and Wilf."
> *CJ*: "To support them? Accepting some form of ongoing responsibility?"
> *Karen*: "That's the issue – when do you stop?"
> *CJ*: "So, when *do* you stop? You need to clarify your role responsibility and unwrap yourself from this involvement. Now the work is for you to close this relationship. Part of closing any relationship is having the opportunity to talk through any emotional issues, particularly as you became so involved with this family that it has left you with a cocktail of conflicting emotions. Can you be gracious and accept their need to love you?"
> *Karen*: "Yes, I can accept that now."

Commentary

As the dialogue suggests, Karen struggled with knowing and managing self. Perhaps it is only through reflection that such knowing can be gained simply because each relationship is complex and unpredictable. There are no prescriptions to apply. It is no good saying to Karen get involved or stay detached. What do these things mean? This question is the focus for Chapter 6.

Re-viewing clinical supervision

My unfolding supervision dialogue with Karen over a number of sessions offers the reader an opportunity to review the clinical supervision process. In particular consider:

- The way I balance the use of Heron's Six category interventions (Box 5.2) to help Karen explore herself within the unfolding situation.

- The balance of challenge and support – is Karen defensive in any way?
- The way I fed theory into the supervision process – have I missed opportunities?
- Have I been judgemental or fallen into any of the line manager–supervisor traps (Box 3.2)?
- What Karen has learnt using the framing perspectives (Box 1.10).

Chapter 6

Knowing and Managing Self within Relationships

My reflection on caring for Stephen in Chapter 4 illuminated my struggle to tune into Stephen's wavelength partly because of his resistance to me and partly because of my resistance to him. Resistance creates a distance between the practitioner and patient that limits the ability to be available to the other. As such, the extent I can be available is determined by the extent the practitioner knows and manages self within relationship (see the 'Being Available' template, Box 2.5).

Without doubt, 'who I am' is my major therapeutic tool and needs to be kept sharp enough to cut the cloth in skilful action. In the following exemplar, consider Simon's existential struggle in the face of Bill's and his wife's suffering. Simon is a charge nurse on a medical ward. His story is a search for meaning in the suffering and joy he experienced, reflecting the deeply emotional aspect of holistic practice and the fundamental need to know and manage self within relationships.

REFLECTIVE EXEMPLAR 6.1 – SIMON'S STORY

"Nursing is a demanding profession. The commitment we invest in our roles provides us with our greatest source of reward – the ability to use our position to aid others. This interpersonal aspect of nursing when encountering people at their most vulnerable is the foundation of our practice and its fulfilment the foundation of our satisfaction even though the price of constant exposure to emotionally challenging situations can be very high. Can we avoid this expense? Or can we grow as nurses through it? Can we become over-exposed to death and dying, resulting in emotional detachment that undermines holistic care and prevents us from using ourselves in a therapeutic way or learning from the experience? By reflecting on my involvement with Bill, a 40-year-old man who died of cancer, I am attempting to discover the factors that influenced my feelings and actions.

Standing at a shade over six feet tall, weighing a muscular 14 stone, the smiling face on the photograph provided a shocking contrast to the image of its owner sleeping in the bed. I use the word shocking in response to how cancer specialises in the distortion of features and expressions more rapidly than a cosmetic surgeon's knife and in a fashion that only first-hand witnesses could believe. When the bones, normally concealed beneath a physique developed through good living and exercise, become not only visible but the dominating feature in Bill's experience, it becomes a cruel irony of nature that many years of development can be so undone at a rate that growth can never equal.

We described Bill as cachexic, a single word to describe so much. As professionals we are very comfortable and familiar with our terminology. It becomes very easy to use and the words can soften their meaning. This is a user-friendly language that cannot portray what it describes. Cachexia is defined as abnormally low weight, weakness and general bodily decline associated with chronic disease, most notably cancer.

In reality, however, it is the image that Jane [Bill's wife] tries to spare her sons Joe and Tim from seeing, fearing nightmares and difficult 'why?' questions. It is the sight of a loving son, a devoted husband and doting father reduced to a living skeleton barely able to acknowledge everything in life that is dear to him and those who love him struggling with their pain.

Bill was admitted to our ward when symptoms of his lung cancer began to overwhelm him and his family. It had been a short disease process typical in its presentation and diagnosis. The dry cough that had failed to respond to linctus annoyed Jane so much that she wore down Bill's reluctance and persuaded him to go to the GP who sent Bill for a chest X-ray. The film showed a shadow that in turn resulted in bronchoscopic biopsy and diagnosis. Simple, systematic and effective intervention. It is the impact that has the medical profession floundering like a bully having its bluff called, 'So what are you going to do now?' You can almost sense the taunt.

Radiotherapy was marginally successful in reducing the size of the shadow. Isn't *shadow* an easy word to use, avoiding the dreaded 'C' word but managing to remain mysterious, sinister, and often, for the patient, ambiguous? But tragically, its postponement of the inevitable was its only consequence. Subsequent community management with the input of Macmillan nurses had kept Bill at home until uncontrollable pain and nausea necessitated admission to hospital. The original plan was to achieve symptom control to facilitate discharge as soon as possible. However, the best laid plans of mice and men. . . .

Bill could feel the pain through his chest wall. A sub-cutaneous syringe driver containing diamorphine and cyclizine to manage his pain and nausea was used. These drugs were initially effective but the diamorphine needed to be increased within hours to achieve adequate pain control.

Bill had lost his appetite and was unable to keep fluids down long enough for them to be of any value. He looked dry and blood tests confirmed this impression. An intravenous infusion was commenced to correct his dehydration. Secondary to his reduced fluid intake Bill experienced oral candida and some painful oral ulcers. Anti-fungal and ulcer medications were prescribed and regular mouth care provided. Bill was nursed on a pressure-reducing mattress.

Over the next couple of days Bill's condition stabilised and improved enough for him to have visits from his sons. They were aged 8 and 12 years old. Jane had protected them as much as possible by shielding them from seeing their father when he had looked so unwell. During this period, over 3–4 shifts, I got to know Bill quite well. He was intelligent, articulate and we shared mutual interests in sport and music. We shared a similar sense of humour and managed to make each other laugh frequently. I wished I had the opportunity to know Bill for longer. Bill and I were disagreeing about England's World Cup chances as I left the ward for two days off. Bill invited me to call round and see him when he was at home as we were aiming for discharge in the next two days. I replied that I would try but I knew deep down that I wouldn't. Not because I doubted that Bill would get home, but once a patient goes home we prepare for the next one. Our busy schedules are exactly that and how much time and involvement should one invest?

On one occasion, whilst completing some paperwork, I found myself watching Bill as his family visited. The indelible image was that of seeing the boys at the foot of his bed and simultaneously touch their dad's feet as their mum hugged him. The boys so needed the physical contact but seemed reserved and hesitant until Bill held out his arms and the boys rushed to him and held him tightly. They seemed scared to let go, and Bill, eyes closed, tried to absorb and retain this very precious moment knowing how valuable time was.

Later that evening, I checked on my sleeping son and cried as I recalled what I had seen earlier. My emotions were a combination of anger at how people's lives are so senselessly destroyed and fear generated where the fine line between life and death is made so visible and where our own mortality is questioned.

Returning from my days off, I noted that Bill had been transferred into the side-room. I immediately asked the nurse looking after Bill what had happened. She informed me that Bill was close to death. He had become increasingly dyspnoeic due to the development of an extensive pleural infusion. A pleural aspiration had been performed which had alleviated some of his breathlessness. However, the effusion was a sign of general deterioration that warranted increased analgesia and a sedative to control his developing agitation. Bill's deterioration was rapid, the disease's only concession to Jane's feelings. 'He's not in pain, is he?' Jane urgently enquired. Before I could respond, Jane continued, 'I wish we could have him home.' I responded by saying that Bill was asleep and peaceful, indicating that the medication was effective and that we were continually assessing his condition. Jane was obviously distressed that Bill had not got home as she repeated her statement to herself shaking her head and crying. 'I think Bill's main concern was to have you all here,' I responded, looking towards the sons, trying to highlight to them how important their presence was to their dad. I continued, 'holding his hand and talking to him is the most you can do regardless of where you are.' Jane forced a smile in my direction and nodded in agreement. She turned her attention to Bill and her sons. Feeling somewhat uncomfortable with the ensuing silence, I asked a typically English question, 'Can I get you a cup of tea or anything?'

Bill's family visited at regular intervals as he slipped into unconsciousness. I continued to let the family know that I was there for them should they need anything. Within an hour Bill died. I stood silently, deprived of the sanctuary of offering tea. I withdrew to allow the family privacy. Jane was very protective of her sons and through her grief she remained strong for them. They were distraught and through their tears betrayed a vacant, disbelieving look; in this instant they were experiencing emotions with demands beyond their tender years. Their sobbing provided a heartbreaking image and I was revisited by the twin impostors of anger and fear and a feeling of frustration at my helplessness.

I offered my condolences simply by expressing how sorry I was and instinctively touched Tim's arm as he stood next to me. Jane took my hand and thanked me for all I had done. I repeated how sorry I was and said how I liked Bill a lot. She seemed to appreciate this and smiled. I was glad that I told Jane this. I felt for some reason that this was important to them as I knew that I would not get another chance to hint at the impact looking after Bill was having on me. The practical aspects were discussed with Bill's brother-in-law and provided a sense of relief that comes with taking refuge in practices over which we have some control.

Bill required a subtle balance of physical and psychological care typical in palliative nursing. But its influence on me as a person, and subsequently as a nurse, was atypical. I found myself experiencing fear, helplessness, inadequacy, anger and levels of distress that I had not felt since my earliest nursing exposure to death and dying. Farrar (1992) recognised these emotions in novices. However, my experience is far beyond novice so why do I seem to be regressing? I initially perceived these feelings to be barriers to effective care as they can elevate stress levels and compromise my ability to carry out clinical care objectively. In providing psychological support I have always felt it prudent to keep some distance between my empathy and my personal feelings, a kind of conditional empathy which is determined by my feelings of discomfort and my emotional self-defence. In short, the experience has exposed barriers in my attitudes that, unless resolved, will impact negatively on my practice.

My reflection illuminates the darkest areas of my practice and reveals the source of my fear, anger and frustration and guides me in my attempts to learn from them and apply my understandings in practice. Bill and I had much in common that stimulated me to empathise to the extent that I was forced to confront my own personal experience of loss and my own mortality. I felt helpless at not being able to alter the course of Bill's prognosis or lessen the impact on his wife and sons. These are perfectly normal human responses but need to be fully understood to turn them into positive emotions, rather than areas for personal conflict and distress. The majority of my nursing practice has been in the care of the elderly environment and my dealings with palliative care in my own age group have been limited. In managing the needs of the older patient, I can see that I could have more easily employed my coping mechanisms that dilute the personal impact and subsequently lessen the felt distress.

This is not to say that terminal disease is any less tragic for the people involved or that it requires any less skill or commitment on the nurse's behalf. But I am able to rationalise the event and see it more objectively. In examining my thoughts related to my own mortality, it is clear to me that it is a subject that I have actively avoided. McSherry (1996) details the importance of discovering our attitudes to mortality in order to resolve our barriers to death and dying. The experience of observing the trauma of Bill's sons brings back memories of my own father's death that I have not allowed to impact on my nursing due to the upset that they still evoke. Reisetter & Thomas (1986) state that these are the very emotions that we need to expose and incorporate into our practice. In avoiding applying my own experience into my practice, I am denying a major source of personal knowing. Utilising this knowing would enhance my care as I could use my subsequent increased capacity for empathy to understand my patients' needs more acutely and view this closeness as a bridge rather than as a barrier.

Applying my own anxiety and fear of death and dying to provide a door to another's actions and thoughts rather than a subject to be dispelled immediately on appearance gives me the opportunity to provide true holistic care. The question, 'How would I feel if that were me?' should not only be accepted but encouraged if holism is our objective. In revisiting my father's illness, I am reminded of the doctors, nurses, and therapists that we came into contact with and the way they made me feel. Whispering at the foot of the bed, head shaking when reading the notes, and being stared at by curious student nurses, are memories that I seldom, if ever, relate to my own ideas of nursing. Do I whisper over my patients, leave patients perplexed and terrified with the shake of my head or the raising of an eyebrow, or forget the individual's right not to be a source of medical curiosity? I wish that I could cast the first stone at these sins but in reality I fear that I cannot. I worry that a lack of true empathy that can prevail when we lessen our humanness leads to a provision of care guided by a form of nursing 'autopilot' that demands little from us. I am equally reminded of the staff who respected my father and our family with their time, skills and most of all their understanding that meant so much to us at the time.

I want to leave a positive impression of my caring on those with whom I come into contact and recognise the factors that reduce this possibility. I hope that Jane's memories of Bill's hospital care are reassuring. I will then have achieved something. At times I feel like a voyeur, impotent, unable to achieve practical goals that would make myself or Bill's family feel better. The danger of containing these feelings is that I carry them around with me into the next similar scenario, immediately creating a barrier.

Through reflection I am now in better shape to use my frustration and anger to enhance my care. Being able to value the care I give reduces my frustration and allows me to accept my limitations, whilst my anger can be channelled into striving to improve in all areas of practice. Anger experienced by patients is often part of the grieving process (Kübler-Ross 1969), but its impact can be damaging if there is no justifiable recipient to direct it at. In harnessing memories of my own anger when experiencing my father's illness, I can detect this in difficult and aggressive people and avoid dismissing them as irritating or their behaviour as meaningless.

The anger I felt at seeing a man deprived of the opportunity to love his sons, enjoy and nurture their growth has to be managed and resolved to avoid extreme levels of stress and potential burn-out. In response to this I am committed to working with our palliative care team to establish a support network for ward nurses to explore, share and hopefully resolve emotional fall-out from our work. I am now a more complete nurse through knowing Bill. Reflection has been enlightening, supportive and rewarding."

Commentary

I feel certain that Simon's story is not unusual for many nurses working on busy medical wards. I know from teaching such nurses on palliative care modules at the university that there is always a deep tension between the prevailing dominant medical model and a palliative care attitude. The frustration at not realising ideal care is strongly felt especially when associated with patients who are dying.

Simon articulates the way reflection helped him to understand his feelings, linking back to his identification with Bill in terms of similar age and interests, having young children and the impact of Bill's death on the children, and his unresolved anger about his father's care and subsequent death. The idea we can separate the personal self from the professional self is challenged by Simon's story.

The X-ray film showed a shadow; the shadow of death that hovered over Bill and his family. How do we learn to live in the shadow of death with its suffering? Simon felt this suffering and suffered himself. As Rinpoche (1992) notes:

> 'Suffering . . . gives you such an opportunity of working through and transforming it. The times you are suffering can be those where your greatest strength really lies. Say to yourself then – "I am not going to run away from this suffering. I want to use it in the best and richest way I can, so that I can become more compassionate and more helpful to others." So, whatever you do, don't shut off your pain; accept your pain and remain vulnerable. And don't we know only too well, that protection from pain doesn't work, and that when we try and defend ourselves from suffering, we only suffer more and don't learn what we can from the experience.' (p. 316)

Such powerful words. Ask yourself, where lies Simon's greatest strength? Benner & Wrubel (1989) argue that burnout is the loss of caring and that the remedy is to reconnect to caring. It is the loss of caring that is truly harmful. And on medical wards such as Simon's ward, caring can be submerged in the pressure of time and cure priorities. Reisseter & Thomas (1986) showed a significant relationship between high quality palliative care, reduced stress levels and the individual nurse's ability to draw on personal experience of death and dying. This would seem to suggest that practitioners who have the motivation and ability to reflect on their experience as a method of development are better equipped to respond effectively to the needs of their patients. In contrast, Atkinson *et al.* (1990) detail the way people deal with personal loss by viewing it in abstract terms that 'prevent us from internalising and personalising questions surrounding our mortality and death.' Atkinson *et al.*'s research indicates that nurses who are able to utilise their own experience to enhance their personal knowing are in a better position to respond to the needs of their patients and the impact upon themselves, and understand the feelings, attitudes and prejudices that influence behaviour.

Simon shared his story in a small guided reflection group consisting of six other practitioners and a guide. The group had been together for several weeks and had developed a strong bond of trust that made it safe for Simon to reveal such deep aspects of self. Simon had not met any of the other practitioners in the group prior to its commencement and the guide was not from his organisation. It is the positive aspect of the 'confessional' – an opportunity to unburden and cleanse self. Sharing his story enabled others in the group to relate with similar stories. As you might imagine it was very cathartic yet through the suffering caring was valued. The whole group felt reconnected to caring. Simon had shifted his energy from dwelling on his suffering to celebrating his caring. Profound energy work.

Simon made the point that he had never been 'taught' how to use himself in a therapeutic way or to deal with feelings that such work evoked. Such revelation gives support to James's (1989) observation that *emotional labour* is generally unrecognised, viewed as unskilled, and as such, not taught. Yet Simon's story reveals that such work is the he(art) of holistic practice.

Involvement

Simon reflects on his involvement with this family. Part of him is drawn into the family's suffering and as a consequence he suffers himself. Through reflection he strives to make sense of his feelings as he positions himself alongside this family. Part of him is also distant, staying on the edge, uncertain of the extent he should become involved.

Simon illuminates that becoming involved is not a rational thing, or a technique to apply, but heartfelt, soul bumping. Involvement is giving the self to the other. Or put another way, the practitioner's depth of involvement, or intimacy with the patient, is a reflection of compassion – for compassion is only possible to the extent the practitioner can loosen herself from her concerns. If a practitioner is wrapped up in her own stuff how can she be available to another? If my gaze is upon myself how can I gaze at the other?

Morse (1991) identifies the risk of 'over-involvement' whereby the therapeutic gaze becomes blurred through entanglement with the other. This is always a risk when the practitioner does not know herself well enough. Becoming over-involved may be a necessary learning journey, for how else can the person come to know herself? Simon noted his fear of 'getting in too deep.' The metaphor suggests drowning, of becoming submerged in another's suffering. Yet, as Simon's reflection illustrates, his willingness to 'go there' and dwell with Bill and his family opened up possibilities for his own learning. In dwelling with the family and letting go of the urge to 'fix it' for them, he could explore the depths of their suffering with them. That he absorbed their suffering and suffered himself is the human nature. None of us are immune from that, but through reflection and guidance he could make sense of his feelings and grow through the experience. He emerges from the chaos of his feelings, wiser, more caring, more able to manage himself in similar situations. If Simon had resisted these feelings then he could only have fled from the situation to save himself. As it was he tuned into the suffering on the different levels of Bill, Bill's wife and children, and flowed with it in its unpredictability.

The practitioner does not set out to 'fix it' for the other person, but to work with the person to help them find meaning in the experience. As many of the stories illustrate, flowing with another in their suffering is not easy work; it is not comfortable. Yet within a caring relationship, caring is reciprocated where the practitioner can express her own humanness. Where caring is reciprocated, the patient or family can care for the nurse – it is a dwelling together along an uncertain path. This reciprocation is inevitable and must be expected and welcomed because in being cared for, the other person has a need to give something back.

By appreciating the person's pattern, the practitioner learns to tune into the patient and family at the appropriate level of involvement within the moment. Resistance to involvement is felt when the patient or family reject involvement or demand an inappropriate level of involvement. It may also be felt within the practitioner; that something about this person or family brings negative attitude or prejudice to the surface and triggers rejection. The mindful practitioner senses and reflects on the rejection and responds appropriately. Leslie, a primary nurse at Burford hospital, projected his need for a high degree of intimacy within his relationships. When this was resisted, he felt rejected and tended to withdraw. Through supervision Leslie came to appreciate his need for intimacy and how he projected this need into his relationships (Johns 1996a).

Reciprocation and resistance

In another published account (Johns 1999), I shared Anna's experience, a district nurse, who was visiting a man at home with terminal illness. His daughter was his main carer who made excessive friendship demands on Anna, which made her feel uncomfortable and she subsequently withdrew from visiting the family. Anna felt extremely guilty at abandoning the patient. In clinical supervision I helped Anna to explore her resistance to the daughter and ways in which she might set limits with the daughter.

All relationships can be viewed along a continuum of reciprocation and resistance.

Reciprocation   ◄─────────────────────►   Resistance

Most relationships fall within a person's 'normal' intimacy boundaries and are not problematic. But as Anna's experience suggests, experience sometimes falls outside normal boundaries, resulting in anxiety. Because of this, practitioners are urged to balance engagement and detachment in caregiving (Carmack 1997). As Menzies-Lyth (1988) notes:

> 'The core of the anxiety situation for the nurse lies in her relationship with the patient. The closer and more concentrated this relationship, the more the nurse is likely to experience this anxiety . . . a necessary psychological task for the entrant into any profession that works with people is the development of adequate professional detachment.' (pp. 51, 54)

The alternative to professional detachment is to know and manage self within involvement. To avoid the situation is a response whereby everyone loses. A more positive response is to 'go there' better equipped because, as Benner & Wrubel (1989) assert, the risk of detachment is a loss of intimacy and a denial of self as caring.

Anna decided to go back into the situation and draw the line, even though the daughter said she would continue to expect more from Anna. However, this time, Anna was less threatened and could resist without fear and loss of relationship.

REFLECTIVE EXEMPLAR 6.2 – JADE AND HILDA

In one guided reflection relationship, Jade, an experienced primary nurse shared her experience of working with Hilda (Johns 1993, 1998a):

> *Jade*: "Hilda told me I was horrid. I asked her why. She said it was because I had made her stand and take a few steps. I reminded her that she had agreed this action yesterday with her primary nurse and her husband. Her response to this was, 'I didn't agree no matter what anyone says!' Hilda implied that we enjoyed bullying her, which upset me. I told her, 'If we wanted things to be easy we would just leave you,' which brought a predictable response, 'Just leave me alone,' which I then did. I felt pressured at the time with the needs of other patients. It made me feel uncomfortable all morning."
>
> *CJ*: "Could you have responded differently?"
>
> *Jade*: "No, it would have been just the same. I had taken the right decision and made the right action based on the chat I had with the primary nurse yesterday."
>
> *CJ*: "You seem angry with Hilda."
>
> *Jade*: "We don't come to work dressed in a suit of armour to protect yourself from all this shit . . . you just feel you are a target for people to fire at." Jade noted that this experience had affected her relationship with Hilda. "I went back to her later to do her dressing and she just pulled away, didn't communicate, closed her eyes to dismiss me."

Jade noted that she had continued to feel awful about this experience for days later, which she rationalised as over-sensitivity. Like Anna, Jade was unable to avoid these awful feelings because she cared deeply about her patients. Hilda's resistance to her also made her angry. In response Jade blamed Hilda, which made Jade feel bad for feeling angry at Hilda! It was as though she was on a merry-go-round of energy sapping emotions. Jade had failed to appreciate Hilda's dilemma; on one hand Hilda hated being in hospital and was anxious to go home but, on the other hand, she wanted to be left alone as she was so tired.

Jade's guilt was a reflection of her perceived failure to care, falling into what Dickson (1982) has described as a 'compassion trap' whereby practitioners get trapped by their ethic of care, as if they have taken responsibility for the way the patient feels. Noddings (1984) noted that the practitioner's sense of being overwhelmed resulting in feelings of guilt and conflict was the inescapable risk of caring. As Jade said, we don't come to work dressed in a suit of armour; armour being a metaphor for detachment. Jade pays a price for her unconditional involvement yet she would pay an even higher price if her involvement was conditional because she would then sacrifice her caring values. Her anger and guilt opened up a learning opportunity to grow through relationship. The idea of professional detachment is like wearing armour. The problem is that the patient can sense the armour and feel rejection, creating a boundary. Reflect on Wilber's (1991) words:

> 'For a line, whether mental, natural, or logical, doesn't just divide and separate, it also joins and unites. Boundaries on the other hand are pure illusions – they pretend to separate what is not in fact separable.' (p. 25)

Depending on the way a line is viewed it either separates or joins. Like the sea meeting the shore, it is simply a flowing moment, sometimes gently lapping waves and at other times a mighty roar of crashing waves, much indeed like relationships. Yet when the waves crash, do I fear being swept away? Like a surfer I must become one with the wave. Resistance is simply the boundary beyond which I fear to surf (Johns 2004).

The reciprocation–resistance continuum (Box 6.1) offers a reflective tool for practitioners to explore the extent they sense resistance within relationships. Ramos (1992) identified embodied impasses or resistance factors within the practitioner that limited the practitioner's ability to realise connected (or what I describe as reciprocated) types of relationships. The first impasse was emotional (over) involvement that reflected the nurse's failure to draw boundaries between self and the other. The second impasse was the nurse's need to control the patient's experience in order to protect the patient and manage the self's anxiety.

Box 6.1 Reciprocation–resistance reflective tool

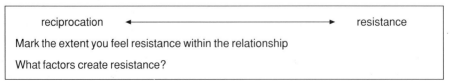

reciprocation ⬅━━━━━━━━━➡ resistance

Mark the extent you feel resistance within the relationship

What factors create resistance?

REFLECTIVE EXEMPLAR 6. 3 – TRUDY'S STORY

Trudy is a district nurse. She shared her experience of working with Catherine and Gary in clinical supervision with me over six consecutive sessions. Catherine has terminal cancer and Gary is her husband. This exemplar gives the reader a good impression of the reflexive nature of guided reflection – the way each session picks up and develops the issues from the previous session. The story also illuminates the nature of wavelength theory (see Chapter 4) in the way Trudy tunes in and flows with Catherine's wavelength but struggles to tune into Gary's wavelength because of her resistance to him.

Session 1

Trudy read from her reflective diary "Catherine is a 47 year old woman with cancer in her bowel and peritoneal secondaries. She has a colostomy. Her husband called the clinic at 17.45 requesting me to visit. The message was 'wife unwell/colostomy blocked?' It was taken by another nurse. My dilemma was, do I visit now or do I refer to the evening nurse? I left it to the evening nurse. I rationalised this by thinking that it would be good for her to make Catherine's acquaintance. On my way home I pass nearby this family's house. I was feeling guilty that I had not responded personally, so I popped in. The curtains were drawn upstairs. Catherine was blind, confused, she had 'gone off her legs'. She was lying in the bathroom. I helped to move her onto the bed and she then commenced having fits. Her two sons who were present could not cope with this. They fled. Her husband was shocked. She was fitting for about 15–20 minutes. I called the general practitioner (GP), who suggested I made a 999 emergency call. I resisted this; I was asking myself, 'do I want her to go to hospital?' I didn't know the preference of the family about managing Catherine's deterioration and eventual death. This had not become a topic of conversation. The GP arrived and gave Catherine some IV valium which worked although she continued to fit intermittently. Her husband decided on private hospital admission. We had to wait two hours for an ambulance to arrive. I stayed with her during this time. Catherine fitted again on the stretcher going into the ambulance. I felt bad because I hadn't spoken to the boys. Was my decision to refer to the night nurse the best decision? I felt I didn't have the full facts of the situation and didn't know the situation well enough to make a good judgement."

I asked Trudy whether she could have rung the husband back to explore what was meant by 'unwell'? Trudy responded, "Yes, I should have done that as Catherine usually managed her colostomy well."

I picked up on Trudy's comment about eventual death and asked her about her relationship with the family and talking about Catherine's impending death. Trudy said, "I have known Catherine for seven months, she knows her condition is terminal. I challenged Trudy on whether she was avoiding talking about this situation with the family. Trudy acknowledged the need to manage hope and whether she should confront Gary's denial at this time, "Gary is uncomfortable talking about these issues and for these reasons I haven't pushed it. I'm sensitive about a right time to discuss Catherine's death and that right time hasn't presented itself yet . . . however I do feel this event marks a crisis within Catherine's illness trajectory. I will explore the meaning of this with Gary and discuss the different options for managing the situation when I visit him on Friday."

I gently probed whether Trudy avoided discussion with Gary and Catherine because of her own discomfort. Trudy said, "My relationship is largely with Catherine. Gary has always seemed on the margins, seemingly uncomfortable with the emotional issues and focusing more on managing the physical. As a result I don't know him very well."

Trudy continued to blame herself for referring to the evening nurse when she should have made the decision to visit herself. I reflected the way in which, with hindsight, we punish ourselves, yet helped Trudy to see that her decision was reasonable at the time, that she couldn't have envisaged the way the situation had unfolded. Trudy challenged herself, "Did I want her at home for my own needs because I would prefer that?"

I suggested that Gary and Catherine had different and potentially conflicting needs. Trudy asserted, "Catherine needs good symptomatic control right now but in a private hospital? I'm left with a sense that Gary just wanted her out of the way." Taking Gary's perspective, I suggested that perhaps he could not cope with what was happening with her right now. Trudy acknowledged the point.

It was nearing the end of our meeting so I asked Trudy what she felt had been significant about sharing this experience? Trudy responded, "Recognising that my sense of guilt is a reflection of the caring trap . . . thinking I should be there for my patients at all times. I seem to get entangled in these types of relationships. And secondly, my sense of unease with Gary that goes against my belief of responding to the whole family."

Commentary

The caring trap, or what Ann Dickson (1982) describes as the compassion trap, is when the practitioner gets trapped by their caring ethic. Trudy takes on responsibility for Catherine's suffering, indeed she absorbs Catherine's suffering as her own. As a result she responds on an emotional rather than rational level to her dilemma – should she visit or ask the evening nurse? She felt guilty when she decided to ask the evening nurse. The trap awaits the practitioner who lacks the ability to know and manage themselves well enough in relationship with the patient or family member. Part of her dilemma is knowing where to draw the line in terms of her shift hours. Drawing rigid lines of work time creates the difficulty for her. Intimacy has no bounds.

Trudy felt the conflict of contradiction within her approach to Gary. She knew she was not available to him, that she resisted him as a threat to her relationship with Catherine. He made her feel angry and defensive. Yet she knew within the scope of holistic practice that she should be available to him, to feel compassionate toward him.

I helped Trudy put these feelings of guilt, distress and anger into the dialogic clearing where we could see them for what they were. Why does Trudy feel like this? Explanations like the 'caring trap' helped Trudy to see herself within the trap and she could see her resistance to Gary. Such visualisations help understanding and shift the negative energy into positive energy for acting on her insights for the journey ahead with this family.

This was my first supervision session with Trudy. It was as if I had held a mirror for Trudy to look at herself. It was a time of connection between us, as I tuned into and surfed her wavelength. It was both emotional and intimate, illustrating how powerful supervision can be. I was mindful of not absorbing Trudy's suffering as my own, modelling how she might, in turn, respond to Catherine's, Gary's and the boys' emotions in the future (parallel process framing, see Box 1.10).

Session 2

20 days later Trudy and I met again. She shared her experience of visiting Gary.

> "He said she couldn't possibly come home as she had a catheter, a syringe driver . . . a stream of problems. I struggled to respond positively to him. I needed to assess Catherine for myself so I phoned the hospital. They were reluctant to give me any information but they said it was okay to visit. Catherine looked really well. If she had been at a NHS hospital they would have discharged her days ago. She had no memory of fitting. She was no longer fitting but had massive oedema of her abdomen and legs. I was questioning her treatment with the staff. She was not on any steroids. I thought the staff had a very limited understanding of Catherine's drugs, for example they thought nozinan in the syringe driver was for the epilepsy (in fact it is a broad spectrum anti-emetic). It was making Catherine sleepy. Catherine said she wanted to go home. She said this in front of Gary when he arrived. I sensed the conflict between them."

I asked Trudy if she could have responded in other ways. Trudy was unsure: perhaps ask the GP to speak with the hospital doctors? I surfaced Trudy's anxiety that Catherine's desire to come home should be respected. I also reasserted Gary's perspective and questioned whose needs are we responding to. Do we understand and respond to Gary on his emotional level or our own? Can he cope with Catherine's illness? Perhaps his difficulty with coping and emotional distress explains why arranging a support package to support Catherine at home was not enough to persuade him to have her home. Trudy was uncomfortable; she felt the hospital was colluding with Gary in terms of his own needs rather than Catherine's, as if

Catherine had become some object to talk about and do things with. We explored Trudy's options and potential consequences. One option was to involve Clare, the Macmillan nurse, more actively in Catherine's care. It felt like bringing in reinforcements to battle Gary.

I asked, "Do you want Clare to respond to or confront Gary?"

Trudy responded, "Clare doesn't know the family well whereas I do. I don't know how Catherine would feel if Clare came in."

I challenged Trudy that what she was really saying was that she didn't know how she would feel if Clare comes in. Will Trudy feel pushed out? Was that her fear? I brought the dialogue back to consider whether it was time to confront Gary with the conflict of needs on an emotional level. I wondered if a cathartic response would be more helpful, for example, 'I can see this is tough for you Gary'. I suggested he might be feeling guilty about not having his wife at home, so such a response might help him face his guilt. It was not merely a stark choice of either hospital or home to die but to take each day as it comes, to leave the doors open. The cathartic response would then make it easier to confront Gary with, "What does Catherine want?" "Should you respect her wishes?"

Trudy responded, "If she came home she could always go back into hospital or the hospice if things deteriorate badly. I haven't really talked with him. I feel concerned that I should be manipulating him toward my views. I accept my sympathies and interests have lain primarily with Catherine."

I suggested that a major issue for Catherine was being in control of her own dying, ensuring that those she left behind could cope without her. There were also issues about her two sons and why she needed to be at home.

At the end of the session, Trudy felt the discussion had helped her to see things differently, most notably paying attention to the husband's needs and how this was central to getting Catherine home. She noted, "It has influenced my future actions and helped me anticipate what Gary may be thinking. I will arrange to meet him again!"

Commentary

Trudy continues to resist Gary yet struggles with this contradiction of her holistic beliefs. Holism is not a rational technique to be applied but an emotional way for being. By empathising with Gary I challenged Trudy to develop her own empathic understanding with Gary's perspective, to tune into his wavelength and to understand his own suffering. This was vital if she was going to shift her perspective of Gary as adversary and become available to him. How do we sense what the other is feeling and thinking at such moments? Only when Trudy has worked through her resistance to Gary can she truly empathise with him. Trudy's emotional entanglement with Catherine is revealed in her anxiety of Clare's involvement. It illustrates how judgement is blurred by her own concerns.

Trudy moves on in her journey with this family. We have re-visited issues surfaced in the first session and yet, just because we can see things differently, does not mean we can easily shift our emotional responses or change our embodied responses. Learning through reflection is a holistic process of knowing and transforming self, rather than a cognitive activity. We cannot simply shrug off who we are.

Session 3

41 days later, Trudy picked up the threads of her unfolding experience with Catherine and Gary.

"I did visit and confront him with the prospect of Catherine coming home. He was uptight. He said 'I know I am being selfish but I've got a life to lead, and the boys as well. If Catherine is coming home then someone has to be here all the time.' He was adamant and said that he had to return imminently to work in Indonesia. I didn't pursue it because I could see it was making him more uptight. I contacted the hospital. They said Catherine could be kept on insurance funding because she had a syringe driver which counted as treatment. I offered to look after her if she came home. But after that I didn't hear from them or Gary. I became despondent about it. Then, this week, she was sent home for the day. Gary informed me and I went to visit her. She was downstairs sitting at the kitchen table. She looked well. No syringe driver, no catheter. She was eating and drinking. Walking up and down stairs. Her legs were less swollen although her ascites remained and made her look nine months pregnant. She said 'I feel really well.' Gary interceded with, 'You're not well, are you?' He was challenging what she could do, getting up and down stairs. I asked her when she was coming home. She said she was working on it, pulling a face at Gary. He said that she was not ready to come home. I asked her what I could do to help her when she did come home.

And today?! I heard she is coming home on Thursday . . . a phone message from Gary. The insurance funding has dried up. He has got to come to terms with it now she's returning home. I have arranged a package of care for her. She's really determined. She said that she had forced herself to eat to make herself better. There was no explanation for the epilepsy. They didn't do a brain scan and she isn't on any epileptic drugs. Perhaps it was a reaction from the nozinan. She was on dexamethasone but now there is friction between them about coming home."

Trudy explored her feelings of involvement with Catherine. She knew it was going to be tough for her when Catherine eventually died. She felt that Gary's comments were off-putting for Catherine. Trudy knew she needed to be supportive toward Gary rather than confronting him with his persistent negative attitude because he may be feeling guilty about not wanting her home. Trudy felt more in tune with Gary, could sense how he was feeling more easily, and hence felt more supportive to him.

She said, "After I last saw Gary, I let it go. I feel guilty about that. I saw him in the shops and I went off the other way rather than face him. I began to feel awkward pushing it for her. Often at home I would think how she was. I couldn't understand why they had kept the syringe driver going. Her body is covered with abscess sites from the driver – they had to change the site every day. She's on MST now."

Trudy reflected on how she had been drawn into this emotional web, entangled and pulled between Catherine and Gary. She felt less entangled now. Even as she talked I got her to visualise me pulling her out of the web. I framed her involvement with Catherine and Gary using the nurse– patient theories of Morse (1991) and Ramos (1992). Trudy immediately identified with the Morse type of 'over-involvement', saying, 'I've been there!'

I suggested we all needed to visit and experience emotional entangle- ment, because only then can we recognise the place. Perhaps entanglement is an inevitable consequence of holistic relationships because it's so hard to resist the suffering of the other. It is like a tidal wave that we must learn to surf and control yet without relinquishing its exquisite intimacy and beauty. It's okay to be vulnerable but like the expert surfer we can ride it. Maybe we do sometimes get swept away, but that's just another experience to learn from. That's why we need clinical supervision.

Session 4

30 days later. Trudy was late as she had been to a funeral that afternoon and then an urgent visit. I wondered if it was Catherine's funeral.

Trudy exclaimed, "No! She's up and well. I'm seeing her twice a week. She's been having some difficulty with her son. He has problems with drugs and also a recent court appearance because of stealing."

Picking up the cue I enquire, "Have you helped the sons talk about what's happening to their mother?" Trudy replied, "No. Gary has not returned to Indonesia yet. He's saying he has got to go next month but he's also said that someone needs to be with Catherine the whole time."

"Is this necessary?"

Trudy was thoughtful. "I don't think so, at least not 24 hours a day because if someone has 24 hour care she can't live a normal life, can she?"

I respond, "If you're waiting to die, can you live a 'normal life'?"

Trudy responded, "Well, she struggles to do the housework but she can wash and dress herself, etc."

I said, "You're responding to her in terms of things she can physically do, what about her responses on an emotional level? Is she coping on this level?"

Trudy: "Maybe she doesn't want to talk on this level although she does give cues such as 'living on borrowed time' . . . it's difficult to talk to her because her husband and sons are often there and they don't want to talk about it."

"Maybe they don't know how to talk about it."

Trudy compared this with another Catherine, who was also dying yet very open to what was happening to her, and who needed to resolve issues such as who was going to look after her five-year-old son. Of course, how people feel and what they think about their impending death can never be predicted. The wavelength becomes a rollercoaster!

I asked, "Perhaps Catherine is ambivalent? As you said, she is not in denial. She accepts she is going to die but she also needs to cope and protect her boys. Perhaps she is trying to be brave? Imagine yourself in her shoes – what sort of things would you need to be doing?"

Trudy said, "Well, sort out my children, put my house in order."

I reminded Trudy of the message from *Final Gifts* (Callanan & Kelley 1992), that the primary task for the dying person was to ensure that those they left behind were able to cope. Trudy again linked this to the other Catherine 'coming to terms' and her actions. Even things like changing internal doors in the house, things that she had wanted to do. She was now quite peaceful with everything sorted out.

I reflected, "Perhaps we can see that Catherine is trying to cope with chaos. Perhaps she does need confronting in order to help her sort things out. Perhaps you are avoiding this for your discomfort and uncertainty about her ambivalence?"

Trudy accepted my challenge. "I just feel with this family they aren't ready to talk about it. I don't feel her physical deterioration has become that marked where her dying has really become an issue. They are a 'difficult' family, I have a number of people who are dying where talking about death is not a problem."

I took Trudy back to the beginning of the session. "All this came out of me asking – was it Catherine's funeral?!" Trudy noted, "We have had a lot of people dying – nine recently. It's stressful. It doesn't help having conflict with the doctors." Trudy then talked through her conflict with a doctor over drug dosage. She sensed the doctor was not listening to her, yet Trudy had not backed down and asserted her point of view. Trudy said, "She was short with me but she didn't bawl me out of the office."

I said, "I've noted the intimidating factor – *being short*."

Trudy laughed. "Some patients have commented on her manner. Her New Year's resolution is to be less short!"

"It's promising she has insight!"

We paused so I continued. "Last session I challenged you to consider the balance of being challenging and being supportive with Gary and Catherine." Trudy said, "My stance towards Gary has changed. I now see their relationship differently. I see that maybe he couldn't go to Indonesia because he couldn't leave Catherine at home and that being with her was an emotional rather than a physical thing. Could he focus on work knowing she was as she was?"

Commentary

Trudy contrasts Catherine with other dying patients she visits in her effort to make sense of her struggle with Catherine and Gary whilst trying to position herself within the tension of confronting the family's reluctance to talk about Catherine's imminent death. What would be for the best? To know is to tune in to the unfolding patterns of shifting wavelengths and sense it. My guidance is to make Trudy more mindful of this tension.

Session 5

21 days later, Trudy says

"I feel that Gary is now letting me in and that I'm responding to my intuition, that the right time has unfolded to talk about feelings and dying. Catherine is now in the terminal stage of her illness. I went in following a phone call from Catherine that her colostomy was obstructed. Up to this time I had been going in twice weekly. She had been self caring so I went in to discuss what had been happening to her. On this visit she was in bed. She said she had great abdominal pain. I sought the GP's advice. The GP had prescribed a suppository but this hadn't worked and had since prescribed Normacol. Because of the pain I advised Catherine not to take this. I also referred her to the night nurse so she could get help if she needed it."

After considering palliative approaches to Catherine's bowel obstruction Trudy continued:

"Gary was downstairs during this visit. I had informed him that the colostomy was obstructed and that this was a sign of things worsening and her imminent death. Gary said it wasn't fair to keep her alive. Why were we giving her all these drugs? That we needed to put an end to all this! I asked him if Catherine was talking about dying. He said that he wanted to look after her at home and not to go back into hospital. I thought he might be strapped for cash but he assured me that wasn't the reason. She didn't want to go back in and he had accepted that. The elder son didn't want to stray too far in case anything happened to mum. No talk of the younger son, he was still having his troubles. I'm now visiting every day."

I challenged Trudy on why she was visiting. Trudy responded, "Because my enrolled nurse is no good at counselling. She 'whips in and out.' Both Catherine and Gary made this observation. She's a good nurse but prefers going in and doing something physical. I need to monitor the colostomy and to respond to her symptoms on a daily basis and to help the family through the crisis."

I noted, "Being there for them?"

Trudy: "Yes, that's right. I had two other patients who were similar to Catherine with obstructed colostomies. One lived for three months after it had become blocked. She would vomit every day. In the end faecal matter, not very pleasant. I have not told them about such possibility. Catherine is struggling to eat just a little. She has requested some 'HiCal' drinks to keep her strength up."

I wondered if Catherine was hanging onto some hope and Trudy was responding on this level. Trudy acknowledged the dilemma of maintaining hope, "I can tell by the look she gives me that she knows she has deteriorated, but she doesn't want to talk about that. She feels the lumps in her tummy, hoping the tumour will still go away."

I responded, "It must be hard for you to see her suffer like that, her grief all bottled up inside . . . when you know it would help her to share it with you." It was a poignant moment to dwell in that truth, in silence for a moment. I broke the spell by challenging Trudy over her team leader responsibilities – what does she need to do when she knows that members of her team are not responding appropriately? Trudy: "I find it hard to tackle such issues because I don't like conflict even when I know it compromises patient care . . . I want to talk more about Gary. Gary is out of control, feeling helpless, very anxious and angry. He tested out the night nurse to gauge her response – which was okay! This is going to be tough, especially when she becomes more physically dependent, vomiting, etcetera. I feel okay, not over-involved. I feel happy because Catherine is quite happy. Things are under control. I enjoy visiting them. Before I wasn't in control."

Commentary

Trudy felt that the dynamics had changed with Gary because he now accepted that Catherine was going to die at home although he clearly struggled with his feelings. The situation is very tense. Focusing Trudy's attention on the situation with her enrolled nurse was misplaced in that her mind was wrapped up with Catherine and Gary. Yet her avoidance of the topic reflects her avoidance of the issue in practice.

Session 6

46 days later, Trudy noted how busy she was and the pressure she felt under just now. She picked up Catherine:

"Catherine . . . her death. She was fighting to the end. She was on a massive dose of diamorphine – 500 mg in her syringe driver. She had another massive fit. I'll read from my diary":

'I visited Catherine Monday morning early; the Marie Curie nurse had rung me to say that Catherine had a very restless night and was not responding to oral commands and there was a steady trickle of black fluid running from her mouth. I decided to assess the situation and rang the GP from Catherine's house. As I entered the bedroom I was shocked by what I saw. Catherine was groaning and rolling around the bed. Gary was trying to hold her onto the bed. She rolled from side to side, legs hanging over the edge of the bed, her catheter tube kinked and twisted around her leg, her tubing from the syringe driver had become detached. Clearly Gary was distressed. Catherine lay across the bed, her huge abdomen hard and contracting, her swollen legs looked heavy and shiny, her face, arms, and shoulders so thin that you see her bones protruding. I sat on the bed, reconnecting the syringe driver and checked the light was flashing. Gently I talked to Catherine, holding her hand. She was calm for a minute, and then she began to groan again, vomited and started to fit. Gary and I rolled Catherine onto her side in the recovery position. I called the GP to come straight away and rang the clinic, asking the reception staff to bleep my nursing auxiliary and ask her to come to Catherine's house urgently. While we waited Gary and I talked; I admitted to Gary that I had never witnessed anything like this before in all my nursing experience.

Catherine's strength was amazing, on occasions rolling onto to her enlarged abdomen. All kinds of emotions were spinning through my head. I felt sad for Gary witnessing this, Catherine's loss of dignity. What an awful death and I was helpless to do anything. I had no valium to stop the fit and no injection available to calm Catherine. I spoke to Gary and said the only good thing about this was that Catherine didn't know what was going on. The GP arrived – he was visibly shocked and passed me a valium enema which I inserted into Catherine's colostomy. Within a few minutes Catherine was calm. I asked the GP for another in case she fitted again and asked him if he had any midazolam 20 mg that I could use to sedate Catherine as she was very agitated and restless. He wrote the medication and Stuart, Gary's son went to collect the prescription. Ann, my nursing auxiliary arrived, and we washed Catherine, talking gently to her, comforting her, cleansed her mouth and put a clean nightie on and clean sheets. By this time Stuart had returned and I could give the midazolam intramuscularly into her thigh. Within ten minutes she was asleep. Gary, Ann and I sat around the bed, emotionally drained, just looking at Catherine. I knew I could not leave Gary alone. The situation was frightening for him. Gary thanked us both and felt reassured that he was not going to be left alone. He was happier that she was asleep.'

Trudy put her diary aside and asked herself
"What was I trying to achieve? My main concern was for Gary who was visibly distressed. Catherine would have been horrified if she could see herself, nightie up around her breasts, legs and bottom exposed, rolling around her bed, groaning, complete loss of dignity. Gary was distraught, unable to restrain her almost falling out of bed. I was frustrated that there were no drugs prescribed that I could have given. When Catherine was asleep and calm, Gary could manage. He rarely touched Catherine – he always stood at the foot of the bed or sat in a chair. I never saw him hold her hand although he always talked fondly of her, I came to the conclusion that he was afraid and it would be less stressful for him if Ann assisted me in all nursing duties.

I've learnt a lot from this but I never did get to grips with Gary. I said to him, 'it won't be long' and queried whether he wanted her family present. He said that they can come at any time but he didn't want them staying. He said, 'I don't think of her death, I think of the future.' He never shed a tear. I went to the funeral. Her father was heartbroken as his wife had died of cancer as well."

I acknowledged Trudy's feelings, "This must have been very traumatic for you . . . you moved a long way to accommodate Gary within your sphere of care."

Trudy responded, "That's been my real learning, to see and respond to the whole family. It's true, I do normally identify with the woman in the situation which often leaves me feeling angry at the spouses, as with Gary, because he seemed to interfere with me helping Catherine meet her needs."

Commentary

Trudy had written a truly astonishing description of Catherine. I felt the power of her writing as she unfolded the events. It is a story of becoming, of coming to know self and the impact of self on the way events are grasped and interpreted. The contradiction between her holistic belief and her practice was evident from the beginning. I was touched by the symbolic moment as they sat around the bed – Trudy and Ann by Catherine, and Gary alone, isolated in his suffering at the foot of the bed. It reflects the impression painted by Trudy that Gary was an intruder, even to the end. So I wonder to what extent she was transformed through this experience. It was not a perfect ending but such situations rarely are. Issues such as supporting the boys were left relatively untouched.

Reflection was a mirror held high for Trudy to reveal herself to herself in the context of her experience with Catherine and Gary. Her honesty was profound and enabled her to find new meaning in being a holistic practitioner, more aware of self, more mindful of her impact on others, and, as a consequence, more able to manage herself within her relationships with patients and families.

Mayeroff (1971) states:

'I am in-place because of the way I relate to others. And place must be continually renewed and reaffirmed.' (p. 69)

As Mayeroff (1971) suggests, Trudy seeks to be in-place within her caring relationships, a place where she can dwell with the other comfortable with her intimacy and vulnerability. Reflection helps her to work out the discomfort so she can know her dwelling place and dwell there more easily.

Blackwolf & Gina Jones (1996) say:

'Perhaps you have begun your path of change and are experiencing the pain of previous pains, as you open the cover to the book of your own life. The cover, which up to now has been carefully sealed up. Like the leaves of a head of lettuce, you are beginning to peel back one blemished leaf at a time, to reveal the you of quiet peace. Hidden beneath your polished presentation to the world, your injuries have been waiting for you to acknowledge their existence. It is time to view your injuries and feel your bruises. Through the experiential [reflective] process, we become real. We really become.' (p. 22)

Trudy did not view herself as injured or bruised because such wounds, as with most of us, are masked by the need to cope. Yet, as the dialogue revealed, Trudy's masks were gently revealed, enabling her wounds to be tended. Perhaps 'wounds' sounds dramatic, yet the metaphor of the wounded healer seems common to most nurses. Trudy not only made connections with her deeper self, she also connected with me, as her guide. I was a clearing where she could unwrap and touch her deeper self. It is a tender process. I must shine a gentle light to help Trudy, and others like her, for we are strongly defended. It was her love for Catherine that allowed herself to reveal herself. In an outcome-oriented health care culture, the temptation may be to shine a bright light that frightens the practitioner caught in the glare. In Chapter 7 I explore establishing an environment that can adequately support practitioners like Simon and Trudy to be available.

Chapter 7

Creating an Environment Where it is Possible to Be Available

The practitioner's ability to be available to work with the patient and family is influenced to a great extent by the conditions of practice. In an ideal world, there would simply be the relationship between the patient and the practitioner. Yet caring takes place within the organisational context that may constrain the practitioner's ability to be with the patient as desired. In this chapter, I explore the practitioner's ability to create an environment where she can be available to work in desirable ways with the patient and family.

There is no such place as an ideal world. Perhaps you have been challenged by earlier chapters to reflect on your vision for practice and whether you realise this vision as an everyday reality. Perhaps you have felt the conflict of contradiction and sensed those factors that do constrain your ability to be available to patients and families. These constraining factors are concerned with tradition, authority, and embodiment, acknowledging that people are essentially historical beings rather than rational beings:

Tradition   A pre-reflective state reflected in the customs, norms, prejudices and habitual practices that people hold about the way things should be.

Authority   The way normal relationships are constructed and maintained through the use of power.

Embodiment   The way people normally think, feel and respond to the world in a normative and largely pre-reflective way.

If people were rational they would change their practice on the basis of evidence that supports the best way of doing something. But even then two people may rationally disagree! This takes us back to Fay's (1987) assertion that in order to be reflective, people need to be open, intelligent, curious and wilful. Three key points to note about constraining factors are:

- Because these factors are normative they are not necessarily perceived.
- Until practitioners become aware of these factors that constrain them they are unlikely to be able to change them.
- Shifting old new norms and moving to new norms congruent with desirable practice goes against the status quo gradient, reflecting that one's actions have consequences for others.

Examples of tradition, authority and embodied factors are evident within the 'influences grid' (Box 1.8) each of which does, to varying extent, influence the way the practitioner feels, thinks and responds to practice. Reflection involves working through the impact of these influences in order to understand and begin to work towards shifting them so the practitioner can respond in more desirable ways to practice situations. However, this may not be so easy when many of these influences are reinforced in normal ways of relating that have become embedded within the organisational culture. For example, nurses may perceive themselves to be subordinate and powerless in the face of the professional dominance of doctors or managerialism. Expectations from others about the way the practitioner should act is a powerful influence because of the need to maintain the status quo, a relatively stable equilibrium of power forces that people accept as normal and which people are attached to because it brings stability and reward.

People are attached to stability because they fear change will disrupt any possible benefit for themselves irrespective of the wider benefit for patient care. Hence when the usually passive person asserts her point of view she creates instability and others are triggered to return her to her normal passive state, 'to know her place' within the order of things. Such patterns of relating are bureaucratic, when knowing your place in the smooth running of the system is more significant than the reason the system exists in the first place (Friedson 1970). As Mayeroff (1971) says 'Sometimes knowing your place may prevent you from ever being in-place' (p. 70) – *in-place* being the therapeutic place to achieve desirable practice.

Without doubt, caring can be difficult to assert within a bureaucratic culture that is driven by outcome targets with limited resources. Such a culture creates a productivity anxiety that is transmitted through successive layers of the hierarchy. One consequence is that nursing, and more broadly, caring, is obscured and regarded as a soft asset to strip because:

- its process and outcomes are marginal to purchasing plans and meeting organisational outcomes
- it has an extensive workforce and represents a significant slice of the budget
- it does not have a strong voice within the organisational culture
- it regulates itself as a subordinate and powerless group controlled by an internalised threat of sanction

As Ray (1989) notes:

> 'The transformation of health care systems to corporate enterprises emphasising competitive management and economic gains, seriously challenges nursing's humanistic philosophies and theories and nursing's administrative and clinical practices.' (p. 31)

Perhaps the answer is for nurses to be chief executives and respond in tune with caring values to the political health care. But of course some nurses are chief executives and they too get caught up in the bureaucratic anxiety trap. As people are promoted into the echelons of management they become socialised to become more like the senior managers and less like the practitioner group they are leaving. So many practitioners have shared experiences of this promotion transition and their struggle to reposition themselves: 'No longer one of us, you must be one of them.'

Roberts (1983) argued that nurses were promoted because they were most like those already in power, and thus could be relied on to maintain the status quo and to ensure the *peasant* nurses were kept in order; i.e. were socialised to know their place. I use the word peasant to emphasise the way Roberts was influenced by Paulo Freire, the Brazilian educationalist who viewed learning as essentially emancipatory. Freire (1972) gives the example of the peasant who is promoted to overseer, and becomes a bigger tyrant to the other peasants than the master himself, because he wants to become like the master himself and share in the rich rewards of the powerful classes. Hence the peasant overseer will sacrifice his peasant values in favour of the values of the more powerful. He is chosen to become the overseer because he most fits the ideal image of those who choose him. Is this how ward sisters are promoted: less for their clinical ability but more for the way they fit an ideal image of management?

The status quo

Reflection is change-oriented and so must always challenge the status quo. As such, contemplating the impact of change on the status quo is a useful strategic focus for reflection (Box 7.1). In using force field analysis the practitioner would first need to identify those forces that either promote or resist change and appreciate the norms that support the status quo.

Breu & Dracup (1976) implemented change in a Coronary Care Unit (CCU) to meet the needs of spouses in response to Hampe's (1975) findings that the needs of spouses of terminally ill patients who were experiencing anticipatory loss were not met by the staff. The CCU had undertaken research which confirmed Hampe's findings for spouses on the CCU. Breu & Dracup used Klein's (1968) eight principles of managing change based on Lewin's force field analysis (1951) to reflect on their success of managing the change process. They concluded:

- There is almost a universal tendency to seek to maintain the status quo on the part of those whose needs are being met by it.
- Resistance to change increases in proportion to how much it is perceived as a threat.

Box 7.1   Force field analysis (Lewin 1951)

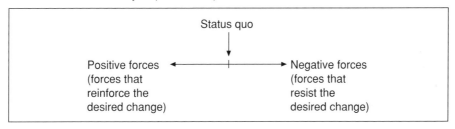

- Resistance to change increases in direct response to pressure of change.
- Resistance to change decreases when it is perceived as being reinforced by trusted others, such as high prestige figures, those whose judgement is respected, people of like mind.
- Resistance to change decreases when those involved are able to foresee how they might establish a new equilibrium as good as or better than the old.
- Commitment to change increases when those involved have the opportunity to participate in the decision to make and implement the change.
- Resistance to change based on fear of the new circumstances is decreased when those involved have the opportunity to experience the new under conditions of minimal threat.
- Temporary alterations in most situations can be brought about by the use of direct pressure, but these changes are accompanied by heightened tension and will yield a highly unstable situation.

These points are food for thought for the reflective practitioner, highlighting that change is a carefully plotted and collective journey rather than an individual journey. It is all too easy to get washed up and broken against an unyielding status quo.

Shifting norms

Norms are the taken-for-granted structures that determine the status quo. When people change jobs, they seek out these norms in order to 'fit in' and be accepted. People who don't fit in are quickly targeted as misfits and pressure is brought to bear on them to toe the party line. Hence conditions of practice or norms are invested with normal power relationships that constitute the status quo, and as such, are not easy to shift. The reflective practitioner understands the forces that constrain her as she contemplates what action to take to realise her vision as a lived reality. To succeed, she must inevitably become more 'politically' oriented, and committed to act in ways congruent with her values. Of course, it would be much easier if she worked with people who shared her vision and were committed to working in collaborative ways. As such, creating the conditions to support holistic caring practices is crucial.

The collaborative team

'It doesn't pay to be assertive here' (Johns 1989a)

These memorable words were uttered by a staff nurse in relation to her concerns about shifting roles in introducing primary nursing. The words reveal the deeply embodied sense that asserting self was against the hierarchical grain and likely to incur retribution. Yet to succeed primary nursing demands a collaborative style of working that goes against the grain of a traditional bureaucratic hierarchy.

Too many people had too much invested in normal ways of relating to let go easily and shift to new norms, resulting in failure to create the conditions that would successfully support primary nursing.

Primary nursing was like a square peg in a round hole.

Hence becoming assertive is not simply an individual effort but requires an organisational effort to create the collaborative team. Central to shifting the culture of the work environment is the shift from transactional to transformational leadership. But here is the rub. If leaders are generally transactional, even unwittingly, then how can they lead the shift to the collaborative team? This is a conundrum that I explore in Chapter 8.

In Box 7.2 I show a set of old norms consistent with a bureaucratic model of health care and a complementary set of new norms consistent with establishing the collaborative team necessary to realise holistic caring practice. In the remainder of this chapter I explore how reflection can enable the practitioner

Box 7.2   The movement from old norms to new norms congruent with establishing the collaborative team

Old norms consistent with a bureaucratic hierarchical team	New norms consistent with the collaborative team
Vision Top-down vision, based on organisational values in terms of outcomes and productivity. Lip service paid to the idea of caring. Sees nursing as supportive to medicine.	Shared vision, based on beliefs and values about responding to people's needs. Sees nursing and other health care workers as complementary to medicine.
Managing work Work is managed primarily on a delegated task-centred approach based on professional and managerial dominance.	Work is managed primarily on the basis of shared vision whereby contribution to realising the vision is understood, valued and based on mutual role responsibility and genuine collaboration.
Transactional leadership Views people as means towards an end reflected in an emphasis on authoritative power (see Box 7.8)	*Transformational leadership* Investment in people reflected in an emphasis on facilitative power and dialogue.
Organisation Emphasis on order, stability, outcome and status quo.	Emphasis on learning and reflection to ensure and sustain effective practice.
Nurses Perceive themselves as subordinate, powerless reflected in a passive mode of being with others and avoidance of conflict.	Perceive themselves as being part of a collaborative team working together within shared vision and shared success, reflected in an assertive mode of being.

to manage conflict in collaborative and assertive ways and to understand and cope with stress in ways that support holistic practice. Leadership is the focus for Chapter 10.

Managing conflict

In my experience of clinical supervision, the majority of shared experiences are grounded in conflict to the extent that I can authoritatively state that managing everyday practice is managing conflict (Johns 1998). From my research I have been able to understand the nature and pattern of conflict to construct a typology of levels of conflict (Box 7.3). At level 1, the conflict is intra-personal, a response to when the practitioner has not responded in tune with her own values. At level 2, the conflict is inter-personal between the nurse–patient/family relationship. At level 3, the conflict is still interpersonal but at the organisational level. As a general rule, conflict will need to be resolved at level 1 before it can be adequately resolved at level 2, and at levels 1 and 2 before it can be adequately resolved at level 3.

Consider the pattern of conflict within the experience Leslie, a primary nurse, shared in clinical supervision concerning Mrs Robinson and the way he responded to the conflict.

REFLECTIVE EXEMPLAR 7.1 – LESLIE AND MRS ROBINSON

Leslie: [expressing his frustration] "Basil is 76. He was transferred to us two weeks ago for rehabilitation following a stroke six weeks ago. He has quite a

Box 7.3   Pattern of conflict (adapted from Johns 1993)

Level of conflict	Manifestation	Level of knowing
1. Intra-personal: Self in context of the environment	Situations of contradiction between the way the practitioner thinks and feels within self (often manifest as a negative feeling of guilt, frustration, distress, anger etc.)	Knowing and taking responsibility for self
2. Interpersonal: Self in context with the patient and family	Situations of conflicting values between the nurse and patient/family (that subsumes situations of conflict within the patient and between the patient and family)	Creating a therapeutic relationship
3. Interpersonal: Self in context of therapeutic work with others	Situations of conflicting values or authority between the nurse and other nurses/health care workers/organisation	Creating a therapeutic environment

severe right-sided weakness. He's very heavy and hasn't made a lot of progress with physiotherapy. He's not communicative with us, although more so with his wife. She decided that Basil would be better off at home than here and therefore wanted him discharged as soon as possible. I said I could see her point of view but felt Basil needed to stay in hospital a further 7–10 days for therapy. She said 'No, I want him home.' I felt she wasn't listening any more to us so I arranged a discharge package and talked this through with the doctor, who felt that the best thing was to go along with her wishes and pick up the pieces if we had to. I felt that I had to put forward formal reasons for Basil to stay in light of some recent experiences when we've been criticised for inadequate or inappropriate discharge. Hence I wanted to ensure the best possible care with agreement from all parties to minimise the risk of failure. Gayle [colleague] said it was defensive nursing."

CJ: "What was your reaction to that?"

Leslie: "I laughed about it and perhaps it was. I had written to the GP summarising the discharge."

CJ: "So the letter served two purposes; from a defensive point of view in light of recent criticism of other recent discharges, 'covering your back'; and from a more positive view, it represented effective communication."

Leslie: "Yes, I felt the letter enabled me to establish effective communication with the home care services although not necessarily with the family."

CJ: "Did you think to send Mrs Robinson a similar letter?"

Leslie: "No, I hadn't thought of that. When I tried to discuss the issues with her she always had a counter argument; physiotherapy – 'I know someone'; speech therapy – 'There is someone in the village'; how heavy he was – 'I have looked after people like him before'. I felt very frustrated at the time and she was not listening to me. I also had a perverse feeling of hoping it would fail. I kept thinking during the days after his discharge, when is it going to fail?"

CJ: "Perhaps that's a natural reaction to not being listened to. You haven't been able to explore her feelings at all?"

Leslie: "No, she was a very abrupt lady. I tried but she shrugged me off."

CJ: "So what do you need to do now as it still seems unresolved?"

Leslie: "I could ring her up and suggest I visit to see how things are."

CJ: "And the consequences, knowing her?"

Leslie: "It would give her a strong message of my concern. I feel I did the best I could in the situation that felt 'distasteful'. I did manage a professional relationship even if I couldn't manage the more personal type of relationship I prefer to develop with families. From an accountability factor I did what was needed. I felt I had been therapeutic without realising it."

CJ: "What does therapeutic mean in this context?"

Leslie: "I think of therapeutic as resulting from developing a warm relationship."

CJ: "You do seem to need this warm feedback from your relationships."

Leslie: "Yes, it makes it easier. It's problematic otherwise."

CJ: "To give yourself within relationship you need to get something back?"

Box 7.4 Typology of the way relatives' construct relationships with caring staff (Robinson & Thorne 1984)

Stage of development	Relative's construction
Naïve trusting	The family (naively) believe that the caring staff view the situation from their perspective and have their best interests at heart.
Disenchantment	The family realise that the caring staff view the situation differently, leading to disenchantment, conflict and potential breakdown of relationship.
Guarded alliance	The family reconstruct the relationship in order to get some of their needs met. They learn to manipulate the system to achieve this.

Leslie: "Yes – I need them to be grateful, but then why should I expect that to be?"
CJ: "You need to put that into perspective."

When Leslie explored alternative ways of responding to Mrs Robinson he acknowledged his need to avoid confrontation with her, "I know I am no good at confrontation." Later in the session I asked Leslie how he now felt about Mrs Robinson. "Puzzled really. A bit sorry that we didn't get through to each other but even though we didn't, I did my best in a professional sense." I suggested that Leslie should reflect on the nature of his relationship with Mrs Robinson within Robinson & Thorne's typology (Box 7.4).

Leslie hoped that any relative's expectations, fears and needs would be identified and responded to appropriately. The Burford model cues are applicable to seeing and responding to the whole family as fundamental to holistic caring. If so, Mrs Robinson's naïve trust would have remained intact. This point highlights the fundamental need to establish and maintain a working dialogue with Mrs Robinson. As it was Leslie found Mrs Robinson abrasive and difficult and was motivated to avoid her, fearing her criticism. The failure to establish and maintain an effective working dialogue led to breakdown and conflict, simply because Leslie failed to tune into this woman's needs, notwithstanding how difficult she made this for him. It was as if Leslie had lost sight of her, and when he saw her again he saw a deeply disenchanted woman.

As a consequence Mrs Robinson was peripheral to the caring situation when she needed to be central to it. She needed to be both informed and involved but felt excluded. But neither did she approach the caring staff, allowing her discontent to fester up to the point of demanding her husband's discharge. Perhaps disenchantment was inevitable. Unfortunately it so often is, as the nurse's 'natural' focus on the patient may obscure seeing the relatives. However, Leslie and Mrs Robinson's relationship became stuck at this level because they were locked into a win–lose scenario that blocked the possibility of developing a working guarded alliance relationship. There were no winners. Leslie felt stressed and guilty, Mrs Robinson was distressed and angry. Her disillusionment can be understood. She was in deep crisis as her normal life had disintegrated.

Commentary

Such experiences of conflict are commonplace, a fact of everyday clinical practice. Perhaps not many spouses would have arranged their husband's discharge as a consequence. More likely they would suffer in silence or complain after discharge. Leslie's interpretation of the situation was misplaced, yet even on reflection he could not see her perspective because he had become so entangled in the conflict. If the conflict could have been surfaced and openly tackled, then Mrs Robinson's disenchantment may have been guided into a guarded alliance relationship, resulting in mutual benefit for all concerned, not least Basil, who seems a pawn in the conflict struggle.

On the level of intra-personal conflict, Mrs Robinson did not reciprocate Leslie's need for a 'warm' relationship. As a consequence, he instinctively withdrew from her, rationalising the relationship as *professional* rather than *personal*. Leslie is in conflict because he is not working in tune with his values. Unwittingly he projects his failure into Mrs Robinson. Instead of working with her, he is now working against her in some covert struggle. In other words his failure to resolve his intra-personal conflict has become an inter-personal conflict between himself and Mrs Robinson.

Thomas & Kilmann (1974) identified five styles of managing conflict: avoidance, accommodation, compromise, competition and collaboration. These styles can be arranged within two axis of being assertive, non-assertive, co-operative and non-co-operative (Box 7.5). Consider what styles Leslie has been using with Mrs Robinson and what style he would desire from a holistic perspective?

He admitted to avoiding conflict – that he is anxious about ensuing conflict. In fact Cavanagh (1991) indicated that avoidance was the most common style of managing conflict by nurses and nurse managers, followed by accommodation, compromise, collaboration and finally competition. Yet the avoidance is avoidance of competition. Leslie could not accommodate Mrs Robinson's wishes because of his own values. She wasn't listening any more: listening to what Leslie was asserting as best or listening to Basil. The other side of the coin is that Leslie was not listening to Mrs Robinson, hence her disenchantment.

From a holistic perspective, the only acceptable conflict management style is collaboration. Conflict cannot be avoided, because people will always see things differently. Yet conflict can be embraced positively within a spirit of collaboration of working together to find the best solutions. Senge (1990) says that conflict is the creative edge. The collaborative mind-set is to think in terms of 'we' – 'How can we resolve this issue'; and to continually re-focus the issue rather than the other person, especially if the situation gets personal and people are losing emotional control. The difficulty with collaboration is that it requires two to tango.

Box 7.5 The styles of managing conflict' grid' (Thomas and Kilmann 1974, as cited in Cavanagh 1991)

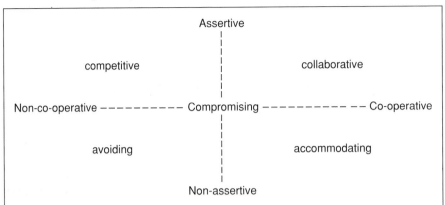

Assertiveness: the degree to which individuals satisfy their own concerns
Co-operation: the degree to which individuals attempt to satisfy the concerns of others

Accommodating
Essentially a co-operative interaction but one in which the practitioner is not assertive – prepared to give up their own needs for the sake of maintaining harmonious relationships and need to be accepted by others. 'Apologetic'.

Avoidance
Characterised by a negation of the issues and a rationalisation that attempts to challenge the behaviour of another is futile.

Collaboration
Involves an effort to solve problems to a mutually satisfying conclusion, a win–win situation; i.e. concerned with needs of self and others. Openly discuss issues surrounding conflict and attempt to find suitable means to resolve the conflict.

Competitive
Pursues his/her own needs at the exclusion of others – usually through open confrontation (win–lose situations).

Compromising
Realising that in conflict situations, every party cannot be satisfied. Accepting, at times, to set aside personal needs in preference to others to resolve conflict.

At the end of the session Leslie retorted that he was human too with human vulnerability and the right not to be abused by relatives. Of course, he has rights, yet his response reflects the way he lost himself within this relationship, highlighting the need for him to know and manage himself within the relationship if he desires to work from a holistic perspective. He was only abused because he failed to read the situation adequately and respond appropriately, locked as he was into his own perceptions of what was best. As a guide or clinical supervisor, my role is not to judge Leslie but guide him to judge himself and yet also to acknowledge that it is a tough world out there and we must not judge ourselves too harshly. The emphasis of clinical supervision is always to create a clearing where people can learn.

Leslie's conflict with Mrs Robinson is a level 2 type conflict. In exemplar 7.2, Cathy is a district nursing sister. Consider the pattern of conflict in the experience she shared with me in clinical supervision about a woman she was visiting and her relationships with the General Practitioners (GPs) she worked with.

REFLECTIVE EXEMPLAR 7.2 – CATHY AND THE GPS

Cathy: "I want to talk about Brenda. She is an 84-year-old woman I have been visiting each week since last summer. I knew her from before when her husband had been ill. She has had stomach cancer for which she has had massive surgery. She initially made a good recovery but then had a blockage that resulted in a stent being inserted. She was a deeply religious lady. Three weeks ago I was talking to her . . . she seemed a bit 'lost' . . . there was something about her . . . I couldn't put my finger on it, perhaps it was the up before the major down. We were chatting about things we normally talk about. I said something like, 'See you next week Brenda.' She put a hand on my shoulder and said just as I was leaving, 'Yes, if God's willing.' She gave me that look. She died later that week after being admitted to hospital. She wouldn't have wanted that."

CJ: "Were there other signs you could pick up on?"

Cathy: "She was more relaxed. She had talked about two of her friends who had died recently. She was quite a brave lady . . . she didn't like tablets and she had pain in her back. We had tried different pain killers that had hardly touched her. I did notice that the lines she had around her eyes had gone . . . her eyes looked bright, I thought."

CJ: "Intuitively you knew what she was saying to you? That she knew she was dying?"

Cathy: "Yes."

CJ: "Could you have responded differently at that moment?"

Cathy: "I didn't because I didn't know what to say . . . I had a cry in the car for her."

CJ: "She was saying goodbye. I suspect she didn't want any fuss about that. Did you go to her funeral?"

Cathy: "No . . . other things that needed to be done."

Cathy cried. I picked up on her tears and suggested that perhaps these were tears she might have shed at the funeral. I named the various emotions I sensed she was feeling: guilt at failing Brenda and her family; anger at the GP for admitting Brenda to hospital against her wishes; and sadness at Brenda's death. A cocktail of energy-sapping emotions.

Cathy agreed she was suffering because of this experience. In response I helped Cathy visualise a 'space' between us where she could place these feelings in order to view and understand them for what they were, to help her convert these negative feelings or energy into positive energy so as to feel more comfortable and to take necessary action as appropriate. I emphasised to Cathy that my role was not to 'fix it' for her but to challenge and support her to resolve as best she could her troubled mind.

"What if you had responded to her cue?"

Cathy was uncertain. "How do you respond to someone like that? Maybe I could have asked Brenda if she thought she was dying . . . and if so to hold her and say goodbye. It's such a difficult scenario to contemplate how I might have responded differently because I felt so emotional."

I asked, "Is closing important for you?"

Cathy felt it was very important. She continued by saying, "I didn't attend the funeral because of a management meeting I was expected to attend."

I challenged her, "Could you have prioritised differently? Could you have said to the GPs, 'Can you please re-schedule this meeting so I can attend the funeral?' or simply given your apologies for not attending the practice meeting? Would the GPs have appreciated your dilemma?"

Our supervision time had finished. The questions were left spinning in the air for Cathy to contemplate. She said she felt better about the situation. As I wrote the session notes I added two further questions:

- Brenda had wanted to die at home. If Cathy had picked up the cue, could she have planned to keep Brenda at home rather than be admitted to hospital or alternatively arranged hospice admission?
- Did you not pick up the cue because you wanted to avoid uncomfortable feelings?

When we met for our next session three weeks later, I drew Cathy's attention to the notes.

CJ: "Did you miss the opportunity to help Brenda manage her death appropriately?"

Cathy: "Brenda definitely didn't want to go into the hospice. Her husband had died there. We had discussed this. She said, 'The hospice is a lovely place but I don't want to go in there because it brings back such memories.' She wanted to die at home . . . she did have a strong family and friends network around her."

CJ: "What were the conditions of her admission to hospital?"

Cathy: "The GP was a bit vague. He admitted her on the grounds of a range of deteriorating symptoms . . . breathlessness. I was thinking of what you said about the 'gap' on the Burford model study day about accepting the inevitable as inevitable, and the way the GP had felt obliged to arrange her admission to hospital rather than accept she was dying."

The 'gap' exists when there is a mismatch of shared expectation between care staff in accepting the inevitability that the patient will die and that further treatment would be futile. The 'gap' represents the potential for conflict.

Accept death as inevitable → focus on caring

Nursing _____ |_____

Accept death as inevitable → focus on caring

Medicine _____ |_____

| Gap = potential for |
conflict breakdown

Cathy felt she had acknowledged the inevitability of Brenda's dying before the medical team. She intuitively felt this and felt her appropriate response was to help Brenda die in comfort. The GP also intuitively knew the inevitability of Brenda's dying yet within the unfolding moment he could not accept this 'failure'. In response to her symptoms he arranged for her to go to hospital where she was admitted for treatment, as futile as that was, rather than arranging management of Brenda's death at home. In the chaos of the unfolding moment the GP's response was a learnt reaction, yet it does suggest how the 'cure' mind-set works. Of course, the GP may have taken the easiest way out. However, the patient's best interests were disregarded and she died in circumstances she would not have chosen for herself.

> *CJ*: "Were there other ways of dealing with this situation?"
> *Cathy*: "Brenda was a strong character but she would have complied with what the GP said."
> *CJ*: "It might be useful to de-brief with the GPs? Perhaps you could have insisted on being called if things deteriorated and you (and your team) could have managed her at home? Are there issues of communication within the care team? I know in the emotional moment it was tough for you to respond to the cues she gave you but we can see how circumstances unfolded that were not in Brenda's best interests, not in your best interests and an expensive alternative for the NHS – the difference between being proactive and reactive?"
> *Cathy*: "We are commencing a new series of meetings on Monday to improve our communication! The idea is to have 'team care plans' where everybody knows what the other is doing."
> *CJ*: "So, should you have attended Brenda's funeral or the GPs' practice meeting?"
> *Cathy*: "For me, the funeral was my priority. In future I would be assertive about going to the funeral and say I would come to the meeting afterwards."
> *CJ*: "Closing seems such important work. Can you find some literature to support that? Knowing the 'evidence' may help you assert your priorities with the GPs – talking the language of the rational mind rather than the emotional mind. Consider how the GPs might respond if you were to inform them that you were going to the funeral and not to their meeting?"

I suggested to Cathy that we used ethical mapping to fathom what would have been ethically the right thing to do (Box 7.6). Framing the dilemma was easy – should Cathy have gone to the funeral or attend the GP meeting?

Box 7.6　Ethical grid considering Cathy's dilemma

Patient's/family's perspective: Attending the funeral would inform the family that Cathy cared for them and be available to support them with their grief	*Who has authority to make the decision?:* Does Cathy have legitimate authority to be self-determining?	*The GPs' perspective:* Attending their meeting was Cathy's greater priority
Is there conflict of values? How might conflict be resolved? Yes	***The dilemma:*** **Should Cathy go to the funeral or to the GP meeting?**	*Ethical principles? What would be the right or best decision?:* Beneficence/malevolence Autonomy Greatest good/justice Virtue
Cathy's perspective: Cathy felt attending the funeral was a greater priority – yet was uncertain if her perspective was reasonable	*How was the decision actually made? (power relationships)* Cathy accommodated the GPs' request and avoid confronting them	*The organisation's perspective?* Cathy felt to keep the GPs happy as they buy our services and make a lot of fuss when they don't get their way

Cathy felt attending Brenda's funeral was the greater need but was this just an emotional reaction? Is closing a significant part of a therapeutic relationship? As it was she felt she had failed Brenda and Brenda's family, which distressed her; feelings she had yet to resolve. She could see the GPs' perspective and that their response was both typical and arrogant. They assumed leadership of the team and expected compliance even though Cathy was not directly employed by them.

In terms of ethical principles we reviewed firstly the ethics of beneficence and malevolence. Beneficence is always acting in terms of doing good whilst non-malevolence is avoiding harm. Certainly Cathy felt harmed, but more importantly she felt the family would have benefited from her being at the funeral. In considering autonomy, Cathy felt that Brenda's autonomy had been compromised with the GP's decision to send Brenda to hospital. However in terms of Cathy's own autonomy we could frame the dilemma in terms of a power struggle between Cathy and the GPs to assert the right for professional autonomy and self-determination. In terms of utilitarianism or greatest good, we could see a tension of Cathy responding to the needs of the individual versus the meeting resulting in benefit for the wider community. In a world of finite resources the tension between the needs of the individual against the needs of the wider community was constant. However, we thought this was a weak argument to support the GPs' insistence that Cathy attend the meeting.

In terms of virtue we could see another tension between Cathy acting on her holistic values and responsibility to the family against the values of the GPs who gave greater value to the smooth running of their practice. As Friedson (1970) noted, the principal aim of the bureaucratic organisation is its own smooth running despite the rhetoric of patients first.

We then considered 'Is there conflict of values? How might conflict be resolved?' The answer was clear that there was a conflict. We could see that conflict manifested itself in terms of conflict of values, failed communication and power interests. Simply put, Cathy perceived the GPs had the power to insist on her attendance. Cathy's authority to act reflected the way she perceived power relationships between herself and the GPs. She perceived that she didn't have the authority to resist the expectation she attend the meeting and anticipated conflict with the GPs if she did resist. As a consequence she accommodated their request rather than risk the anticipated consequences. We then used the 'influences grid' to consider the factors that had influenced Cathy in making her decision to accommodate the GPs' demand. I have summarised these in Box 7.7.

Power

Cathy's decision to attend the GP meeting rather than Brenda's funeral represents a triumph of patriarchal power. One discourse of power relationships is to view nursing and caring as feminine struggling against a dominant patriarchal view of medicine and managerialism. Gilligan (1982) makes the distinction that men and women differ in ethical priorities; women lean towards an ethic of caring whereby primary responsibility is caring, whereas men lean towards an ethic of justice whereby primary responsibility is to ensure order.

Feminine (Brenda)		Masculine (the GPs)
Ethic of caring – giving priority to attending the funeral	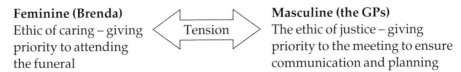 Tension	The ethic of justice – giving priority to the meeting to ensure communication and planning

The 'team' meeting is a ritual of power flexing and control where the dominant voice of the patriarchy (both male and female doctors) and power pattern of relationships with subordinates is reinforced, provided subordinates attend. Not attending the meeting to go to a funeral may seem an innocuous event in itself, yet from a power perspective the decision is a symbolic challenge to the status quo. Brenda is making choices which, if tolerated, undermine the patriarchal dominance. The power game is to diminish her perceived autonomy to act on her own judgement. Batey & Lewis (1982) describe this type of autonomy as discriminatory autonomy, i.e. the degree of autonomy the practitioner believes herself to have. Roles overlap and there is always a degree of competition to 'own' the overlapping ground, a competition that nurses are ill-equipped to win because of their internalised sense of subordination.

Box 7.7   Factors that seem to influence Cathy's decision

Influence	Significance
Expectations from self about how I should act?	Cathy felt her expectations of how she should act were fundamental to her dilemma.
Conforming to normal practice?	Cathy's normal practice would have been both to attend the GP meeting and to go to Brenda's funeral.
Expectations from others to act in certain ways?	Cathy certainly felt the GPs expected her to be compliant with their wishes and 'know her place' within the 'team'.
Need to be valued by others?	Cathy said she did not need to be valued by GPs but on reflection, she realised she did like positive feedback and did want to be valued by the GPs, and that this might have been a subtle influence she did not want to acknowledge.
Doing what was felt to be right?	Cathy felt that attending the funeral would have been the right thing to do, more so than attending the GP meeting, even though both were 'right'.
Misplaced concern? Loyalty to staff versus loyalty to patient/family?	Cathy felt 'forced' to be loyal to her GP colleagues rather than Brenda and her family although in her heart her primary loyalty was to her patients.
Emotional entanglement/ over-identification? Negative attitude towards the patient/family?	Cathy had a strong involvement with the patient and family. Indeed, she might have been accused of being too emotionally involved which blurred her perception of what was best. In exploring this influence Cathy revealed her unresolved distress about her father's death. As a consequence Cathy felt she became entangled in the suffering of dying patients although she did not experience this as conflict. On the contrary she felt this made her more sensitive to the needs of her patients and families whilst recognising she still had some grief work to do for herself.
Limited skills/discomfort to act in other ways? Lack of confidence?	Cathy admitted she was not very assertive and felt she would have been humiliated if she had challenged the GPs more strongly. She recognised herself as someone who avoided or accommodated conflict.
Time/priorities?	Cathy's NHS Trust had significantly reduced the number of district nursing sisters (G grade), forcing her into a team leader role to manage more junior staff that had reduced her direct care role contact. Hence managing priorities and role conflict had become an increasing dilemma for her.
Anxious about ensuing conflict? Fear of sanction?	Cathy's fear of sanction was the crux of her dilemma: what sanction might ensue if she defied the GPs' demands? She recognised that she had internalised a sense of subordination and fear that had made challenging the GPs a very uncomfortable prospect. She knew that they would likely report her to her managers.
Information/theory/ research to act in a certain sort of way?	Cathy was unable to make a good argument to support her decision to attend the funeral rather than the GP meeting.

Patriarchy

Watson (1990) noted that patriarchy presents a potent barrier to nursing's realisation of its holistic vision:

> 'Caring as a core value cannot be forthcoming until we uncover the broader, more fundamental, politic of the male-oriented worldview at work in our lives and the lives of people we serve.' (p. 62)

Reverby (1987) explored the way caring has been viewed as an extension of being a woman; indeed, as a woman's duty in contrast to her work. Reverby asserted that nurses' lack of power stems from this relationship between womanhood and caring and the subordinate relationship of nurses to doctors.

Lawler (1991) and James (1989) both noted how caring in nursing is largely invisible, often de-valued by nurses themselves, and seen as largely unskilled, being the natural extension of women's social roles. Lawler's research, entitled *Behind the screens* was concerned with body work, whilst James's work entitled *Emotional labour* was concerned with emotional work. Perhaps then it is not surprising that nurses have tended to delegate this work to unqualified staff, valuing instead more medical-type tasks.

Buckenham & McGrath (1983) highlighted the way nurses have been socialised into passive, subordinate and powerless perception of self *vis-à-vis* medicine; a perception that renders them incapable of fulfilling their self-perceived role of patient advocate. Buckenham & McGrath noted the way nurses rationalised compliance with medical domination because of the need to be valued. It is natural for dominant professions such as medicine to re-inforce subordinate behaviour in other health care professions, such as nursing (Oakley 1984). In other words doctors are always motivated to maintain the status quo and resist any rivalry for power.

Chapman (1983) suggested that doctors reinforced nurses' subordination through humiliation techniques which become a normal way of relating between them. The aim of the game is to keep nurses 'in their place'. Stein (1978) illuminated the nature of the doctor–nurse game whereby the nurse suggests to the doctor what to do in such a way that the doctor can claim credit for the idea. The point of the game is to ensure the doctor does not lose face. The game also reinforces the nurse's subordination. The game is also import-ant for the doctor to play because he or she realises the significance of the nurse's knowledge. The pay-off for the nurse is the doctor's patronage. Stein argues that failure to play the game is 'hell to pay'. Cathy knew that sanctions would be taken against her.

Perhaps the situation has changed since 1978, but then you, the reader, will know these things for yourself.

Power within bureaucratic systems such as the NHS has a typical authoritat-ive pattern to ensure a docile and competent workforce; docile to the extent that its subordinates do not disrupt its smooth running. This power is reflected in the prevailing use of positional, reward and coercive types of power in contrast with facilitative types of power that characterise leadership of the

Box 7.8   Leadership and sources of power (adapted from French & Raven 1968)

Authoritative sources of power	Facilitative sources of power
• Positional (legitimate): Based on the subordinate's perception that the leader has a right and authority to exercise influence because of the leader's role and position in the organisation.	• Relational (referent): Based on the subordinate's identification with the leader. The leader exercises influence because of perceived attractiveness, personal characteristics, reputation, or what is called 'charisma'.
• Coercive (sanction): Based on fear and the subordinate's perception that the leader has the ability to punish or bring about undesirable outcomes.	• Expert: Based on the subordinate's perception of the leader as someone who has special knowledge in a given area.
• Reward: Based on the subordinate's perception that the leader has the ability and resources to obtain rewards for those who comply with directives.	

collaborative team (see Box 7.8). To act differently and resist the GPs Cathy must shed her fear of sanction and become assertive within an organisational culture that is likely to perceive her assertiveness as a threat and hence respond in a hostile way to ensure that Cathy knows her place.

Becoming assertive

Cathy, like many practitioners, was unable to be assertive with the GPs with whom she worked. Guided reflection had helped her to see herself within this situation. Cathy knew that to realise desirable work, in this case attending Brenda's funeral, she needed to assert her perspective in ways that would be accepted. When I asked her what she needed to do now about this situation, she balked at the idea of confronting the GPs but did say she would assert going to the funeral given the situation again. She has explored the likely consequences and shed her fear of sanction. Of course, whether she would respond differently is uncertain but is vital to be positive.

In helping Cathy to look at her assertive self I asked her to place herself within the assertiveness stereotype map (Box 7.9) comprising four stereotypes (Dickson 1982). Instinctively Cathy knew she was a 'Dulcie' – she laughed that the GPs walked all over her. When I asked who she would like to be, her answer was 'Selma'. She knew she could never be like 'Agnes', it just wasn't her personality. She could see the risk of becoming an 'Ivy': back-biting and manipulative responses to her frustration. However, she knew people like this, even at the surgery where she worked and sensed how destructive these people were. Being an 'Ivy' is the antithesis of collaborative ways of working.

Box 7.9　The assertiveness stereotype map (Dickson 1982)

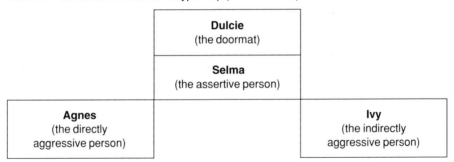

Box 7.10　Asserting rights scale (Dickson 1982)

	Right	Score 1–10
1	I have the right to state my own needs and set my own priorities as a person independent of any roles that I may assume in my life.	
2	I have the right to be treated with respect as an intelligent, capable and equal human being.	
3	I have the right to express my feelings.	
4	I have the right to express my opinions.	
5	I have the right to say 'yes' or 'no' for myself.	
6	I have the right to make mistakes.	
7	I have the right to change my mind.	
8	I have the right to say I don't understand.	
9	I have the right to ask for what I want.	
10	I have the right to decline responsibility for other people.	
11	I have the right to deal with others without being dependent on them for approval.	

So how can Cathy move from being 'Dulcie' to being 'Selma'? The most important factor is to help Cathy to see that she has the right to be treated with respect in her role and express her point of view. These two points are included within Dickson's (1982) eleven 'rights of women', which offers a reflective tool for Cathy to see herself (Box 7.10).

I ask practitioners to score themselves out of 10 for each point. They can then re-score at later times to give themselves feedback that they have become more assertive and to reinforce their rights as women not to be oppressed. Cathy did not score herself, although she felt she wouldn't do very well if she did. The scale made her feel inadequate. It was painful for her to see herself like this because she felt, by and large, that she was a competent practitioner who got on well enough with the GPs. She didn't want to make a mountain out of a molehill and rock the boat, that she would soon get over it and move on. The 'rights' scale had rocked her confidence. It was too challenging so we had to back-pedal to a safer place.

The assertive action ladder

It was more constructive for Cathy to reflect on being assertive through using the assertive action ladder (see Box 7.11). I constructed the ladder by analysing the pattern of coaching practitioners in clinical supervision to take assertive action. The ladder consists of ten steps, each step a rung to realising effective assertive action.

Applying the model to Cathy's experience

(1) Having felt the need to assert self (the motivational self):
    Cathy felt a strong responsibility to Brenda to attend the funeral and guilt when she did not attend. She knew this was an unsatisfactory state

Box 7.11   The Assertive action ladder

10	Being able to tread the 'fine line' of pushing an issue and yielding	(the controlled self)
9	Keeping self and other in 'adult' mode	(the managed self)
8	Being adept at counter-coercive tactics against more powerful others	(the empowered self)
7	Being adept at interaction skills	(the skill to assert self)
6	'Taking the plunge'	(the resolve to assert self)
5	Creating the optimum conditions to maximise effectiveness	(the scheming self)
4	Being able to make a good argument	(the knowledge to assert self)
3	Understanding the boundaries of autonomy and authority in role	(the right to assert self)
2	Having a focused vision for practice	(the ethic to assert self)
1	Having felt the need to assert self	(the motivational self)

of affairs that reflected a pattern of working with the GPs that could no longer be tolerated.

(2) Having a focused vision for practice (the ethic to assert self):
Cathy held a strong vision of holistic practice whereby attending the funeral was significant in terms of her relationship to Brenda and responsibility to support the family.

(3) Understanding the boundaries of autonomy and authority in role (the right to assert self):
Cathy was helped to see that she had the authority to decide to attend the funeral. She was not employed by the GPs, although she did perceive the GPs had authority over her and was helped to re-define the nature of this relationship. Their attitude was confronted as inappropriate although fear remained that if she upset them then she would 'pay for it'.

(4) Being able to make a good argument (the knowledge to assert self):
This is the crux issue. How can Cathy convince the GPs that attending the funeral was more important work than their meeting in language they would accept? Two key theoretical points need to be emphasised; first, the significance of closure within the therapeutic relationship; and second, the support for the family. Is there research to support these points?

(5) Creating the optimum conditions to maximise effectiveness (the scheming self):
To see GPs as a group or as individuals? At a meeting or in the course of the day? Mornings or afternoons? How best to tackle the GPs given the situation again: a more proactive approach might be to take the initiative and think upstream and inform the GPs that she will be attending the funeral.

(6) 'Taking the plunge' (the resolve to assert self):
Cathy has now thought the issue through and come up with her plan of action, but can she carry it through? The coaching role was to reinforce her sense of responsibility for taking action, infuse her with courage and deflate any sense of fear.

(7) Being adept at interaction skills (the skill to assert self):
Cathy is now in the midst of asserting herself and needs to be skilled in communicating her message, for example being adept at using Heron's Six-category intervention analysis (see Box 5.2).

(8) Being adept at counter-coercive tactics against more powerful others (the empowered self):
Possible tactics might include:

- Cathy needs to be in 'collaborative' mode for managing conflict – trying to keep the situation on the issues rather than conflict becoming a battle of wills. Hence, think 'we' – 'we' have a problem.

- To confront the GPs with their caring values. It is often the organisation's Achilles heel to be revealed as uncaring, what I term as 'taking the moral high ground'.
- To give the GPs' behaviour back to them if they assert power over Cathy – 'asserting your power does not help solve the problem'.
- To reduce their power by visualising them as bully boys trying to get their own way.

(9) Keeping self and other in 'adult' mode (the managed self):
To stay in adult mode Cathy must be aware of and manage her own anxiety, especially the urge to flee into child mode in order to cope with the parental onslaught of Cathy being viewed as difficult and irresponsible. The key is to keep the issue in focus rather than let it degenerate into competitive mode and into a win-lose battle that she is ill-equipped to win. It is vital Cathy is not afraid of any threat of sanction or loss of reward.

(10) Being able to tread the 'fine line' of pushing an issue and yielding (the controlled self):
At the end of the day, Cathy may need to give way because the GPs are more powerful than her and refuse to accept her perspective. She could still exercise her authority and go against the GPs' wishes, although that might undermine the collaborative team. But you might argue, what collaborative team? because it doesn't actually exist. Yielding is retreating with dignity, with one's integrity intact. She hasn't so much lost but retreated. The mindful practitioner will sense this line and realise that to overstep the line may risk being marginalised as difficult or actually being punished in some way.

Yielding

Yielding to the situation is a strength not a weakness. To compete needlessly is to exhaust yourself and feel defeated. As Blackwolf & Gina Jones (1996) note:

> 'Learn to yield. Yielding is not being passive. It is being sensitive to energy flows and extending wisdom. Allow the winds of change to flow through you rather than against you. Be flexible with what is happening today. Yield to the circumstance, yet be rooted with who you are.' (p. 281)

It is perhaps rather obvious to conclude that conflict is stressful. In the following two exemplars Helen is a clinical nurse specialist (CNS) for nutrition. Consider her experiences with two patients she shared over two consecutive clinical supervision sessions about ward staff whom she felt acted inappropriately toward the patients she was supporting. We have met Helen before in Exemplar 4.3 when she reflected on the impact of using the Burford model on her relationships with patients.

REFLECTIVE EXEMPLAR 7.3 – HELEN'S STORY

Helen: "Am I just a technician! This lady I saw last week, she's about 80, a lovely, lovely lady. She was admitted to one of the elderly care wards in early December. She had ruptured her oesophagus – this carries an 80% risk of mortality. Later she had a femoral embolus that required a right above knee amputation. She was referred to me for Total Parental Nutrition (TPN). The aim was for the oesophagus to heal spontaneously – it can happen. But not with this lady! She had a massive leak into her mediastinum. The doctors with hindsight had some regrets about the amputation; she was not fit for a thoracotomy. They inserted a gastrostomy tube for feeding. I went to visit her on the ward for 'technical things' – checking up that she had a good care plan, etc. I was really going there to be supportive. It should have been a two-minute visit but it wasn't. I went in there and asked myself the cue, 'How must she be feeling?' I pulled up a chair and asked her. She talked about vomiting."

CJ: " The ward staff had been dealing with this?"

Helen: "Yes, but not appropriately. She was encouraged by our chat and then I asked her how she was feeling. She just cried and cried. She then apologised for crying, saying that it would have been better not to have survived at all. She talked of her feelings of loss – eating, independence, her leg, her total feelings of being dependent. I let her talk about these things. I just had to 'be there' for her and out it all came. She became calm again, began to talk about possible futures – talking about her leg rather than her stump. It felt really good to spend time with her in this way, almost nothing to do with her 'tube'. That was just a by-line."

CJ: "Well, it was your reason for visiting her – to maintain her tube . . . however you put the tube into a holistic perspective: you saw her rather than the tube."

Helen: "Yes, I can see what you mean . . . I felt overwhelmed, humbled to get a sense of what she has lost. She doesn't have a lot of family. My next challenge is to go to the nurses and talk about how we are going to deal with it."

CJ: "In terms of her rehabilitation?"

Helen: "Up to now she has been too sick. She's also isolated in a side room because of MRSA. People spend as little time as possible with her because of that."

CJ: "The leper colony mentality."

Helen: "She would have been on the MRSA isolation ward if they had had a bed."

CJ: "The paradox – someone who needs a lot of time gets very little."

Helen: "Yes . . . have you heard the 'pizza' jokes about that? – sliding them under the door so the staff don't have to go in there."

CJ: "Do you confront such attitude?"

Helen: "No . . . but I am going back there today to follow it up. I want to talk to Vera, the ward sister about it."

CJ: "Did you feel angry towards the nurses?"

Helen: "Initially I did but I can see how it happens. If I challenged them they would say something like, 'It's alright for you swanning about all day, we're getting the job done'."

CJ: "You were angry for a short time and them you rationalised it?"

Helen: "It's not their fault. They were generally ignorant of the issues. My anger would have been a waste of time, it would have achieved very little. It happens everywhere. I want to use my anger positively rather than chew myself up."

CJ: "Can you do that?"

Helen: "Yes, by confronting people."

CJ: "You just said you couldn't confront the nurses? Do you mean at the time you couldn't confront them but now perhaps you can?"

Helen: "Yes, I realise I am avoiding it to some extent."

CJ: "Yes, it's tough to confront people under these emotional conditions. You would probably get sucked into a competitive mode of managing the conflict. So you've been carrying this anger around with you?"

Helen: "I think I have. I said to Melanie, my colleague, 'Sometimes I really love my job. I'm doing a good job, it's exciting and then something happens likes this that makes me feel totally de-motivated, upset, angry and like a very small cog in a very large wheel that doesn't give a monkey about me at all. I seem to have been going round this circle for years and now I need to break out of it'."

We explored Helen's options for taking action. Using the conflict management grid (Box 7.6), Helen could see the way she was avoiding confronting the staff nurses and the way she had rationalised her non-action. In contrast she felt she usually accommodated doctors. However, she was resolved to act with integrity to fulfil her responsibility to ensure the patient was better cared for despite her fear of upsetting the nurses.

Commentary

As noted in Exemplar 4.3, Helen had implemented the Burford NDU: Caring in Practice model into her clinical practice, shifting her 'technician' approach to the patient into a whole person focus. Through dialogue Helen gives herself feedback that reinforces her holistic values and how these values are in conflict with others. She cannot easily put aside her own values or tolerate un-caring by others.

As her guide I confront her avoidance and the way she rationalised not taking appropriate action: 'My anger would have been a waste of time.' Yet does Helen fail the patient? Where does her primary responsibility lie? Perhaps confronting them when her own anger is high will only lead to an ugly and unproductive confrontation of mutual destruction within the competitive battlefield. She acknowledges the collaborative way forward: 'My next challenge is to go to the nurses and talk about how we are going to deal with it.' But can she break through the avoidance norm that constrains her? We pick up the story in her next clinical supervision session:

Helen: "Picking up our last session, I feel better about the limits of my responsibility by making the nurses on the ward aware. I tried to focus on my role responsibility and the relationship between seeing the tube and seeing the whole person, seeing the tube as part of the whole person, but I did feel I was getting into a mess. I can link this with my subsequent experience with Thomas. I'll read from my diary. 'Thomas has pancreatitis. He's very sick. He was having TPN through a Hickman line. I knew him from ten years ago when he had cardiac problems. He latched on to me as "his nurse", off-loading anxieties onto me. My visit to the ward was apparently "routine" to monitor the technology.'"

CJ: "What do you mean 'apparently routine'? Has this changed?"

Helen: "It's changed already. It now includes, 'Who is this person?' – listening to the person – what is he asking or not asking me? And it includes knowing, 'How is this person feeling?' and, 'How does he view the future?' His pain was not being adequately dealt with. He was also frustrated at sitting and waiting for something to happen – that's the nature of his treatment. He's on a diamorphine pump for the pain – the technological response. Yet he was uncomfortable and unable to rest well enough. He was angry at the nurses for their handling skills. He felt they yanked him about. He was also frustrated at the nurses' comments and platitudes towards him. I tried to help him consider less technological approaches to his pain management but he reacted against these. He had been socialised into technological responses and so he couldn't see beyond them. He was venting his frustration at me. I didn't feel rejected. I went to see the ward staff. They were irritated at my interruption as they were trying to finish handover, trying to hurry up. I had a sense of them being upset about something else. I acknowledged this feeling. They acknowledged that the ward was heavy at the moment, and their own distress: lots of young people with cancer and in particular, a young girl who had been sexually abused by her father."

CJ: "In other words, the ward staff were not available to you to talk about Thomas?"

Helen: "I sympathised with them but asserted I was trying to make it easier for them to nurse Thomas, who they already viewed as a difficult patient."

CJ: "Are you always sensitive to ward nurses' concerns?"

Helen: "No, not always [laughs] . . . I am trying to be though . . . they were obviously concerned about something."

CJ: "Were they surprised at your concern for them?"

Helen: "Yes they were and pleased that they had the opportunity to off-load a bit. I responded by helping them talk through their feelings concerning the sexually abused girl being discharged into an abusive environment. They were distressed and felt helpless about this and other ways to help the girl."

CJ: "This is an example of having to deal with 'what's on top' before we can deal with our own agendas; otherwise the ward staff may have simply rejected you and Thomas. To them, at that moment his needs were not as significant as the girl's and your concerns not as great as their own."

Helen: "Most resistance to my ideas about Thomas came from the most newly qualified nurse. She used his 'anxious' disposition to account for his pain! She said things like, 'He's always asleep when you go in so I don't see how he can be in pain', all the kind of things that Thomas told me that irritated him so much."

CJ: "What happened?"

Helen: "I discussed other ways of dealing with his pain, although I didn't go far enough such as suggesting pain charts. Afterwards I thought I should have done that. I was feeling irritated with them. I responded by telling them that they could prevent unnecessary complaint but perhaps that was not the best way to do this."

CJ: "I suppose you even quoted McCaffery (1983) to them? About pain being what the patient says it is?"

Helen: "Funnily enough I did! The staff nurse knew this quote but I don't think she believed it."

CJ: "It exposes contradiction between theories we hold and how we practice. That was the confession bit for you – 'feeling irritated' . . . is this uncomfortable for you?"

Helen: "Not uncomfortable but knowing the best way to deal with it is difficult."

CJ: "I think your intervention was valid. You were responding to help them see the consequences of not listening to you and Thomas."

Helen: " I wrote his kardex as a narrative and told the staff I had done that."

I guided Helen to explore the possibility of involving Thomas's named nurse in writing the notes with her, highlighting how such collaboration has a number of distinct benefits that improve relationships and potentially improve patient care by:

- making visible and legitimising Helen's nutrition role within the caring and treatment process
- fostering a collaborative relationship with the named nurse and other ward nurses, leading to mutual decision-making, a positive approach to conflict, and mutual support
- improving communication and continuity of care
- fulfilling Helen's CNS teaching and supportive role and role-modelling a holistic approach
- confronting negative attitudes and getting the patient's voice heard
- positive action converts her 'irritation' into positive energy

Picking up the last point, I challenged Helen to consider why she felt so irritated with the situation. She was uncertain, so I suggested she was irritated for two reasons: the ward staff were not accepting her 'expert' advice, and second, she had absorbed some of Thomas's frustration at the nurses as if an outraged mother whose child had been hurt by these careless people.

Helen felt the first cause of her frustration was true but she hadn't perceived the second reason. However, she could see this possibility. She could see the parallel with the way the ward staff had absorbed the abused girl's suffering and suffered themselves. Helen had managed her irritation, containing it so it did not affect her appropriate response to the ward staff. By listening to their concerns she was able to support the staff with their own problems and in doing so, create the space for her to assert her concerns. She trod the proverbial 'thin line' of pushing an issue yet being prepared to yield – the hallmark of the assertive practitioner. From a clinical supervision perspective, Helen demonstrated how she had applied insights from one experience into a new situation. She role-modelled being available and collaborative ways of managing conflict.

The harmonious team

The ability of practitioners to collaborate in resolving conflict may be jeopardised by what I have termed *the harmonious team*. The harmonious team is concerned with maintaining a facade of togetherness or teamwork. It does not talk openly about difficult feelings or issues between its members and seeks to protect itself from outside threat. Conflict is brushed under the carpet. As a consequence, conflict is inadequately resolved and continues to simmer under the harmonious surface (Johns 1992). The harmonious team is vividly evident within Hank's complaint. Karen is an associate nurse who reflected on an incident involving Hank's complaint, with me in clinical supervision.

REFLECTIVE EXEMPLAR 7.4 – HANK'S COMPLAINT

Karen: "One night last week Hank complained to me about the actions of one of the night staff. He was very angry about it, so I wrote about his complaint in the notes, really to cover my own back because if something had happened because of that . . . if he had got worked up and had a heart attack. I didn't state who was involved or the nature of the incident. Christine [a night associate nurse] picked up what I had written in the notes and said that she felt 'very sad I had to write that, that some things were better said, not written.' She didn't deny the incident but criticised my documenting it."

CJ: "The way you handled it?"

Karen: "Right. I re-read my notes of the incident because I had written them in a hurry. I realised I had used a word that could have been replaced by a better one."

CJ: "An antagonistic word?"

Karen: "Yes. I made a comment further on in the notes and replaced my initial note to make it clearer to people reading it."

CJ: "Less volatile?"

Karen: "Yes, but what got me was Christine's criticism of my way of documenting it when *The Nursing Times* goes on about 'whistle blowing' and how complaints should be documented. I felt she was trying to cover for the person involved although she acknowledged that the event had happened."

CJ: "And now?"

Karen: "I pointed it out to Leslie as he was the primary nurse. He commented, 'I'll have a word with the person involved.' I went home and worried about it all night, worried how she would take it, what she would say. So I need feedback."

CJ: "What would you do differently given the same situation again?"

Karen: "Only thing I could have done was to ring her and ask her to explain from her point of view."

CJ: "Think of the response you might have got from this."

Karen: "From my perspective, if it was me . . . I would have appreciated it."

CJ: "And knowing the person involved?"

Karen: "I can't say . . . she could nearly be my grandmother."

CJ: "How do you normally get on with her?"

Karen: "I see her in the evenings and nights when she works . . . but I don't have much to do with her . . . superficial."

CJ: "Do you think this action against Hank was out of character for her?"

Karen: "I think it was an exaggeration of her normal character."

CJ: "You think?"

Karen: "I don't work with her. It's difficult to know how she is with other patients. The event itself was quite trivial, it's Hank's anger that got to me."

CJ: "Do you think Hank's anger was reasonable?"

Karen: "I felt at the time that if it had been me then I would have been upset and angry. She was inflicting her values on him, not respecting him."

Karen and I explored her options. We agreed she should talk this through with the care assistant. This was not possible face to face but she could ring her at home. I asked Karen if she still wanted Leslie to deal with it. She suggested that he didn't want to. Karen felt she hadn't wanted him to do it in the first place, it was because he had offered. We also rehearsed Karen's response to the associate nurse, acknowledging that what Karen did was morally correct although perhaps a little insensitive in the way she reported the event. The key factor was to keep the situation grounded in the therapeutic situation rather than it becoming a secondary situation of interpersonal conflict (as it indeed, had already become). I urged Karen to live the supervision maxim – tough on the issues, soft on the person, and take action because of her integrity even though she was fearful of this prospect.

In our next session, three weeks later:

Karen: "I went home and phoned her!"

CJ: "How did you feel when you picked up the receiver?"

Karen: "Terrified! She was angry but she didn't get as angry as she possibly could have done."

CJ: "Have you learnt that it pays to belong to the harmonious team? If so, if a similar situation occurs you will think twice before confronting it?"

Karen: "Yes."

CJ: "What can you do about it?"

Karen: "I don't know. I'm really dejected."

CJ: "Can you share this experience with your colleagues, to secure their support and to assert the therapeutic team to off-set this malignancy?"

Karen: "I felt like a chicken at the prospect of Leslie acting on my behalf. I'm now truly humbled. I didn't stop to think. I'm feeling very stupid. Why did Hank wait to see me?! He was probably just thinking about it when he saw me."

CJ: "How do you think Mandy [the care assistant] might be feeling now?"

Karen: "I hope she thinks I had the courage to ring her."

CJ: "Be positive about this. Your phone call to Mandy was a cathartic intervention – you enabled her to vent her anger at you, yet she was also confronted with the fact that she did not act appropriately towards Hank. Her angry reaction was to being exposed. You can rationalise her anger in this way. It's imperative that you do not see yourself in the wrong."

Commentary

As the dialogue reflects, the issue of Hank's complaint at being treated badly by a nursing assistant had degenerated into a secondary issue of Karen breaking the norms of the harmonious team. It was Karen who was in the wrong rather than Mandy. The issue had twisted from being a patient-related issue to an interpersonal one where loyalty to the 'team' took precedence over loyalty to the patient.

Karen's distress was the outcome of vilification – a reflection of the power of the harmonious team to regulate its members. Karen was motivated to limit the damage by accepting her villain role. As she noted, she was learning to play by the rules. Leslie forgot to give Mandy feedback about the incident, reflecting his own avoidance of conflict and his failure to exercise his primary responsibility to the patient.

The rules of the harmonious team are not made explicit yet it seems as if it is socialised into the very fabric of practice. As such it is not easily shifted despite espoused claims to value the therapeutic team. In other words its existence is a contradiction within holistic practice.

Perhaps Karen didn't handle Hank's complaint in the best way. Yet writing a report in the notes is a correct way of reporting patient distress. Perhaps discussing the situation at shift report would have been better but by then the night staff had departed. Reporting the incident to the primary nurse is again good practice and it is not unreasonable to have expected Leslie to deal with it – but he is a coward and conveniently forgets about it – or put another way, he brushes it under the carpet. Perhaps Karen might have reported it to the senior nurse. If I had been Karen's line manager I would have intervened and confronted both Christine and Mandy with this incident, but perhaps at a de-briefing session rather than a formal confrontation. By making it public the conflict would have been brought into the open and hopefully led to more collaborative ways of managing conflict and tackling unacceptable clinical practice.

As it was, Karen did not report the situation, again keeping the complaint contained within the team. Altering the notes was unprofessional, and perhaps should have been picked up by other staff, but it wasn't because it was righting a 'wrong' rather than being seen as 'wrong' in itself. It was Karen making good her crime.

But I was not the line manager at this time. I was an external supervisor. The dialogue reveals the way I urged Karen to take action – pushing her against a gradient that threatened her. To her great credit she acted responsibly but was wounded in the process. My role was to help her lick her wounds and gather strength to tackle such issues more positively in the future. You can imagine what might happen on another occasion. Yet despite Karen's distress, she said that she enjoyed going through the situation in supervision. She hadn't wanted to come to the second supervision session because she thought it was going to be too hard. She had a slight residual fear about retribution from the night staff but at least the care assistant had gone on holiday for a month!

Horizontal violence

Hank's complaint reveals the way staff can be violent to each other when threatened. Perhaps it is nature's way, triggering the fight or flight response. The norm would have been for Karen to get Hank's complaint under wraps and stew in her juices, doing violence to herself rather than violence to others, or at least how others perceived her actions as being violent.

The idea of *horizontal* stems from bureaucratic–hierarchical systems, whereby the subordinate person (the nurse) is unable to project her anger or frustration at her more powerful oppressors. She can only fire at those on her own level. Yet, even on her own level, this violence is muted within the harmonious team perhaps because people are motivated to be partially invisible, to keep their heads down to avoid criticism (Street 1992). Hence *harmony* is a collusive strategy to paper over the team's potential violence. Perhaps because nurses are expected to care, to hold hostile feelings towards others is unacceptable. Yet if people do bottle up feelings and stew in their own juices then from time to time people will erupt and blow their top, as explained within the water butt theory of stress. Yet being partially visible to each other (as Karen says she does not know the night staff) people are isolated and unavailable for mutual support.

Stress and coping with work

The exemplar stories suggest that work can be very stressful for many reasons embodied in self or embedded within the social norms of practice. Drawing particularly on the work of Munley (1986) and Vachon (1988), I have

Box 7.12   Stress factors in palliative care

Stressors evoked by patients or family members	Stressors occurring in practitioners' own inner experience	Stressors emerging from or affecting the hospice work environment
Sadness evoked by awareness of patient's or families' spiritual or emotional distress.	Burdened by the responsibility for the quality of life experienced by patients.	A subtle pressure to create ideal hospice deaths or be an 'ideal' nurse.
The cumulative impact of dealing with many patients declining/dying at the same time.	Being saturated by grief.	Over-investment of self leading to burn-out conditions.
To continually form attachments that were certain to be broken by death.	Patients who die 'too fast' before staff could be of much help.	Sense of not having the time to meet the 'ideal.'
Trying to stay supportive to patients/families who were manipulative and by the subtle drain of being a scapegoat for frustrations and anxieties of patients and family members.	Psychic exhaustion during lingering death watches.	Staff interactions due largely to the high expectation staff have of each other in a work context that values sensitivity.
Feelings of failure when suffering not eased or a good death not achieved.	A feeling of loss or being cheated was especially salient when a favourite patient died or some unfinished business.	Inter-disciplinary tensions and role ambiguity. Administrative work.
Some deaths hard to watch especially emaciation, mutilation or external tumours.	Sense of not being effective.	The 'niceness' culture and the harmonious team.
Patient's family who were not 'coping well' or 'not facing reality'.	Identification with patients as well as an awareness of own mortality.	Perceived lack of support or conflict of values between managers and nurses. Emotional labour not being visible or not being valued.

summarised the noted causes of stress for palliative care nurses (Box 7.12) that offers a reflection on stress and its causes. It emerges that the major causes of stress were more related to organisational tension rather than therapeutic work with patients and families.

One potential stress factor is the burden of expectation to work toward creating an environment where being available is possible. Clearly, such expectation can be tough for the individual practitioner. Commitment to caring values can carry a heavy price. Being committed to her values, the practitioner cannot easily turn her head aside when her values are compromised. Neck and shoulder muscles ache from the burden. I have felt so many practitioners' shoulders where the muscles are taut, knotted and ache. Stress accumulates without realising it, giving headaches and sapping energy to balance the body. Perhaps it is easier to sacrifice the caring values in order to survive. Yet this will only worsen the situation, leading to a downward spiral towards burn-out because caring sustains the caring quest.

Perhaps the task is too much for individual practitioners like Karen. Perhaps it needs leaders who understand the need to create practice environments that nourish practitioners. Yet human systems can be shifted by individuals with determined political action simply by role-modelling caring behaviour – in the way the practitioner works with patients, in the way she talks and writes about her patients, in the way she responds to her colleagues; by keeping her integrity intact others will notice and respond. It will ripple like the soft breeze of a butterfly's wings in flight – vulnerable, yet beautiful, and yet tough to withstand the storm, not torn apart by conflict but embracing conflict towards unifying her colleagues towards a better world.

Water butt theory of stress

If people are vulnerable to express their feelings or deal positively with conflict, then stress is likely to accumulate within the individual person. Like a tinder-dry forest it needs only a careless remark or incident to ignite.

The person might blow their top or blow inside. In the water butt theory of stress imagine I have 100 points of energy. If I am 30 points stressed then I need another 30 points to balance that stress, leaving me only 40 points of energy available for therapeutic work. If I have 40 points of stress then I can barely cope. My remaining energy will evaporate and it will feel as if I am drowning. I can then only blow my top. Yet blowing my top creates a mess that others will be uncomfortable with. No one likes overt displays of anger or despair; people are motivated to clear the mess up and pretend it didn't happen – again the harmonious team, sweeping up and brushing the mess under the carpet and pretending that everything is okay on the surface of things.

Having blown my top, my stress levels drop to a manageable level and slowly drip, drip, drip, it begins to fill up again, because the cause of the dripping has not been addressed. Sometimes a violent storm fills my water butt quickly and like lightning itself I snap and blow my top and rage at events or people (Parker 1990; Pike 1991; Wilkinson 1988). Pike (1991) notes:

> 'Moral outrage ensues when the nurse's attempts to operationalise a choice is thwarted by constraints. The outrage intensifies when these constraints not only block action, but also force a course of action that violates the nurse's moral tenets.' (p. 351)

I guess we all feel this outrage from time to time, but the water butt does have a drainage tap. The mindful practitioner can monitor her stress levels, draining stress off and converting the stress (or negative energy) into positive energy necessary to take appropriate action to resolve the sources of stress. In doing so, like the gardener drawing off water from the water butt to water the flowers and nourish their growth, so the practitioner can be watered to grow through experience. However the tap might be blocked, requiring help to unblock it – the value of guided reflection. The water butt is a powerful metaphor for learning through experience.

Box 7.13   Feeling light–feeling drained scale

Week commencing: 20th May 2002.
Day: Wednesday

Please score on the scale the extent you feel either light or drained at the end of the work day.

| *I go home feeling* ⟵————————————⟶ *I go home feeling totally drained* | |
| *light*   1 2 3 4 5 6 7 8 9 10 | |

What stress factors contribute to your sense of feeling drained?	*Arrived in the morning to a horrible phone call from a patient's relative who held me personally responsible for his wife's wait in A&E when I had already advised him that there were no beds in the hospital.*
What satisfaction factors contribute to your sense of feeling light?	*Did teaching session. I always enjoy teaching. Also put together a bid for further training in the hospital. Didn't think I would be able to do it this quickly.*
What can you do to go home feeling more light and less drained?	*I confronted the relative and listened to his worries. He apologised to me for being rude. Problem resolved.*

Feeling light–feeling drained scale

To help practitioners reflect on their stress I conceived the feeling light–feeling drained scale (Box 7.13). Being drained is having no energy left at the end of the workday. I am sure every reader has experienced that feeling of near exhaustion after a 'heavy day.' At the end of the workday, the practitioner scores the extent they feel either light or drained. The questions ask them to explore factors that might have contributed to feeling either light or drained and what they can do to improve the light score. Like all reflective models, the scale is designed to focus the practitioner on resolving contradiction, i.e., knowing and managing their own stress in order to be more lightened and less drained.

Practitioners become sensitive to both stress and positive events. Stressful events become less stressful because the practitioner learns to become better equipped so situations are no longer perceived as stressful. Light situations are also acknowledged, and in doing so enhancing their value. It is all too easy to get locked into negative perceptions rather than positive perceptions.

In Box 7.13 I give an example of one practitioner's score. This practitioner's normal score was around 7, suggesting a relatively high residual level of stress. On a very good day this might drop to 5. In the example, her score is 10. This is due entirely to an altercation with a patient's relative despite its successful resolution. Such was the stressful nature of the situation it submerged her feeling light factors. In clinical supervision, she was able to explore the situation in more depth, her response to it and ways of resolving it, so if she faced a similar situation it wouldn't take so much of her energy away.

Burnout – the failure to sustain caring

Failure to realise desirable work or manage anxiety in constructive ways may result in burnout. Cherniss (1980) describes burnout as a process in which 'the professional's attitudes and behaviours change in negative ways in response to job strain' (p. 5). Maslach (1976) suggested that the major negative change in those experiencing burnout in people-centred work was 'the loss of concern for the client and a tendency to treat clients in a detached, mechanical fashion' (p. 6).

McNeeley (1983) observed that when practitioners felt they had lost the intrinsic satisfaction of caring, they became focused on the conditions of work, for example, off-duty rosters and workload issues, characteristic of bureaucratic models of organisation. McNeeley believes that bureaucratic conditions are antithetical to human service work and strongly advocated that such organisations needed to move to collegial ways of working with staff in order to offset the risks of burnout.

Taylor (1992) noted a theme within the literature of how nurses have been dispossessed 'of their essential humanness as human beings and as people, by emphasising their professional roles and responsibilities' (p. 1042). Taylor draws attention to the fact that nurses are human too and, as such, are vulnerable to the same issues that face their patients and families. The lack of recognition of humanness in nursing through a focus on roles and responsibilities has led practitioners to strive to be something they were clearly struggling to cope with. Taylor noted that practitioners didn't recognise or understand their own ordinariness as human beings. Consequently, they become alienated from themselves in their efforts to cope with and live with the contradictions in their lives. Jourard (1971) noted that such striving damages 'the self' and reinforces the need to cope in a vicious downward spiral of self-destruction towards burnout and a state of anomie.

Ironically, being patient-centred may perpetuate a denial of self and re-inforce contradiction and ultimate self-destruction. As Jade, one of the primary nurses at Burford Hospital said, she didn't come to work dressed in protective armour. Dewey (1933) observed:

> 'Unconscious fears also drive us into purely defensive attitudes that operate like coats of armour – not only to shut out new conceptions but even to prevent us from making new observations.' (p. 30)

Dewey believed that anxiety limited the practitioner's ability to learn through experience. The professional is closed to protect self rather than open to possibility. 'Armour' is akin to professional detachment.

Benner & Wrubel (1989) believe that the answer to stress and burnout is not the development of an adequate personal detachment as advocated by Menzies-Lyth (1988), but the reconnection of the self with caring. Burnout is the descent into a black hole when the caring self has been scrapped away on the uncaring sharp edges of systems despite rhetoric to the contrary. The contradictions are no longer tenable. The bonds that contain snap. It is as if nurses are dispensable. There is little sensitivity to the profound nature of journeying with another person to help ease that person's suffering.

Yet burnout can also be viewed as a healing space, whereby the nurse can descend into herself and discover her self. It may be dark, lonely and painful but it can still be a healing space. Such healing is a journey to discover self, rather than recover, because recovery suggests returning to what she was before – a self hurt, only for the hurting to start all over again.

Nicklin (1987) observed that 85% of managers considered stress to be only a moderate problem which they had no specific policy to deal with. The Briggs Report (DHSS 1972) identified that services supporting nurses are rare, inadequate, fragmented and not targeted to those most in need. There is no evidence to suggest this situation has improved since 1972. In fact, the situation may have deteriorated due to the persistent stripping of nursing resources since the development of the business culture prompted by NHS Trusts. To say the least, it is profoundly ironic that a caring service should care so little about those who care. The emergence of clinical supervision is an acknowledgement of the need for formal structures and the failure of informal support systems. The cynics amongst you might consider that support is not the real agenda of supervision but a means of surveillance however it is wrapped up. Whatever the case, clinical supervision is no substitute for the therapeutic team.

Support

Caring is a reciprocal relationship. Facing loss or grief alone is liable to exacerbate vulnerability and suffering yet the word 'professional' creates an expectation of being able to cope and isolates one from one's colleagues. Therefore, if nurses and other health care practitioners care, or are expected to care, then they need to work in caring environments whereby they are both challenged and supported to care. Practitioners need to be able to share their suffering otherwise they will suffer loss of emotional and spiritual integrity. Distress or sadness are natural triggers for reflection and open up the possibility to talk about such feelings and healing. If the practitioner is suffering it is most likely that other colleagues also suffer – so rather than a collusive silence, we need ways to penetrate the silence to support each other. Remen (1996) puts it like this:

> 'Whatever we have denied may stop us and dam the creative flow of our lives . . . avoiding pain, we may linger in the vicinity of our wounds . . . without reclaiming that which we have denied, we cannot know our wholeness or have our healing.'
> (p. 70)

So consider the following questions:

- are adequate support systems in place?
- are people stressed or, worse, burnt-out?
- if so, why do you think that is?
- do you see seeking help as a strength rather than weakness?

- do you explore your anxiety as a learning opportunity?
- are you truly available to support your colleagues?

In Helen's story, Helen deals with her frustration in two ways; first by talking to Melanie, her colleague, illuminating the importance of having support available within everyday practice; and second, by being available to the ward staff to listen to their grief. In supporting the ward staff Helen did not avoid her own conflict. She gave the problem back to the ward staff yet in a way that was not perceived as overtly confrontational. Ask yourself, are you skilled at being supportive to your colleagues? Can you manage your own frustration and suffering to respond to the needs of your colleagues? Without doubt, if nurses are to care for others then they must care for self and each other. Anything less is a contradiction of caring that compromises the realisation of caring. As the stories vividly illuminate, guided reflection is one significant way to connect with caring.

De-briefing

At a recent clinical audit meeting at the hospice, it was felt that staff needed to be mindful of de-briefing as a group at the end of each shift, in recognition of the emotional impact of caring for some patients and issues of misunderstanding. Staff had occasionally de-briefed following particular incidents, but de-briefing as a daily ritual acknowledges that work can be stressful and that staff have a responsibility to be mutually supportive. De-briefing has a number of obvious benefits:

- It acknowledges that sometimes, for whatever reasons, practice can be tough, where practitioners can safely reveal their feelings; where it is okay to be distressed, angry; cutting across a culture where practitioners have hidden their feelings in the (misguided) belief that 'good nurses cope' or not to burden their colleagues.
- It allows practitioners to be heard above the din, to be recognised and valued as persons with human needs and human frailties.
- By constructing the therapeutic team, bringing staff together to create a new culture of mutual support in their caring quest; bringing vision into clear view.
- To understand the nature of conflict.
- By confronting inappropriate attitudes, behaviours, assumptions and defence mechanisms that disrupt therapeutic ways of working with patients and colleagues.
- For leaders to role-model the disclosure of feelings and to encourage and facilitate reflection with colleagues.
- For promoting the morale, self-esteem and motivation of colleagues, with organisational consequences of retaining staff, enhancing quality of care and reducing staff sickness.
- To realise the learning organisation.

Postscript

So, do you work in an environment that makes it possible to be available to work with patients to realise desirable practice? Do you truly work in collaborative and supportive ways? These are the key issues.

I have not explored more physical environmental aspects such as the colour of walls, the use of plants, noise and smell, opportunities for privacy, in fact everything about the physical environment. Neither have I dwelt on resource issues such as staffing numbers, staffing mix, shift patterns, equipment – all those things that make it more possible to be available to patients. Perhaps many of these issues have emerged in the stories so far and will be picked up in the next chapters that look at more organisational aspects of reflective practice.

Chapter 8

Reflective Communication

Introduction

Communication weaves together practice to ensure that care is continuous, consistent and congruous within and across practice settings. Using reflective techniques the reflective practitioner communicates to ensure:

- continuity of care over time despite changes in personnel
- consistency of care between different care workers
- congruence of care between care workers in tune with shared vision and best practice
- collaboration between care workers to ensure the above points

Communication is both verbal, through language, and non-verbal, through body posture, senses and intonation. Communication is both formal and informal. Formal verbal communication takes place via writing notes and reports, through shift reports, ward rounds and various care meetings that may include patients and families. Informal verbal communication takes place in the way practitioners relate to each other and with their patients and families through the day; corridor conversations, passing remarks, the sluice room conference, coffee chat, etc. I am sure the reader can coin up many euphemisms for such informal verbal meetings, all accompanied by a vast range of non-verbal communication that convey positive, negative and power messages.

Talk

The way practitioners talk with patients, families and with each other is a caring act. What we say is a reflection of our values. Therefore if I espouse to be caring, compassionate and work in collaborative ways with my colleagues, you might expect my speech not just to reflect those values but in fact be caring, compassionate and collaborative. Anything less would be a contradiction that the mindful practitioner would acknowledge and work towards resolving. Talk is both a process – an act in itself, and an outcome – it aims to achieve something. Hopefully it is both of these, but talk can also be uncaring; tongues can be sharp, and venomous. It is also having a deep connection with nature and harmony within the cosmos. Only when practitioners can communicate consistently at this level is communication effective.

Dialogue

From a reflective or mindful perspective all speech acts are viewed as dialogue. The essence of dialogue is collaborating with others, either patients or colleagues, in order to move the community toward the realisation of a shared vision, yet always holding the vision and ways of realising it open to scrutiny. However, as Isaacs (1993) notes:

> 'Unfortunately, most forms of organizational conversation, particularly around tough, complex, or challenging issues, lapse into debate (the root of which means 'to beat down'). In debate one side wins and another loses; both parties maintain their certainties, and both suppress deeper inquiry.' (pp. 24, 25)

There is nothing collaborative in the patterns of talk that Isaacs alludes to. Such talk reflects patterns of power relationships and rivalry, where people jostle for control typified by people lining up to get their point across and win the argument. Very little genuine listening takes place. People partially listen to what they want to hear, seeking feedback to reinforce their position rather than be open to new possibility through dialogue.

$$\boxed{\text{Fundamental to dialogue is to listen}}$$

To listen; it sounds so easy. We probably all claim to listen, but do we listen carefully? Or do we listen to what we want to hear, or distort what we hear in order to fit into our own scheme, to confirm our own assumptions? To listen it is necessary to know and suspend one's own prejudices, concerns and assumptions. It is the empathic listening and connecting with the patient as discussed in Chapter 4. Yet communicating with colleagues seems to be an altogether more difficult form of dialogue than with patients, because issues of power and different agendas infest the communication space. Unresolved conflict simmers beneath the polished tables.

Isaacs' (1993) notion of dialogue as the 'free flowing of meaning' suggests a liberation of energy previously trapped within people's defence of assumptions and the struggle to emerge triumphant in debate. People can only move forward when there is common understanding and subsequent shift of the forces that sustain the assumptions that sustain a particular state of affairs. Too often people review problems with the same mind-set that created the problem in the first place. Of course the problem does not get resolved. Within dialogue there need not be consensus, just the commitment to move towards it. Within the dialogical process there is a shift from problem solving towards acknowledging and resolving paradox that requires thinking about the way people think about things. Mezirow (1981) calls this critical consciousness – the ability to be conscious of our consciousness; alert to one's mental models and how these influence the way one is thinking and feeling within the unfolding moment. In other words being mindful. Only then can people transform their perspectives to see things differently.

Reflective hand-over

Traditionally, nursing has been communicated through an oral culture typified by the hand-over or shift report. The function of the hand-over is literally to communicate relevant information to ensure the smooth transition of care from one shift to another and hand over responsibility of care to the next shift of nurses. The practitioner may use the patient's notes to communicate care although these, in my experience, rarely adequately reflect the patient's care or treatment patterns simply because of the shifting nature of treatment and care, the prevalent oral culture and because models for writing are generally inadequate. Given the general inadequacy of written notes, the verbal hand-over might be considered the most significant form of communication to ensure continuity of care.

Using my own practice as an example, the new shift nurses gather in a room for the 'report' by nurses from the current shift. Conscious of confidentiality, the door is most often closed to prevent others over-hearing what is disclosed. The nurses report on the patients, with the patient notes in front of them to refer to if necessary, although rarely. The emphasis is on the nurse reporting – the new shift nurses write notes of what is said on scraps of paper. Some exchange of views takes place but this is usually in the form of opinions rather than dialogue around decision-making or care dilemmas. Nurses rarely express their personal feelings, especially if these feelings are problematic in some way. The report usually lasts for one hour, which for 6–10 patients is longer than most units engage in this activity.

I have often discussed this format with the nurses involved, suggesting we might move to a more reflective format with a greater emphasis on dialogue, creating the opportunity for people to reflect on the way we think, feel and are responding to care issues around the patients and their families. Most practitioners agree this would be helpful but practice does not change, as if we are locked into a habit. Why do nurses write notes on scraps of paper when the patients' notes are available? In response I am told that 'it's handy' to have a list in the pocket rather than keep referring to the notes.

Writing such notes is a distraction from dialogue; indeed it is a means of avoiding dialogue. I have challenged the senior nurses to role-model dialogue by revealing their own thoughts and feelings and to challenge others to respond. A dialogical approach shifts the culture of the report from essentially information-giving to reflection. This does not mean information will not be given, but the emphasis has changed. The notes can be read either before or after the report, and considered in light of the hand-over dialogue.

Bedside hand-over

Sitting around in a room discussing patient care can be challenged from a holistic perspective of involving the person and their family in their care (Ward 1988). Yet do patients want to be involved in decision-making and taking responsibility for their health? A considerable literature emerged in the 1990s

Box 8.1   Involving patients in decision-making and walkround hand-over – literature sources

Ashworth P. D., Longmate M. A. & Morrison P. (1992) Patient participation: its meaning and significance in the context of caring. *Journal of Advanced Nursing* **17**: 1430–9.

Biley F. C. (1992) Some determinants that affect patient participation in decision-making about nursing care. *Journal of Advanced Nursing* **17**: 414–21.

Jewell S. E. (1994) Patient participation: what does it mean? *Journal of Advanced Nursing* **19**: 433–8.

Matthews A. (1986) Patient centred handovers. *Nursing Times* **82**(24): 47–8.

McMahon R. (1990) What are we saying? *Nursing Times* **86**(30): 38–40.

Refearn S. (1996) Individualised patient care: its meaning and practice in a general setting. *Nursing Research* **1**(1): 22–33.

Rowe M. A. & Perry M. (1984) Don't sit down nurse, it's time for report. *Nursing Times* **85**(26): 42–3.

Trnobranski P. H. (1994) Nurse-patient negotiation: assumption or reality? *Journal of Advanced Nursing* **19**: 733–7.

Ward K. (1988) Not just the patient in bed three. *Nursing Times* **84**(78): 39–40.

Waterworth K. & Luker K. A. (1990) Reluctant collaborators: do patients want to be involved in decisions concerning care? *Journal of Advanced Nursing* **15**: 971–6.

Watkins S. (1993) Bedside manners. *Nursing Times* **89**(29): 42–3.

that explores the idea of patent participation in decision making (Box 8.1). Yet like many innovations in practice, the topic has seemingly faded from public interest. Perhaps, like the hospice in which I work, they tried it and it didn't work. The idea was resisted, and ultimately rejected, because nurses did not feel comfortable with this shift in the pattern of communication and the constant threat to patient confidentiality by disclosing information in public areas.

Working with and negotiating decision-making is fundamentally an 'attitude'; whether patients are able to or want to be involved is another issue. For many reasons patients may resist taking responsibility for their own lives. The mindful practitioner will appreciate these dynamics and judge whether to accept the other's dependency or confront it. However, if practitioners do value patient involvement in decision-making, then it is incumbent on them to create space where this can happen. What better opportunity than the shift report rather than sit in a closed room?

The approach to implementing bedside hand-over at Burford hospital in 1990 was written as a protocol (Box 8.2). The 'walkround' involved visiting each patient before moving into 'the office' to complete the report. We anticipated that this approach would enable:

- the nurse to say hello and greet the patient (and family)
- the nurses to invite patients to reflect on their care and care decisions
- the patient to give their perspective first
- care values and processes to become more transparent
- the nurse to make better sense of information having seen and spoken with the patient beforehand

The protocol emphasises the primacy of written notes as the means for continuing care, written as narratives rather than in nursing process format.

Box 8.2   Protocol for bedside hand-over

Stage	Action
1	The nurse who orientates the person/family to the unit draws attention to the style of communication practised by practitioners with patients (as stated in the Unit booklet), emphasising the patient's right not to be involved in hand-over and for confidentiality/consent to participate.
2	Times for hand-over are noted.
3	Hand-over commences with nurses involved visiting the patient at the bedside. This approach is referred to as 'the walkround.' The intent is to invite patients/families to reflect on their care.
4	The patient's right to confidentiality during the 'walkround,' as advised by the NMC is respected. As such, nurses act to enable the patient's control over the disclosure of information. The nurse leading the 'walkround' may sensitively cue the patient to prompt disclosure as appropriate. (Standard of care on confidentiality)
5	Following the 'walkround,' the nurses continue the report in the staff room to fill in gaps of information and understanding.
6	The primary means of communicating care is the patient's notes written as caring narratives. (Standard on ensuring continuity, consistency, and congruence of care)
7	Following the report, the nurse continuing care assures herself of patient care by continuing the patient's narrative (pattern appreciation): updating the narrative as necessary.
8	The patient's notes are clearly marked and stored by the patient's bed within the storage basket.

Stage 8 of the protocol refers to the storage of the patient's notes. We decided to store these with each patient simply because we viewed these as belonging to the patient. The idea of patient-held records is well known in community settings, again reflecting the philosophy of working with the patient in terms of their health. This practice really challenged practitioners to become very mindful of what they write knowing that what they write might be read by the patient or the patient's family.

Confidentiality

The crux of appreciating confidentiality was to determine the meaning of 'public space' as set out in the UKCC code of professional conduct on confidentiality

(UKCC 1987). Shared ward areas are public spaces and hence the nurse could not say things about the patient or family without the patient's permission if others might overhear (Johns 1989b). As such, any patients unwilling or unable to engage in the report, were not talked about at the bedside. The nurse would cue the patient to self-disclose, for example, 'How are things this morning?', encouraging participation. In this way it was the patient who would disclose information about themselves. At least in principle.

One morning I observed the night associate nurse and primary nurse communicate at the bedside of one lady in the three-bed ward. They stood at the foot of the bed as the night nurse informed the primary nurse. The primary nurse was a little deaf – and so the night associate nurse spoke loudly – loud enough for me to hear at the end of the ward and loud enough for the other two patients to hear what was being said. The woman in the bed was also deaf. She was sitting up trying to listen to what was being spoken. However she was not involved in the discussion. Clearly the protocol had failed and confidentiality had been broken.

We had a teaching session whereby each nurse was talked about in public as per the observed incident. The staff's reaction was a revelation: they felt very uncomfortable. As a consequence we wrote a standard of care: 'Patients do not have confidential information disclosed about them accidentally' (Box 8.3). We invited students to shadow the walkround hand-over and feedback their

Box 8.3　Standard statement: Patients do not have confidential information disclosed accidentally

---

1.0　*Structure criteria*

1.1　Patients' rights for confidentiality set out in hospital information booklet
1.2　Orientation for new staff to include teaching session on confidentiality and communication
1.3　Notes stored in holders at foot of each bed

2.0　*Process criteria*

2.1　The primary nurse discusses with each patient/relative the way nurses hand-over care and rights of confidentiality on admission
2.2　All staff act in such a manner to maintain each patient's right of confidentiality:
   - Nurses hand-over according to walkround protocol (see Box 8.2)
   - To avoid careless talk inside and outside the hospital
   - Mindful of inquiry and to whom information about the patient's care and treatment is disclosed
   - Leaving notes open

3.0　*Outcome criteria (see scan sheet)*

3.1　Patient controls disclosure at bedside
3.2　Patients feel involved in the hand-over
3.3　No accidental breach of confidentiality occurs at any time

Box 8.4 Confidentiality scan sheet

Standard statement: Patients do not have confidential information disclosed accidentally Scan sheet				
Date............................ Hand-over observed by...				
1	Patients are involved in the hand-over of their care	Yes	So-so	No
2.	Patients control the disclosure of information concerning themselves	Yes	So-so	No
3	The nurses do not talk about the patient outside the patient's listening	Yes	So-so	No
4	No accidental breach of confidentiality takes place	Yes	So-so	No
5	Patient's notes are not left open in a public space	Yes		No
6	Ask each patient: *"Do you think your nurses have always treated what they know about your health/illness in a confidential manner?"* [Sinha and Scherera 1987]	Yes	So-so	No
Score 3 for Yes, 2 for So-so, 1 for No				

observation using the scan sheet (Box 8.4) to ensure we both involved patients in the hand-over as appropriate and did not breach confidentiality. As you might expect, such scrutiny of practice helped staff to become more mindful of patient involvement and confidentiality. It was also an excellent learning experience for students. The nature of standards of care is explored in Chapter 9.

Patient notes

In the first edition of the book I gave this section the heading 'the nursing process'. I like to think that the nursing world has moved on just a little to think beyond the nursing process to more creative and reflective ways of thinking about and writing patient notes. For most practitioners since the late 1970s, the nursing process has dominated the approach to thinking and writing about patient care. Essentially the nursing process is a linear problem solving approach that structures thinking through four stages:

Goal setting an interpretation of assessment in terms of identifying specific actual or potential problems/patient needs and goals to be achieved in responding to the problem/need

Planning establishing the best response to solve the problem/need

Intervention   carrying out the planned care
Evaluation   determining whether the set goal has been met, including re-defining the problem or goal as necessary in light of events

The care plan is designed as a table consisting of these four columns. In theory, a practitioner should be able to pick up the care plan and continue the patient's care as a seamless activity. However, most aspects of care cannot be prescribed in advance, at least not without reducing the patient to an object to be manipulated. Some aspects of care may be more amenable to prescription, for example technical solutions to medical problems such as wound dressings and responses to pain and nausea. Yet these responses are better framed within a protocol based on evidence of best practice as guidelines to inform the mindful practitioner. Aspects of care concerned with the human–human encounter are almost impossible to prescribe given the uniqueness of each individual and each caring encounter.

The nursing process has attracted much adverse criticism (Howse & Bailey 1992; Latimer 1995; McElroy *et al.* 1995; White 1993). Although the nursing process was intended to promote a culture of individualised and negotiated care (De la Cuesta 1983), ironically the opposite tended to happen when it was accommodated with the prevailing nursing culture in the UK characterised by allegiance to the reductionist medical model. Rather than change practice, the nursing process was accommodated to fit within this existing culture, resulting in a minimal or lip-service response to the ideology of individualised care (Latimer 1995). It is easy to see why, because the splitting up of the patient into problems mirrored the medical model. The nurse was now able to diagnose problems. The patient became a set of problems or needs (problems being viewed as too mechanistic) based on complex systems advocated within an accompanying array of nursing models. These models were almost exclusively from the USA. These models were theory-driven and, as in the nature of any model, sought to find a comprehensive representation or conceptualisation of nursing.

The nursing diagnosis movement (NANDA) has been a natural development from the nursing process within the USA yet, in my view, is a process fraught with difficulty because it imposes abstract meanings on 'nursing' concepts in the futile effort to ensure consistency of diagnosis. In this respect this movement mirrors medicine's approach to diagnosis. Practitioners might find common understanding of what a grade 4 glioma is, but can practitioners find common meaning in using the word suffering, spirituality or agitation? Of course not. It is a positivist illusion to think otherwise.

So pause for a moment and ask yourself: what does individualised care mean to you? Do patient's notes reflect the wholeness of care?

These are profound questions. Yet is it necessary to put the adjective 'individual' in front of care? How could care be anything other than individual? The opposite might be termed institutionalised care. Ray (1989) coined the expression 'bureaucratic caring' as a reflection of the way the individual might become obscured within the layers of bureaucracy. The human within the machine becomes a contradiction. As Wilber (1998) puts it, systems are the language of 'it' and 'it' is a stark colourless landscape of labels. The individual's cry can be difficult to hear amidst the din. To compensate we need to say 'individualised' to remind ourselves that we care for unique human beings and that we carers too are unique human beings. We can only find meaning in the unfolding moment and respond with our humanness . . . humanness at risk of being buried beneath an avalanche of concepts and prescriptions. The nurse becomes a technician.

As practitioners begin to respond within a holistic perspective, they realise the nursing process is a contradiction, making little allowance for holistic and intuitive processes that are acknowledged as significant in the way experts make decisions about complex caring situation (Cioffi 1997). The Dreyfus & Dreyfus (1986) model of skill acquisition indicates that the expert practitioner intuitively makes clinical judgement based on grasping the whole situation. The model sets out five characteristics of intuitive judgement:

- *Pattern recognition*: A perceptual ability to recognise relationships without pre-specifying the components of the situation.
- *Similarity recognition*: An amazing human ability to recognise 'fuzzy' resemblance despite marked differences.
- *Common sense*: A deep grasp of the language culture so that flexible understanding in diverse situations is possible.
- *Skilled 'know how'*: The practitioner can respond without resorting to rule-governed behaviours.
- *Deliberate rationality*: The expert practitioner has a web of different perspectives that causes them to view a situation in terms of past situations.

The inadequacy of the nursing process in guiding patient care means that practitioners do not use it, at least in any meaningful way. Clearly communication systems need to be based on the way the expert practitioner thinks. Anything less will be absurd. Does a skilled carpenter choose a blunt spoon to chisel wood? Of course he doesn't – he chooses a sharpened chisel of the right width.

In an observational study of the impact of primary nursing on the culture of a community hospital (Johns 1989a), one practitioner commented, 'Much of it is just nursing, you don't have to write that down.' This comment reflects the pattern recognition and common sense knowing that this practitioner and her colleagues possessed, and their struggle to write down what was so obvious to them. Another practitioner commented, 'Patients we know well don't need care planning' – a comment that again reflects all elements of intuitive knowing.

I asked one staff nurse on her return from holiday if she had read her patients' care plans. She commented, 'I haven't had time because it's so busy.' The response reinforces the comments above, symbolising the way the nurses on the unit did not use care plans as part of their daily planning. However, I sensed that this intuitive knowing was not based on appreciating the patient's life pattern, but from knowing the patient in terms of the nurse's perspective.

In other words, patients did not need care planning because we know them as a group of similar patients. This was reflected in the notes that had a strong focus on medical and physical care issues with very little focus on emotional, psychological and spiritual aspects of care.

As one of the primary nurses said, 'When I deliberately change something on the care plan, I come back from my days off and it hasn't been carried out. Is it because they disagree with what's been said or are they too busy to read the care plans?' Other nurses countered this comment by saying they resented less-experienced nurses telling them what to do, or that they disagreed with what was written and therefore disregarded it, that is, if they had read it in the first place.

Completing patients' notes is often thought of as a task to be done at the end of the shift. Practitioners recognise this task as generally meaningless and yet feel anxious about writing something, possibly motivated by an internal censor that if nothing is written, then care has not been carried out. The fear becomes reinforced when audit systems are constructed around the completion of patient notes. Hence, what is written tends to be descriptive rather than evaluative, and meaningless in terms of communicating the essential nature of continuing care. If the nursing process is meaningless then, as Batehup & Evans (1992) have challenged, 'Why do we keep this sacred cow?'

The nursing process is an inadequate form of communication for the reflective practitioner because it does not represent how she views and responds to situations. It constrains thinking simply because practitioners no longer think that way. Most practitioners know this, yet have been unable to move beyond this deeply embodied worldview because the nursing process comes to dominate the way nurses conceptualise their practice. Even when practitioners acknowledge the absurdity of the nursing process they seem powerless to move to more meaningful and practical ways of communicating care.

So what alternatives are there, given that a holistic approach eschews any reductionist and deterministic approach to nursing practice, yet values the idea of best practice?

Narrative

The reflective practitioner constantly pays attention to what is unfolding, hence being reflective is a constant process of assessment or appreciating the shifting patterns of people's experience. In noting the shifting pattern, she compares what is unfolding with what has gone before. Has the analgesia made a difference? Is Mrs Jones more restful? Is the wound healing? Is Alison better able to breast feed? Has the new bed for Mr Smith been delivered to his home? Assessment and evaluation are two sides of the same coin – what is unfolding now and what has happened before.

In writing, the reflective practitioner is mindful of being meaningful and pragmatic. At Burford hospital, given the inadequacy of the nursing process, practitioners embraced the idea of narrative as a more adequate form of communication (see accounts by practitioners in *The Burford NDU Model: Caring in Practice*, edited by Johns 1994).

Narrative intends to capture the unfolding experience of working with or journeying alongside the patient through their health–illness experience, illuminating the way care issues emerge and are responded to using the Burford cue questions. Narrative should always be concise, reflective, evaluative and capture the drama of the unfolding story.

Contemplating the cue *'How do I feel about this person?'*

I have often been asked how the practitioner can write about her responses to this cue. First, the practitioner needs to remember that it is only a cue to tune the practitioner into her own thoughts, feelings and concerns that may interfere with being available to the patient and family. If the feeling is negative, then the practitioner is challenged to confront and work through the concerns. If the negative feeling is triggered by something about the person's family's behaviour or attitudes, then the best way of dealing with this is to acknowledge the difficulty using a cathartic response, 'I sense you're anxious?', 'You seem angry?', 'I sense this is not going well?'. This is also cathartic for the practitioner as she responds to her own anxiety in understanding the significance of the event and cautions her against absorbing the patient's anxiety as her own.

The practitioner might write something like: 'Sheila is very anxious. I acknowledged her anxiety and enabled her to surface and talk through her fears . . . (list). The practitioner's emotional reaction might be: *Sheila's anxiety manifests itself as demanding and abusive*. The practitioner may initially have felt abused and defensive as these darts of anxiety were fired at her, but she does not write it. In other words the practitioner writes about what she has done with her concern rather than about the concern itself. She acknowledges the patient's feelings as valid and converts her own anxiety into positive action, acknowledging that Sheila may be overwhelmed and bewildered by events and possibly angry at the way things have unfolded, especially when she faces a life threatening illness, and has experienced a lack of caring prior to transfer from another hospital.

REFLECTIVE EXEMPLAR 8.1 – REG SIMPSON'S NARRATIVE

In Reg Simpson's narrative note the presence of each of the Burford reflective cues and the way the cues help to weave the narrative form. If you are used to filling in boxes, for example as per the Roper *et al.* model, then your natural inclination might be to respond to each reflective cue as a question to answer. That's fine as long as you are mindful of seeing the whole person. With time, as with all models of reflection, you internalise the cues and construct your own internal model that emerges as your narrative style.

Date	Narrative	sig
6/11	Reg was admitted this morning for one week's respite care. He has been attending Day Care for the past 4 months (see attached notes). He is 93. He has cancer of prostate gland with bony spread. He lives alone although his daughters live close by and provide support for him on an ongoing basis. However, as Reg says, he is not managing so well. He feels very tired and uncoordinated. Pain well controlled – on MST 20 mg bd. (see pain chart). This morning he got himself into a real mess getting dressed. He feels he will need more support. His daughter needs a break from caring, hence this admission.	

Reg wears a hearing aid and requires people to speak loudly to hear. He is very philosophical about this admission and indeed about his eventual death. He was tearful when talking about his wife who died 27 years ago. I asked him if he anticipated being reunited with her? He laughed and said 'no'! He has no strong faith – he thinks he will simply return to the earth from whence he came. He still enjoys the *Guardian* newspaper, doing crosswords and watching TV. He has been a very keen angler but fears he may now lose this – so dependent on help to continue fishing. He enjoys company, chatting – was appreciative of my chat with him, especially talking about philosophical issues. Worked in a bank for all his working life.

Reg presents with a number of issues; difficulty with sleep, has a catheter which he dislikes, poor appetite, fatigue, fragile skin – small break, loss of mobility and dependence, anxiety about future support. No pain. He is on a wide range of medication for his heart (see list) – he has some lower oedema for which he wears tubigrip. He also takes an antidepressant.

How can we help this man?

Symptom management – stable but observe.

Difficulty and anxiety with sleep. He commenced sleeping tablets six weeks ago. These have been helping. He was waking up at 04.00 and becoming distressed as he lay awake for the remaining five hours before he got up. He goes to bed around 22.00 – 22.30.
Action – monitor sleep on visual analogue scale (Box 8.5).

Poor appetite and loss of taste. He enjoys soups. He says he has lost a lot of weight over the past months. However, he takes this in his stride.

Date	Narrative	sig
	Increasing loss of mobility. He has stopped using his electric scooter at home – because he was getting his feet mixed up! He walks with a zimmer frame – in fact walked with one nurse to eat lunch at the table. Lacks confidence. **Action – refer to physiotherapist.**	
	Fragile skin – he has a small break on left hand after an accident with his grandson. No other breaks. Will need pressure relieving equipment (see Waterlow score/lifting-handling assessment) **Action – monitor pressure areas. Wound is 2 cm × 1 cm. Stage 2 (see wound care protocol)**	
	Catheter in situ – he doesn't like it but it is working okay. **(protocol care)**	
	Reg says he is prone to constipation – bowels last opened two days ago. No discomfort, that's not unusual for him. He usually takes lactulose when it becomes a problem. **Action – monitor using bowel chart (Box 8.6)**	
	Support for the future **Action – to discuss with daughters the current situation/to support his daughters**	
	Assistance with personal hygiene **Action – negotiate best way with him on a daily basis (see standard of care)**	
	Consider self-medication, to ensure he maintains his competence with drug taking. He enjoyed his soup for lunch and managed some pudding!	
	Arrange delivery of *Guardian* newspaper.	
7/11	New wound noted on outer side of right leg (size 1 cm × 4 cm. Stage 2). He knocked his leg on the side of the bed (see wound care plan). Seen by physiotherapist – he can walk with one person safely – need to encourage mobility but remember he is also fatigued! He really enjoyed 'jacuzzi' bath this morning.	
	Sleep: Reg woke as usual at 04.00 and lay restless until breakfast. Medication is currently temazepam 10 mg. Sleep assessment (using VAS) did not reveal any particular factors that disturbed his sleep. **Action: can we review our approach as it distresses him?**	

Date	Narrative	sig
	This afternoon he was dozing in his chair as he does at home. He asked me the time. I said 4 pm – he groaned, 'Oh no – when is dinner time?'. He is clearly bored, he structures his day through meal events (even though his appetite is poor). I asked him how the crossword went yesterday – he said he hadn't been in the mood. I found him the *Telegraph* for today. (We need to order the *Guardian* for him!). Hazel will help him later with it as he enjoys company.	
	Seen by Dr Webb – he is booked for thyroid function test on Monday. Also to review use of sertraline (antidepressant). Does he need this? (depression assessment) **Action: Offer Reg day care to engage him?**	

Bowel chart

While it feels almost heretical to contemplate a return to the bowel chart, mapping or charting is a practical and meaningful approach to monitoring patterns of care, such as bowel care. At a glance the pattern over time is revealed alongside the response to shifting patterns and the efficacy of the response in bringing care back into a desired pattern.

The chart (Box 8.6) was designed at the hospice where constipation is a particular and often difficult symptom for many people: patients, families and nurses! Before the bowel chart was used, the hospice used a standard care plan with the ubiquitous goal that 'the patient should have their bowels opened every 1–3 days' (depending on what is normal for that person). The care plan also stated the (almost) universal first line of action, 'if patient uncomfortable suggest one *bisacodyl* and one *glycerine* suppository.' Whilst this response may, for many people, be the best response, it may not always be. The risk with standard care plans and protocols is that they impose a 'best' response rather than be perceived as a guideline to inform the response. This is more so, when best practice is prescribed through research such as National Institute for Clinical Excellence (NICE) guidelines. Protocols help to ensure consistency of response by practitioners based on best practice and therefore there must be good reason for deviating from the guideline. In Box 8.6 I leave the reader in suspense to consider the response to Reg's diarrhoea.

Box 8.5 Monitoring sleep

Sleep VAS	Reg Simpson	6/11/02
Complete satisfaction with sleep	←————————*————→	No satisfaction with sleep
Mark perception on scale What factors influence this mark? NB: pain, position, hunger, drink, temperature of room, environment, noise, bed, bedclothes, anxiety, emotion, usual sleep pattern, sleeping tablets, full bladder, other?	Reg says he slept worse than he has been doing at home despite maintaining fairly normal sleep pattern. He felt being in the hospice was okay, although it was strange being in another bed – not so comfortable as his bed at home. Comforted by nurse spending time with him in the 'early hours'. No pain. Action: ? increase night sedation	

Sleep VAS	Reg Simpson	7/11/02
Complete satisfaction with sleep.	←————————*————→	No satisfaction with sleep
Mark perception on scale What factors influence this mark? NB: pain, position, hunger, drink, temperature of room, environment, noise, bed, bedclothes, anxiety, emotion, usual sleep pattern, sleeping tablets, full bladder, other?	Sedation not increased. Yet Reg seemed more dissatisfied with his sleep than last night. I sat with him and he talked about his wife and the prospect of not being able to manage at home anymore. Even had half cup of tea. He seemed more settled afterwards.	

Sleep VAS	Reg Simpson	8/11/02
Complete satisfaction with sleep	←————————*————→	No satisfaction with sleep
Mark perception on scale What factors influence this mark? NB: pain, position, hunger, drink, temperature of room, environment, noise, bed, bedclothes, anxiety, emotion, usual sleep pattern, sleeping tablets, full bladder, other?	Reg more satisfied with sleep although he was awake again – he said he enjoyed day care, took his mind off things. I gave him hand massage with some lavender and he managed to doze for another hour.	

Box 8.6   Bowel chart

Assessment of bowel habit.

Assessment of bowel habit Reg Simpson 6/11	Prone to constipation. Last went two days ago. Reg is not uncomfortable
Threats to bowel habit?	Morphine – would he be better on fentanyl patch? Poor mobility and fatigue, poor diet and fluid intake
Plan	Monitor

Date	Shift: am/ pm/ night	Open? y/n	Assessment/description	Response/evaluation
7/11	am	n	Doesn't take any laxatives and eats a low fibre diet	Encourage Reg to drink more
	pm	n		
	night	n		
8/11	am	n	Again he says it isn't a problem	Reg declined bowel massage. He is reluctant to drink Prescribe movacol
	pm	n	He says he feels uncomfortable (maybe movacol?)	
	night	n		
9/11	am	n/y	Reg accepted offer of suppositories (see protocol)	Small hard stools passed. He felt better.
	pm	n		
	night	y +	Diarrhoea ++ Probably overflow??	

REFLECTIVE EXEMPLAR 8.2 – GERARD'S NARRATIVE

I visited Gerard at home to appreciate whether he would benefit from complementary therapy. My appreciation is written as an unfolding story based on the Burford cues. Unlike Reg Simpson's narrative I have boxed the Burford cues in order to guide other practitioners unused to working with the Burford model cues despite my reservation that the cues might be viewed in a reductionist way. I have incorporated two visual scales into the narrative: 'relaxed – tense' and 'positive – gloomy' to appreciate Gerard's emotional and psychological being. His scores suggest he is not as relaxed as he makes out.

In scoring Gerard I am mindful because it may be perceived as insensitive and that I am concerned with the outcome rather than the process. Gerard was in free-fall towards his inevitable death. He clung to hope and exploring his feelings and thoughts would have been too painful. As it was, when I sat on his bed waiting for the doctor, his tears and fears spilled out. There was no longer any point in evaluating whether reflexology or any other therapy was enhancing his sense of well-being. The scales also enable an evaluation and audit of treatment.

Gerard and Lisa narrative notes

Name: Gerard Hanwell	Address: 9 The Havens, Ludborough
Age: 43	GP: Dr Candice Main
Meaningful others: Lisa – wife, Jessie aged 7, Greta aged 3 Both sets of parents	District nurse/Macmillan nurse Amy – District nurse Esme – Macmillan nurse
Diagnosis/ synopsis of illness: **Wednesday October 16th**	Cancer tip of penis surgically removed one year ago. Lymph node involvement in his left groin – lymph node excised but the cancer has invaded the left leg and groin areas. Poor response to chemotherapy. Wound now extensive and spreading rapidly through the leg and pelvic areas. Very offensive smell – being treated daily by district nursing and pads changed about every two hours by Gerard or Lisa due to heavy exudate. Charcoal being used to combat the smell although Gerard finds the edge of the dressing press on the wound causes discomfort.

• Who is this person? • What meaning do they give to this health–illness experience? • How do I feel about this person?	Gerard is pale and apprehensive. He is pleased to see me – and quickly tells me his history and the way he and Lisa are exploring alternative treatments – currently taking an exotic bark diet. Gerard knows he has cancer spread. His openness and Lisa's despair, seeing the pictures of his children on the window sill, I feel a strong connection with him and his family – I want to help them if that's possible.
How is this person feeling? *mood/stress/anxiety/fears/body image*	Relaxed $\xleftarrow{\qquad\qquad\overset{2}{\quad}\qquad}$ Tense 5 4 3 2 1 Positive $\xleftarrow{\qquad\overset{3}{\quad}\qquad\qquad}$ Gloomy 5 4 3 2 1 On the surface Gerard seems relaxed and philosophical. Lisa is more anxious, a point Gerard picks up – that it is harder for the onlooker. They are both positive and expectant about my involvement, that it fits in with their chosen alternative approach at this time.
How has this event affected their usual life pattern and roles? • *Sleep* • *Eating/drinking* • *Mobility* • *Pain* • *Elimination* • *Work/play* • *Relationships* • *Energy/fatigue*	Gerard finds difficulty getting comfortable at night with the movement and pain in his left leg. Need to review his analgesic pattern? Lisa is not sleeping and still working. Diet – Gerard on his special diet – needs to drink 5 L water each day. The diet is very challenging but he is determined. Gerard can just about get up/down stairs – pain increases significantly with movement. No comment on bowels at this time. Gerard was working up to a week ago. He worked as a computer software engineer in a small firm – his work very supportive, but Gerard anxious about this as his work is crucial to firm's success. Gerard was a very keen footballer, supports Charlton – fanzine on floor. Enjoys music very much – Queen – had to cancel concert at week-end to see Tribute band due to leg.
What is important for this person to feel comfortable?	Pain control and position for leg. Hope!! Support for Lisa.

What support does this person have in life?	Lisa – although her work have given as much time as she needs to be at home. Both sets of parents live nearby and support Lisa with the children. District nursing and Macmillan support.
How does this person view the future for them-selves and others?	Gerard understands he has the option of further chemotherapy if the alternative approach fails to respond. Both he and Lisa are positive that he will beat the cancer.
Contra-indications	None.
How can I help this person?	Offer reflexology weekly using essential oils (patchouli for positive thinking/frankincense as blend to calm emotions/one drop of juniper berry). Help with odour and rid toxins. Suggest lavender on wound gauze as deodorant and analgesic. Suggest lavender and bergamot in aroma-stone to fragrance room. Possibility of therapeutic touch?? teach Lisa to give this.
Evaluation	Gerard very relaxed and enthusiastic following reflexology. He would like me to visit again they are going on week's holiday for half-term, so make appointment for two weeks (30/10).

Wednesday October 30	Amy, district nursing is leaving as I arrive. She reports the wound has worsened. Jessie, the 8 year old opens the door. She's off school with a cold. Gerard cheerful. Good break. He feels the wound is stable and the smell less offensive. Lisa allergic to lavender and bergamot! (she has asthma) They have stopped using charcoal because too painful cutting into his wound! Gerard's legs have swollen – tumour must be constricting blood and lymph flow.

Reflexology treatment – Gerard asleep – says it was 'fantastic' afterwards. |

Suggest seeing lymphoedema nurse at hospital – but can he get there? Gerard's legs very dry – leave some grapeseed oil for Lisa to apply.

Gerard and Lisa are going to Lourdes tomorrow with his parents. As Gerard says 'who knows what might happen, I'm not particularly religious but maybe a miracle?' I wonder if that comment reveals how darkly Gerard and Lisa are thinking as they try and maintain a surface sense of hope.

**Monday
November 4**

The first thing I notice is the smell – not as bad as my first visit but still hangs like a cloud.
I ask 'How was Lourdes?'
They did not go as Lisa's passport had expired!
His father had brought some holy water back and poured it on Gerard's leg. He says, 'It felt warm'. Hope high.
Gerard describes the way his wound continues to spread. Leg remains swollen although had gone down after my last treatment – now swollen again. He continues with alternative approach.
I ask, 'Do you ever contemplate that you won't beat this thing?'
He responds 'I'm hopeful it will get better but sometimes it does cross my mind that I won't.'
Lisa says Gerard had 'disturbed' weekend – not sleeping, confused, restless. Lisa is exhausted.

Reflexology – Gerard quickly asleep. Again, he says the treatment was fantastic. I finish with TT. Lisa asks if this was what I was going to teach her. I wonder if reflexology may help twice-weekly. Appointment for Friday.

**Friday
November 8**

Speak with Esme before visit – she is on phone to Lisa. Things have deteriorated ++. Esme saying to Lisa that Gerard will die, need to tell the children. The wound now solid black necrosis, infected and had haemorrhaged. I feel as if I am walking into a cauldron. Blood transfusion arranged for Hospice next Monday.

Arrive at house – children blank faces, shocked. Lisa brave. Gerard in bed – he is shocked, devastated with the news. I sit with him, helping him to talk through his tears and fears. Waiting for GP 'any moment' – so he declines a treatment. Downstairs I comfort Lisa – and break the children's despair by doing Greta's feet – Jessie joins in. Children bounce easily.

Wednesday November 13

Big mix-up. District nurse comes at 11am – give Lisa and Gerard more time in the mornings. Gerard in bath – he shouts his greeting down the stairs. Children back to school after 'colds'.
Gerard's pain control improved – especially at nights enabling everyone to sleep better!! Still some pain on movement.

Arrange visit for Friday 15/10.

Friday November 15

Gerard back downstairs in his 'usual' chair. More colour in his face after the blood transfusion. He is cheerful and looking forward to his reflexology. Continuing with his alternative diet.

Reflexology uneventful yet Gerard says it was relaxing and that he was transported to another place beyond fear. He can't explain it but it was profound. Lisa comforted listening to him say this – I give her a reflexology to relax her. She is very stressed although tries to be calm on the surface. It works well – 'at one point I was conscious that I did not have one thought in my head.'
Appointment made for 25/11.

Monday November 25

Gerard admitted to hospice – deteriorated last week. Children also sick – Lisa's mother at house with them.
At hospice Gerard not conscious. His sister, Leanne, has arrived from NZ. I stay with family. I greet Gerard and he stirs. Lisa jumps in expectation. I sit with them as Lisa unfolds the story of Gerard's deterioration. His breathing is very erratic; it bothers her listening to it. It also reflects Gerard's distress underneath the midazolam.

I use Therapeutic Touch for about 20 minutes shifting his breathing pattern from Cheyne-Stokes to normal rhythm. I take the heat out of him – he is

	more settled, more relaxed. Lisa says his hands are warmer – she is so grateful. She can sit easier with him now. I also give Lisa reflexology as she holds Gerard's hand – help relax her. She actually falls asleep for a short time. She feels relaxed and energised afterwards.
Wednesday November 27	Gerard died yesterday in Lisa's arms with children present. Very emotional. The staff are deeply affected by his death.

Integrated care pathway

Integrated care pathways are becoming in vogue. In theory, pathways plot the 'usual' pattern of treatment and care for a particular medical condition. In this way both cost and use of beds can be better predicted and managed, reflecting the integrated pathway's roots in American insurance companies! The practitioner then follows this pattern unless deviation or variation occurs for whatever reason. The pathway documentation consists of treatment and care outcome statements, supported by protocols to guide best practice. Variance is documented with action taken to return the patient to the normative path.

The treatment and care statements are quality statements that can be evaluated on a daily basis, for example 'Reg is comfortable with his pain.' In this way quality becomes part of everyday practice and that is the real benefit and excitement of this approach providing the pathway is viewed as a guideline for best practice rather than as a cost-management prescription.

Chapter 9

Assuring Quality

In this chapter I explore an approach to assuring quality congruent with reflective practice. In Box 2.9 (see Chapter 2) the final assumption for a reflective and holistic model for health care states:

> 'Caring in practice is a responsive and reflexive form in context with the environment in which it is practised.'

Put another way, do practitioners realise desirable practice as a lived reality? The notion of *reflexive* is to look back and seek feedback to inform (whomever is interested) whether actions have resulted in desired outcomes. If not, why not? Is it faulty vision, faulty judgement, faulty actions or a mixture of all these? Or perhaps the conditions of practice are inadequate for excellence to flourish? Are the quality indicators inadequate? In other words, feedback to ensure effective performance is complex and can be viewed on two loops (Argyris & Schön 1989) or even three loops (Isaacs 1993):

Loop 1   Do practitioners' clinical judgement and skilled responses realise desirable practice?
         Do the conditions of practice hinder realising desirable practice?
Loop 2   Is the understanding of desirable practice flawed?
         Are the indicators for realising desirable practice adequate?
Loop 3   Is thinking flawed?

Loop 3 picks up the significance of dialogue. It takes reflection to its most sophisticated level by challenging the *way* people think about issues. Quality assurance is the dialogue between the way things are and the way things would like to be. It is the creative tension necessary for learning.

Shifting tides

I work in a hospice funded as a charity. Each year, the National Care Standards Commission Inspectorate visits to monitor the hospice's quality of service against a set of standards. Up until 2003, the Inspectorate collected their own evidence. From 2003 the Inspectorate requires the hospice to provide evidence of meeting the standards. So how best can the hospice, or indeed any organisation, respond to the quality challenge?

Clinical governance

In the UK the quality agenda is centred in the development of Clinical Governance, defined as:

> 'A framework through which all NHS organisations are accountable for continuously improving the quality of their services and safeguarding an environment in which excellence can flourish.' (NHS consultation paper *A first class service* 1998)

In the UK, the emergence of National Service Frameworks (NSFs) and the National Centre for Clinical Excellence (NICE) has begun to both indicate and dictate the quality agenda. Groups such as Commission for Health Improvement (CHI, soon to become CHAI) make quality judgements, and yet at the end of the day, the responsibility for creating this environment in which excellence can flourish is dependent on practitioners. Practitioners must take ownership of quality and live quality as part of everyday practice. Quality must become central to their lives, not be a peripheral notion that is essentially someone else's business. If so, then quality is imposed and reactive; an imposition that seeks to bring organisations and, ergo, practitioners to heel. If practitioners do not take control of the quality agenda then quality systems will impose conformity and compliance rather than be creative opportunities.

Feedback systems include clinical supervision, standards of care and clinical audit that collectively provide a comprehensive response to realising an environment in which excellence can flourish. Each of these learning opportunities is grounded in reflection, highlighting the organisational value of reflection as a process of professional development and assuring quality.

Clinical supervision

The nature of clinical supervision was explored in Chapter 3 and its impact on clinical practice highlighted throughout the exemplars presented in the subsequent chapters. The great value of clinical supervision is to create the space for reflection within the business of everyday practice. And yet, paradoxically, it is for this reason that clinical supervision has struggled to gain a foothold because space is already compromised by other pressures. Locally more and more NHS Trusts, influenced by the clinical governance agenda, are viewing supervision as mandatory for all practitioners. As such, the NHS Trusts need to prioritise practitioner development rather than view it as something tagged on the end of everything else.

As a quality assurance tool, clinical supervision can highlight situations where desirable practice has been or has not been met. Yet it only offers snapshots of practice rather than a systematic approach to managing quality. Its real value is to enable practitioner development whereby an emphasis on judging performance is likely to compromise its developmental potential. Yet it can be assumed that if the aims of clinical supervision are met then quality of care will improve.

Standards of care

Standards of care offer a reflective approach to managing quality by focusing on discrete aspects of practice. Although standards of care can be imported from a validated external body, I am interested in developing standards of care constructed by practitioners themselves. This approach generally follows the development of standards of care at Burford Community hospital between 1989 and 1991, an approach based on the Royal College of Nursing Standards of Care project (Kitson 1989).

A standard of care reflects a local practice situation that is professionally agreed, and both desirable and achievable. It reduces the practice situation into structure, process and outcome criteria which are able to be monitored.

A local practice situation is a statement of practice sited to the particular practice unit, for example 'Patients are cared for in a safe and therapeutic environment.' A midwifery unit may interpret this standard in a very different way to a surgical unit, yet both will pay attention to research and policy that determine what is therapeutic and what is safe.

Professionally agreed involves all people involved in meeting the standard of care: nurses, doctors, paramedical staff, cleaners, cooks, pharmacists etc. The idea of professionally agreed goes against the grain of setting patient-centred standards of care – can professionals and ancillary staff adequately set standards for patients and families? Do patients or patient representative groups need to be involved? At Burford, we invited Age Concern to 'vet' our standards as most of our patients were elderly. At the Hospice where I work, we involve volunteers who have experience of caring for dying relatives as part of the shadow clinical governance committee that oversees the quality initiative.

There is a natural tension between *what is desirable* and *what is achievable* that captures the essence of quality. Quality is what is real, what is in front of you. You can feel the fabric of a shirt and sense its quality. However quality is also something relative or comparable with other shirts – i.e., that quality has a desirable element to it. Clearly, standards of care have to be achievable other-wise they would never be met and the hospice would fail its annual review and be closed down. Yet standards also need to reflect desirability, as some-thing to move towards. Senge (1990) describes this tension as creative tension, a dynamic state of affairs that fuels learning that I explore deeper in Chapter 10, in relation to developing the learning organisation.

Criteria

Box 9.1 sets out the nature of structure, process and outcome criteria with some examples. Practitioners often get confused between structure and pro-cess criteria and to some extent they do overlap. Structure criteria are things that need to exist for the practice situation to be met. A policy is an example of structure, as is the Organisation's vision and mission statements. In contrast, a

Box 9.1　Standards criteria and examples

Criteria	Examples
Structure criteria describe resources that are necessary to exist to enable the standard statement to be achieved.	Staffing levels. Attitudes and skills of staff, e.g. the complementary therapist ensures 12 hours of professional development yearly. Number of syringe drivers. Colours of walls. Number of single rooms. Maintenance contracts.
Process criteria are actions by care workers necessary to achieve the practice situation.	The nurse assesses each person's usual sleep rhythm on admission. The doctor sees the person within 20 minutes.
Outcome criteria are relevant indicators of patient actions or behaviour that indicate the standard statement has been realised.	Patient's unsolicited expression of satisfaction with their meal. Patient is comfortable with his pain.

formulary or protocol is an example of process – actions that practitioners must take usually in a specified order of action, for example mouth care:

The practitioner assesses and responds to each patient's mouth as per mouth care formulary.

The formulary would be appendixed to the standard. One might argue that the existence of the formulary is a structural issue, but it is really just a summary of various process criteria. A process criteria in a standard for wound care might state:

The practitioner is informed by the protocol (appendixed) *for wound healing in deciding how best to respond to each wound.*

Nutrition

One of the standards of care we wrote at Burford hospital concerned nutrition. The standard statement was 'Patients can enjoy a nutritious meal.' This standard statement recognises two elements of eating – nutrition and enjoyment. For many patients at Burford and, indeed, for people everywhere, meals structure the day. It is a social event. For people who are ill, nutrition is an important ingredient in getting well. Yet often when people are ill, their appetites are diminished, hence the significance of nutrition although the quality of hospital food and service has often been criticised. I am sure that most readers will have firsthand experience of hospital food, either as a patient, friend or care worker.

So, what might be relevant indicators to inform practitioners that the standard statement, 'Patients can enjoy a nutritious meal' has been met? List your indicators *before* turning to Appendix 2 to reveal a potential scan sheet. The scan sheet is internalised by the practitioner as a reflective framework and so, at meal times, the practitioner is both more sensitive about care but can also spot if the criteria are not being met for whatever reason. If appropriate, use the scan sheet in your practice and see what aspires. Obviously writing the standard on nutrition would involve the catering staff and the dieticians. It may develop into situations where patients are unable to eat for whatever reason to include protocols for parenteral nutrition.

Relatives

Consider the standard statement, 'The family are informed, involved and supported within the caring process.' What relevant indicators might inform you that this standard statement has been met? At Burford, in response to this challenge, we secured a small research grant and surveyed families. We identified a number of process criteria alongside which I suggest a number of questions that might be asked to get feedback that the process criteria have been met. I like to think that these questions are caring cues that can be unobtrusively slipped into dialogue between the practitioner and family member rather than as a formal questionnaire that demands the family's judgement:

The caring team inform the family who they are and how they can be contacted.
Q: Do you know the caring team and how to contact them at any time?

The nurse on duty initiates a 'concerned interaction' with the family each time they visit.
Q: Do the nurses approach you when you visit and ask how things are or do you have to approach them?

The nurse responds positively to the family's request for information and nurse informs the relative where she/he, for whatever reason, is unable to disclose information.
Q: Are you adequately informed about the patient's condition and progress?

The nurse is aware of how the family is thinking and feeling about the patient's care.
Q: Do you feel the nurses knew how you thought and felt about [the patient's] care?
Q: To what extent were you consulted and listened to in making decisions?

The nurse has explored with the family their desired involvement with the patient's physical care and setting the limits of care giving.
Q: To what extent did you feel welcomed and involved in caring for [the patient]?

The nurse identifies and responds to the relatives' (holistic) support needs
Q: Looking back, could the care staff have supported you more in any way? (physically, emotionally, psychologically, spiritually, culturally, socially)

The logic of monitoring process criteria is simply that if the process is right then the outcomes will be right. Of course nothing is predictable, and the vagaries of the human condition suggest that some family members will never be involved, informed or supported enough.

Value of standards of care

Standards of care are a true quality assurance tool because they do not just monitor quality but seek to develop quality. In summary standards of care offer practitioners/the organisation:

- a framework for developing specific aspects of clinical practice
- a change management model
- a way of connecting values with practice
- a process for group reflection and team learning
- a resource management model – the focus on structure creates the opportunity to reflect on resources available and the way resources are utilised
- a means for practitioners to demonstrate professional accountability
- a quality assurance tool
- a means to respond to quality agendas
- a way to integrate quality as part of everyday practice

A means for practitioners to demonstrate professional accountability

Quality needs to be lived as part of everyday practice whereby practitioners take responsibility for ensuring their own performance. The responsibility of organisations is to create the conditions whereby practitioners can realise their responsibility – the essential role of clinical governance. Perhaps health care practitioners have been passive about quality seeing it as someone else's business. As a result, quality measures have been top–down and imposed on practitioners rather than engaging practitioners in responding to the quality agenda.

The effective (reflective) practitioner takes responsibility for ensuring her own effectiveness and working collaboratively with others to ensure best practice. This is the bottom line. There can be no compromise with this expectation. Indeed, practitioners should welcome and embrace this challenge as the hallmark of professional practice.

A way to integrate quality as part of everyday practice

Again, to re-iterate – quality is something lived. It should not be viewed as something outside everyday clinical practice but viewed as something integral to everyday practice. In other words, quality is something that practitioners need to be mindful of within practice. As such, it is important that monitoring tools are designed to be integral with caring, as part of everyday practice. Of course, whether the tools are perceived as caring is a reflection of the person who uses them. As I shall illustrate in the examples of standards

Box 9.2   Key points in developing a standard of care

(1)   Identify an appropriate topic for writing a standard of care, for example, 'Patients are comfortable with their pain'. This topic may be a reflection of a current issue or part of a comprehensive list of standards that need to be developed, for example to respond to the National Care Standards Commission's core and specialist standards of care.
(2)   Write the topic in the centre of a flipchart.
(3)   Engage the group to brainstorm ideas that relate to this aspect of practice and cluster on the flipchart.
(4)   Accept all contributions non-judgementally.
(5)   After approximately 10 minutes discuss each brainstormed idea led by initiator.
(6)   Reflect on the experiences of patients around the brainstormed ideas, grounding the activity in actual practice rather than as an abstract idea.
(7)   Consider all relevant sources of knowledge that might inform the standard (theory, research, policy, etc.) This will almost certainly require a literature search and review at a later date.
(8)   Draw relationships between the brainstormed ideas.
(9)   Reformulate ideas as structure/process and outcome criteria.
(10)   Write the definitive standard statement.
(11)   Tick off 'check list for writing standards'.

of care following, monitoring tools are observational or asking the patient or family specific questions. Observation tools include scanning and spotting. Scanning is a planned monitor of the standard of care using a designed scan sheet, usually a set of criteria that can be observed. Spotting is simply opportunistic observation of criteria during the course of the day, for example, noticing an immobile patient does not have a drink within easy reach at meal time.

The standards group

At the hospice, the standards group meets for one and a half hours each month to manage the standards of care programme by reviewing existing standards and developing new ones[1]. The group is open to all multidisciplinary staff and is chaired by the standards of care facilitator. In the spirit of the learning organisation, all nursing staff are expected to manage at least one standard of care around a topic of interest. This person then becomes the hospice resource person for that aspect of clinical practice, setting up and maintaining a resource file containing relevant information and research. The resource person is also responsibility for ensuring the standard is monitored as designed and reports to the Clinical Governance group. Key points in writing a standard of care are set out in Box 9.2.

Setting a monitoring schedule is always tentative, especially in the first instance. Perhaps begin with weekly or monthly depending on the particular

---

[1] As at October 2003, 26 potential standards have been interpreted from the National Care Standards Commission care and specialist standards for development. The full list is set out in Appendix 3.

standard and the extent it is 'spotted' as failing its criteria. Who should monitor? As I suggested with the relatives standard, monitoring techniques that involve asking patients or their families are best slipped into normal conversation as part of caring, for example:

- Did you sleep okay last night? (sleep standard)
- You seemed restless in your sleep last night? (sleep standard)
- How was the meal today? (nutrition standard)
- What is this drug for? (self-medication standard)
- (to a relative): How do you find Bill today? (relatives standard)

Obviously questions that suggest judgement on care processes require sensitivity. Visitors may be especially reluctant to give negative feedback when still visiting (Nehring & Geach 1973). As such, questions are better designed as open questions than closed questions. In Box 9.3 I set out a checklist for writing a standard of care. The last point is rather hopeful because although practitioners are positive about quality as an ideal, in practice they struggle to accommodate this approach with issues of owning quality, time and technique. It sounds easy but in practice standards are a difficult concept to embrace, difficult to write, and even more difficult to monitor because of time. Hence the organisation must invest in a standards of care facilitator and create the space for this work to be accomplished. It is vital work.

In summary, standards of care are a reflective and versatile approach to managing quality that contribute to developing the learning organisation by creating an opportunity for focused multi-professional group reflection around specific aspects of clinical practice with the intention of understanding and realising best practice.

Box 9.3   Checklist for writing standards

- Reflects agreement by all practitioners/workers involved in meeting the standard statement.
- Reflects consumer rights and needs.
- Reflects optimum quality, i.e., the tension between what is desirable and what is achievable within resources but always have a creative edge.
- Reflects organisational outcomes.
- Reflects professional values and ethics.
- Reflects relevant theory and research (evidence–based practice – ensure an index of literature explored).
- Resource file established.
- Monitoring strategy designed and review date set (agenda for standards group).
- Avoidance of ambiguous statements or unnecessary jargon.
- Has identified pragmatic monitoring tools (usually observation or questions to ask) and set monitoring schedule and review dates (this will be tentative in the first instance).
- Subsumes relevant policies.
- Has converted process criteria into protocols or care pathways for 'best practice'.
- Has been lots of fun!

Clinical audit

Clinical audit, like standards of care, offers an opportunity for multi-professional group reflection around specific patients with the primary purpose to answer two fundamental questions:

- Did the patient/family receive best care?
- Do we know what best care is?

Clinical Audit in the NHS (1996) states that:

> 'Clinical audit is a clinically led initiative which seeks to improve the quality and outcome of patient care through structured peer review whereby clinicians examine their practices and results against agreed standards and modify their practice where indicated. The future development of audit would aim to achieve:
> - A clear patient focus – through patient experiences that clinical quality and clinical outcomes become more meaningful
> - Greater multi-professional working across the different clinical and managerial disciplines which contribute to the patient's episode of care
> - An intersectoral approach where a patient's care is managed across primary, secondary and continuing care
> - Professional self-development
> - Better integration of effectiveness information.' (pp. 3, 4)

While clinical audit has a powerful impact on those who take part in it, many practitioners remain uninvolved. Consider this question for yourself: if you are involved, what factors have influenced your involvement? If you are not involved then why not?

It is the same question as to whether practitioners are involved in quality, although clinical audit is a very practical approach to assuring quality, more so than standards of care because the process is simply reflection on experience keeping the two clinical audit questions in the foreground. Practitioners are only likely to become involved where they retain a clear sense of ownership of the process of audit and feel it is a safe environment for discussing sensitive details about their professional practice without the fear of provoking management sanction or civil litigation (Clinical Audit in the NHS, NHS 1996, p. 4).

As standards of care are developed they are integrated within the clinical audit process (in the example given as a check list) creating another opportunity to review standards of care. At the hospice clinical audit meetings, a practitioner prepares and presents an overview of the patient and family's care and treatment. The patient/family is usually chosen because their care has challenged the caring team in some significant way and highlighted areas of practice that are problematic. The practitioner then summarises recommendations for future practice which are subsequently audited and presented to the Clinical Governance Group. Recent topics have included:

- Appreciating the nature of agitation in terminal illness and knowing how best to respond.

- Patients who are 'off-hand' and with whom it is difficult to create 'good' relationships.
- Conflict with aggressive and demanding relatives.
- Seemingly intractable pain.
- Patients who did not 'die well'.
- Very poignant or emotional deaths where staff have become (over) involved or felt they have 'failed' in some way.

What has been most interesting to note is that these issues have no definite solutions. They are complex and indeterminate, what Schön (1987) described as the swampy lowlands of practice. It is only through reflection that the nature of these topics can be grasped and alternative ways of responding surfaced. Of course each clinical situation is different and learning cannot simply be transferred from one situation to the next. But through reflection a deepening of appreciation is becoming evident. Clinical audit, like standards of care, is a learning opportunity, as indeed are all reflexive quality systems.

Chapter 10

Clinical Leadership and Nurturing the Learning Organisation

In Chapter 2, I set out the explicit assumptions that underpin a reflective model for nursing and health care. One of the assumptions states that *practitioners accept responsibility for working toward creating the learning organisation* (Senge 1990). As discussed so far, reflective practice offers the practitioner an opportunity to learn through everyday practice toward realising a vision of desirable practice. In doing so, the vision itself is developed and factors that constrain realising the vision are exposed, understood and worked towards shifting. However, in Chapter 2 I identified the conditions necessary to exist in order for reflection to be successfully accommodated into clinical practice. Of most significance is clinical leadership. In this chapter I intend to highlight the nature of reflective or transformational leadership: the way that reflective leadership can be nurtured through guided reflection, and the role of leadership in facilitating the learning organisation using clinical supervision as an example, by using two exemplars from students undertaking the Masters in Clinical Leadership programme at the University of Luton.

A key role of clinical leadership is to nurture an environment whereby the organisation can learn, what Senge (1990) describes as the learning organisation:

> 'One where people continually expand their capacities to create the results they truly desire, where new and expansive patterns of thinking are nurtured, where collective aspiration is set free, and where people are continually learning how to learn together.' (p. 3)

Senge (1990) writes that the state of being a learning organisation never actually exists, since the more that is learnt the more acutely aware we become of ignorance. Organisations are continually journeying and practising the disciplines of learning with varying degrees of success. Senge (1990) describes five component technologies – personal mastery, mental models, shared vision, team learning and systems thinking – that do not *create* the learning organisation, but when converged can facilitate experimentation and advancement (Box 10.1).

Sally is a deputy ward manager working within a NHS hospital. She strives to know and realise herself as a clinical leader. In her reflection *A little voice in a big arena* she reflects on the meaning of leadership within the context of a particular situation that brought her into conflict.

Box 10.1 Senge's five component technologies that converge to innovate the learning organisation

Systems thinking	Systems thinking is being able to perceive the whole pattern of things and the ways systems or parts inter-relate with each other, even when apparently invisible. This system is not confined in time.
Personal mastery	Personal mastery is the discipline of continually clarifying and deepening our personal vision, of focusing our energies, of developing patience and of seeing reality objectively. People with a high level of personal mastery are able to consistently realise the results that matter most to them – in effect, they approach life as an artist would approach a work of art. They do that by becoming committed to their own lifelong learning. (Senge 1990, p. 7)
Mental models	Mental models are deeply ingrained assumptions or images that influence how the practitioner understands the world and how they take action. The discipline of working with mental models starts with turning the mirror inward; learning to unearth our internal images and assumptions of the world, to bring them to the surface and hold them rigorously to scrutiny. It also includes the ability to carry on 'learningful' conversations that balance inquiry and advocacy, where people expose their own thinking effectively and make their thinking open to the influence of others. (Senge 1990, pp. 8, 9)
Building a shared vision	The practice of shared vision involves the skills of unearthing shared beliefs and values about the nature of practice that fosters genuine commitment rather than compliance. In mastering this discipline, leaders learn the counter productiveness of trying to dictate a vision, no matter how heartfelt.
Team learning	The discipline of team learning starts with 'dialogue' – the capacity of members of a team to suspend their individual assumptions and enter into a genuine 'thinking together' and recognising the patterns of interaction in teams that undermine learning.

REFLECTIVE EXEMPLAR 10.1 – A LITTLE VOICE IN A BIG ARENA

With an ever-demanding society, the National Health Service (NHS) endeavours to provide modernisation and change to meet the needs of society. Policies and protocols are multiplying, targets and deadlines are everyday phenomena and 'budgets' have become the new buzzword. Front line staff struggle to maintain the focus of a patient-centred service where, every day, there is the constant battle with the system to provide holistic care. I work as a deputy ward manager within an elective orthopaedic unit in an acute hospital trust. This reflection exposes issues of conflict that arise within my role and how I am learning to respond in ways congruent with my values as an emerging clinical leader.

As a deputy ward manager my role can be one of confusion and difficulty. I am viewed as a leader but not completely let off my reins to explore. When those reins are sometimes dropped I find I'm pulled back with the understanding I wasn't ready to go it alone! My role is ward-based, which enables me to maintain patient-centred contact whilst experiencing management and leadership within the NHS. I work along side my ward manager and aim to maintain high standards of care in a professional and organised environment.

Within my role I come up against daily issues of conflict. The pressures placed on the NHS today are filtering down to ward level where the cracks are beginning to show and leadership within this environment is becoming an uphill struggle. As Cope (2001) notes:

> 'Within organisations we see managers struggling to come to terms with new demands on their managerial and leadership style. We have shifted from a position where control is managed by virtue of a formal badge of office (manager, patient, director, etc.) to one where we have to lead people through the use of more intangible and flexible forms of leadership.' (p. 1)

Following on from Cope's view, I feel leaders of today find they have to focus not only on themselves and the workforce but the surrounding issues, where difference and non-conformity are beginning to become valued, where expression can be an open forum and vision is developing into a natural phenomenon. The NHS is experiencing a change in leadership styles and moving forward from the transactional forms of leadership, which Schuster (1994) discussed as being hierarchically driven using status and influence to abuse power. Leaders find themselves developing many strings to their bow; Senge (1990) felt that learning organisation leaders became designers, stewards and teachers. They were responsible for developing the organisation allowing people to expand their skills and clarify their vision. Reflecting traits of transformational leadership that Burns (1978) cited by Dunham & Klafehn (1990) can be expressed as:

> 'being committed, having vision of what could be accomplished and empowering others with this vision so that all would accomplish more with less. The leader meshes with followers on deeply held values.' (p. 28)

As a deputy ward manager I am a puppet with many strings providing quality to my work, as a teacher, adviser, supervisor and expert. I work alongside my colleagues supporting, focusing and respecting them and the organisation as a whole. We acknowledge protocols and policies in our everyday work and strive to create and maintain a vision for our future.

With new government initiatives being continually developed there are ever-more pressures placed on the organisation to meet targets and deadlines and deliver a cost effective health care, contributing to a rapidly changing environment. Leaders have to balance the reality of maintaining quality of care on a reduced budget with reduced resources. This view is shared by Klakovich (1994) who expressed:

> 'for some time, staff nurses have been pressured to do more with less, that is, to maintain high productivity without sacrificing quality.' (p. 42)

Because of the pressures being placed on the health service and each department managing their own resources issues of conflict arise. Barriers are erected, protocols and policies are barraged around and common courtesy becomes a thing of the past.

Taylor & Singer (1983) suggest that through tension, companies' capacity could grow as long as the people involved can survive the stress. They discuss that without a certain amount of tension within the working environment barriers for change would not be broken down. However tension can cause upset and barriers to be extended not broken down, the staff can become de-motivated, demoralised and unsatisfied. I feel this is reflected within the work of Benner (1984), who discussed that pressures placed on nursing teams can cause the nurses to originally cope with the challenge but in reality they are providing 'too little too late'.

Through one such lived experience I became entangled in a conflict situation involving the placement of a patient arising from pressure within the organisation. Since the government introduced the traffic light system for bed management, 'red alert' has become an everyday event in my hospital. Working within an elective ward environment we have a rapid turn around of patients and on some occasions are left with an empty bed. We often assist the organisation by accepting non-orthopaedic elective admissions and minor trauma admissions to assist with the tight bed management of the hospital. We have strict guidelines on what we accept due to our rapid pace of work, the experience of our team and the infection risk to our elective patients.

On the occasion in question, the bed manager approached me regarding a gentleman who had been admitted to the accident and emergency department with severe head injuries. He had been brutally assaulted and the police were treating it as attempted murder. His condition was unstable and he required a nurse to specially look after him. As the assailant had not been being caught he was deemed at risk and would also have a police guard.

I was surprised at the bed manager's request to place this gentleman (who shall take the pseudonym of George) within our ward environment. I felt the environment to be inappropriate, the staffing was already tight and there was no room for movement to create a special nurse. The ward was busy and there were several acute postoperative patients being monitored and there was also the very real issue, due to the open ward environment, of risk to the patients and staff. I expressed my concerns and stated my case in a professional manner to the bed manager, who accepted the situation and the admission was refused.

Two hours later I received another phone call from the bed manager. This time in a uptight and forthright manner he stated, 'There is nowhere to place George and pressure is now being placed on me to have George moved from accident and emergency. It has been discussed with the hospital manager and hospital administrator and George will be admitted to your ward!'

The wind was taken from my sails. I took a deep breath and restated my case detailing the ward policy and stating the ward would be unsafe in the event of George's admission. I was outraged that discussions had been held without my input and decisions had been made without one of the managers entering the ward to see the environment, the workload and the staffing levels. There had been no respect for myself and my staff, no reasoning or compromise, just a very dictatorial attitude.

An assembly of senior management then appeared on the ward, the bed manager, the hospital manager and the hospital administrator. I was approached and told that George would be brought to the ward shortly and they had been able to provide a nurse from another area for George for the shift. I felt in awe and overpowered by the situation but did manage to question why it had been handled in this way and why there had been no discussion with myself and my team over the appropriateness of this patient's placement. My questions were not directly answered; the hospital administrator stated the ward staffing had not been affected as they could provide cover for the next twelve hours and the situation would be reviewed in the morning. Although I could see it was to no avail, I expressed that I was unhappy with the situation, the lack of communication involved and still believed this to be an inappropriate placement. The managers left the ward and George arrived with his nurse and police guard.

An hour later, which was late evening, the chief executive of the hospital appeared on the ward and approached me. She acknowledged the situation that had occurred with George's admission. She explained the difficulty in finding an appropriate placement for George and acknowledged the issues I had raised. She expressed thanks for the cooperation of my staff and myself and asked to be made aware of any problems. I was left feeling bruised by the situation but the chief executive had just applied the first band-aid. Because she had gone out of her way to visit the ward and acknowledge a difficult situation I did not feel so alone. It may have just been clever and kind words but it gave me an inner strength to review the situation.

Conflict situations surrounding bed management and appropriate placement of patients continue. The situation I experienced touches on issues of conflict manipulation, 'focusing on getting away from what we don't want rather than creating what we do want' (Senge 1990 p. 157). The hospital managers saw that George's admission to the accident and emergency department had caused disruption and once George's condition had been stabilised their priority was to move him to a more isolated environment. George was viewed as a problem which needed to be fixed!

I perceived the need to provide George with a more secure environment but had real concerns that the area of elective orthopaedics was inappropriate and I felt little would be gained from this transfer. Cavanagh (1991) discussed that competitive style of conflict management usually occurs when a person follows their own gain to the detriment of others. This can lead to frustration, anger and arguments, creating damage to relationships and not viewing the situation as a whole but with tunnel vision.

Using Johns' (1998a) ethical mapping framework [see Box 1.9] enables the practitioner to view a situation from a variety of different concepts.

'The map helps the practitioner see different and often contradictory perspectives of any situation and to examine the factors that determine which perspectives prevails' (Johns 1999, p. 118). Envisaging the ethical map and placing the patient's, doctor's, nurse's and organisation's perspectives to the forefront, it quickly became apparent to myself that the only gain of George being admitted to the ward was that the organisation managed to place their problem patient. I feel George would have received a short-term gain from being placed within a more secure environment. The high dependency nursing environment that was required for George was unacceptable and inappropriate within a busy ward.

Abiding by the Nursing and Midwifery scope of professional practice, as a nurse you need to have competence and confidence with the care you provide to your patient. 'Acknowledge any limitations in your knowledge and competence and decline any duties or responsibilities unless able to perform them in a safe and skilled manner.' As the ward's deputy manager I felt I had failed within my duty to act as an advocate for the nursing team, expressing their limitations and knowledge to care for such a highly dependent patient. I felt overpowered by the organisation and had been told what I was to do rather like a naughty school girl rebelling against her teacher.

This transactional form of leadership had left me feeling angry and frustrated. I feel the managers involved were working from a negative short term vision and not considering all the components involved within their decision. Cope (2001) discussed this as map conflict: conflict occurring when two people viewed the same situation from different perspectives. Map conflict can lead to tense situations, lines of communication can break down, leading to little or no resolution. Theorists in the past have believed that conflict situations have a positive effect on ourselves and the organisation. Deutsch (1971) cited by Cavanagh (1991) discussed how conflict could be 'highly enjoyable' as you gain experience of your own capabilities. I feel we have to be aware that a conflict situation does not turn into a game for one or both parties' enjoyment and self-development and we keep the problem in the forefront of our minds otherwise it could develop out of control. Cope (2001) discussed the fantasy ladder [Box 10.2] where a factual problem becomes modified and distorted turning into fantasy, which then has a potential for conflict. Both parties can end up being on the fantasy rung of their ladder causing a gap to develop between them (fantasy canyon). 'The fantasy is built on both sides; the conflict is no longer about anything

Box 10.2   Fantasy ladder (Cope 2001)

↑	Fantasy	Now has little relation to the original fact and has turned into myth or story
	Fiction	The story has its roots in fact, but critical details have been modified
	Faction	One person has put a spin on it, so it's still basically true, but now has a personalised edge
	Fact	All people involved in the experience would agree on the details

substantial – it is simply about ego, beliefs, political position and power' (Cope 2001, p. 116). Conflict then becomes a battle of wills and casualties develop. The opportunity to solve the problem becomes reduced and only concludes because one party intimidates or shouts the loudest.

Very quickly I became the child within the situation with the parent telling me what I was going to do. Although parent–child situations can at times be comforting, this situation became one of a critical response to a rebellious non-conforming child. Taylor & Singer (1983, p. 71) touched on this view when they discussed a bureaucratic organisation; they expressed a feature of such an organisation 'is that people should obey rules and should know their place.' However, they went on to say, 'contacts with staff in other departments are limited and these people are often seen as competitors for resources or even enemies who do not understand the difficulties and needs.'

Although I do not feel staff are always viewed as competitors and I do not believe this was the case in this situation, I *do* feel I was viewed as not understanding the organisation's needs as a whole, which went on to incite the parent-like attitude of the hospital administrator. If I had been approached in a collaborative way, then I feel certain a compromise would have been reached. I was trying to maintain a 'professional' or adult approach but the response was parental. My 'outrage' reflects my shift into a rebellious child digging her heels against an overbearing parental attitude. When the pattern of communication is not reciprocated then lines literally become crossed and communication breaks down.

Once George had been placed on the ward my focus was on the staff as I felt I had let them down and allowed the ward to be placed in an unacceptable position, I saw myself as the parent, comforting and nurturing the staff around me. I became a teacher, mentor and coach, ensuring the staff remained focused on George and his needs and not the negative energy felt towards the situation that had occurred. Dunham & Klafehn (1990) expressed the dilemma that leaders can feel trying to show alliance to two separate groups who expect them to take two different forms of action. Although I had a feeling of guilt for not 'fixing' the situation, I feel that the staff around me showed me allegiance, they were disappointed but did not take the view that my action should have been any different. However my self-esteem had taken a big knock.

I became accountable for the situation that had developed and I refocused on the position, trying to ensure no harm was to come to George and aiming to provide a good quality of care. I had an inner fear regarding the situation and the way my position had been viewed. I felt anxious and unconfident in my abilities; I had become a shell of the deputy ward manager who had started her shift. I was trying to save face with my staff and function as if the situation had never arisen:

'Anxiety is our biggest enemy; it holds us back, makes us doubt our worth and ability, makes us worry about losing approval.' (Dickson 1982, p. 147)

I found myself within a coat of armour, protecting myself from possible further conflict from the ward staff. I was afraid of criticism for accepting George's admission from my colleagues. Instead of being impulsive and strong I became concerned that I had placed us in an unacceptable position and the ward was at risk. All health care workers live out the daily tension of balancing what is therapeutic against what is safe. Perhaps practitioners err on the side of safety for the fear of criticism if the people in their care come to some harm.

Balancing therapeutic care against safe practice became a real issue; I understood the need for George to be placed within a ward environment and his therapeutic needs but I was fully aware of the ward policy and the issues of safety. The issues of maintaining his safety and the safe practice to my other patients were paramount. I was scared of criticism; I was scared of making the wrong decision but I wanted to protect George and my other patients from coming to any harm. This became an underlying factor within my decision and my reaction to the situation. I envisaged the results of my actions and chose the action which, I believed, would provide benefit to my patient over harm that might have been caused; Tschudin (1993) explained this as the 'teleology theory'. Tschudin explained that the difficulty with this theory was to what extent one can decide what is good and what will do harm. My intentions were to create a safe environment for George, my patients and other staff. I wanted to avoid harm being done (non maleficence) complying with my code of conduct with respect and a professional stance.

Klakovich (1994, p. 42) emphasised, 'to preserve the caring practice of the nursing profession in today's healthcare environment, a new leadership theory is needed.' Transactional leadership can have a damaging effect on the caring values, which was the effect within my situation. Leadership roles should aim to enhance the caring values of the nursing team in order to gain and provide the optimum care available. Burns (1978, cited by Dunham & Klafehn 1990) felt this had been found in transformational leadership, however following the work Kerfoot (1996, p. 433) who talked of connective leaders, 'as those who connect instead of conquer, collaborate rather than compete, entrust and empower rather than control, contribute rather than demand.' I feel connective leadership could be the next stepping-stone up from transformational leadership.

Transformational leadership and connective leadership follow many similar traits. However connective leadership steers its focus more closely on the 'preservation of care' (Klakovich 1994), nurturing and cultivating the caring attitude of the NHS alongside change management. Although the transformational leadership acknowledges the importance of maintaining care, Klakovich (1994) believed there was still some emphasis on competition and conflict.

There are only minimal comparisons made between the two leadership styles within the literature I obtained. This may be due to the fact that the leadership styles are so similar they are viewed as one and the same.

So I propose, does the connective leader develop from a transformational leader through experience or possibly due to the human traits they already hold? We can only wait and over the next few years this may become evident within the changing world of the NHS.

Reflecting on the conflict surrounding George's admission and the involvement of the chief executive has opened my eyes to the leadership styles involved. The hospital administrator approached the situation with a transactional leadership style showing a dictatorial attitude oozing negative vision. This clashed with the transformational leadership style with which I had approached the situation. I felt I needed to empower my vision on to my colleagues to allow us to approach the situation together and complete the task ahead. The chief executive approached using a connective leadership style, she visited the ward late in the evening and not on an official time-table. She expressed her understanding of my concerns and the needs of the organisation. She offered her support and acknowledged my dedication to my role, she expressed thanks to myself and my team for assisting in George's admission, she showed warmth and empathy throughout our conversation. This created an uplift of my confidence and my self esteem, maintaining and cultivating my caring attitude. Effectively she was bridging the gap between the organisational leaders and myself. Seden (2003) notes that:

> 'Managers now have responsibilities within boundaries of their own workplace and also within new organisational arrangements, networks and partnerships. This means that managers need clear understanding of their own organisation remit and that of others and the way in which such structures and culture impact on each other.' (p. 103)

The art of communication and respect for each other is vital to visualise the wider picture. This should enhance a positive vision to go forward as an effective leader, bridging gaps for the future.

Footnote

With the ever-growing pace of the NHS, conflict situations occur on a daily basis. How we deal with these situations has an impact on how we develop professionally and personally. When I was a newly qualified nurse I would shy away from conflict situations, unconfident and naive in many situations that occurred. I quickly became burdened with others' unwanted jobs, unable to complete all the tasks to my high standard and I became unsatisfied and exhausted as my time management collapsed. Through past experience I have learned to question and say no in order to hand the task back to the appropriate person. My time management remains questionable and is an ongoing evaluation at my appraisal, however as my confidence has grown my career has grown with it and I have emerged as a leader. Reflective practice has played a major role within my development, using clinical supervision and ethical mapping techniques to challenge others and myself. I still learn through new experiences and challenges, people's reactions and effects of the conclusions reached. Dickson (1982) expressed:

'As women develop more familiarity with the skills, they learn how to be more reflective in situations instead of reacting only to the other person. Thinking and consequently acting with more clarity improves self confidence at a deep and fundamental level instead of muddling along, feeling generally burdened with worries and concerns, they learn to decide on priorities and to sort out who and what really does matter in their lives.' (p. 159)

Following the work of Dickson (1982) and gaining an understanding of the different behaviours that people can present with has opened my awareness of the way a situation is approached leading to successful conclusions.

Through the lived experience of conflict I have discussed, and the review of the leadership styles involved, I have become aware of the muddy puddle that exists within big organisations with several leaders working through differing agendas to reach one goal. The use of different leadership styles leads to clashes, breakdown in communication, resulting in a bad atmosphere and a negative working environment. Effective communication is the key, a leader who can inspire others to follow and belong to their vision, ensures a team approach and conflict remains minimal. I feel that Senge (1990) expressed this poignantly stating:

'If you can cut a photo in half, each half shows only part of the whole image. But if you divide a hologram, each part, no matter how small, shows the whole image intact. Likewise when a group of people come to share a vision in an organisation, each person sees a individual picture of the organisation at its best . . . the component pieces are not identical. Each represents the whole image from a different view . . . When you add up all the pieces of a hologram . . . the image becomes more intense. When more people come to share a vision, the vision becomes more real . . . people can truly imagine achieving [the vision].' (p. 212)

Although I feel that I am a little voice in a big arena, through embracing, empowering and inspiring others with my vision a little voice can forever grow bigger. This will not happen overnight or in a week's time but through continuous reflective practice, self regard and respect I will develop and grow. The leader inside me will be unleashed and continually embrace the changing world of the NHS.

Transformational leadership

Sally draws attention to the tension between transformational and transactional leadership. As a reflective practitioner she is mindful of her leadership and works towards realising the values of transformational leadership. Yet she works in an organisation that is deeply transactional. In her work she understands the tension and positions herself to safeguard her values whilst accommodating the demands of her managers. Sally's situation is not unusual. Indeed, it is a scenario played out daily across the health care arena, leaving nurses like Sally bruised and battered. The metaphor of 'band-aid' is very apposite. Sally needn't have been hurt in the first place within a transformational leadership culture.

Box 10.3   Transformational versus transactional leadership

Transformational leadership	Transactional leadership
Essentially mindful: leading towards realising values	Essentially mindless: reacting to resolve organisational objectives
Reliance on facilitative power – relational and expertise	Reliance on authoritative power – positional, coercive and reward
Invests in people towards shared vision and shared success	Views people in terms of tasks to be done
Views problems as a learning opportunity	Views problems as threats to order and control
Emphasis on process	Emphasis on outcomes
Seeks both negative and positive feedback to promote and develop the learning organisation	Seeks negative feedback to promote and protect the status quo
Grounded in collaborative relationships with colleagues	Grounded in bureaucratic relationships with subordinates

'round table'   'pyramid'

In Box 10.3 I set out a comparison between transformational and transactional leadership. As Sally highlights, transformational leadership is espoused as desirable within health care organisations, yet a transactional culture cannot accommodate transformational leaders because of the bureaucratic nature of health care driven by productivity anxiety. Transformational leadership is grounded in collaborative relationships with colleagues as symbolised by the 'round table', whereby each person within the team or organisation has an acknowledged significant role within the whole guided by shared vision. Each member respects and values each other's contribution and accepts responsibility to work collaboratively to realise the shared vision.

In contrast, within the transactional model as symbolised by the 'pyramid', the vision is set on high and imposed on those below. Because the vision is so lofty it is not easily visible and even the leaders lose sight of it as they become embroiled in the daily transactions to ensure the smooth running of the organisation. Transactional leadership is represented by the triangle with levels of status. At each level, the triangle repeats itself, a self-perpetuating system that seeks negative feedback to maintain control. Parental-child patterns of communication are the normal pattern of relationship and exaggerated (as illustrated in Sally's reflection) when there is a threat to control. These patterns are one-way, reflected in Sally's metaphor of having only a 'little voice'. Yet she did hold to her guns and her 'voice' was heard along distant corridors prompting the chief executive's band-aid response. When she was acknowledged and valued it was immensely surprising and healing. First, it should not be surprising, that only reflects the way Sally was perceived as a spanner in the works disrupting the system. At the moment she needed to be supported, she was made to feel more stressed and ultimately distressed by the anxiety of others. Wake up Chief Executives everywhere before it is too late. Effective support needs to be modelled through the system to combat the endemic anxiety.

In contrast, the transformational model is represented by an oval with the vision at the centre to guide the collaborative effort towards its realisation. In this model, each person values each other's unique input, reflected in the dominance of relational and expertise types of leadership power. Patterns of relationship are adult–adult, yet such pattern demands that each person accepts responsibility for both self and for the team.

And there's the rub. Consider again Cathy's story (Chapter 7) and envisage how differently her experience might have been if she worked within a transformational leadership culture.

The learning organisation

In exemplar 10.2 Susan Brooks reflects on her understanding of the learning organisation and the way she acts to create it through the role of a clinical supervisor within the wider ethos of transformational leadership. Susan's exemplar involves supervising a colleague in another clinical area to her own, thus contributing to the learning organisation on an organisational rather than her own local area. The reader might like to revisit and refresh the organisational issues of clinical supervision explored in Chapter 3.

REFLECTIVE EXEMPLAR 10.2 – CREATING AND SUSTAINING AN EFFECTIVE LEARNING ENVIRONMENT

The 1990 NHS and Community Care Act placed on organisations the statutory duty to provide effective quality care. In response NHS organisations have in recent years implemented a programme of clinical governance as a framework to fulfil this duty (Halligan & Donaldson 2001). Individual practitioners are expected and required by their employers to play an active part in such local clinical governance arrangements (Donaldson 2001). Individual learning, which may contribute to the emergence of the learning organisation, appears therefore to be a prescribed duty and nurses are particularly aware of their required commitment to the concept of lifelong learning and the statutory duty to maintain professional knowledge and competence (Department of Health 1999; Nursing and Midwifery Council

2002). Garside (1999) notes a natural tension between the necessary regulatory and professional surveillance culture in the NHS and the equally necessary developmental elements of learning where innovation and risk are welcomed. Garside (1999) admits that this tension between regulation and surveillance and learning and development is unlikely to disappear, but she does suggest that they can co-exist. It seems it is the task of the transformational leader to manage such tensions both proactively and creatively.

As a transformational leader, my task is to synthesise the five technologies that constitute the learning organisation: personal mastery, mental models, shared vision, team learning and systems thinking, as an integrated ensemble (see Box 10.1). The desirability of the creation of a learning organisation is widely supported in the literature, and Garside (1999) suggests that the application of the concept of the learning organisation is so patently self evident that it is merely a collision of theory and common sense.

While the desirability of the learning organisation appears incontrovertible, operationalising the concept is arguably problematic. Statutory and regulatory documents seem to assume an innate desire in individuals to learn, and indeed Senge (1990) writes that not only is it our nature to learn but we love to learn. Such assumptions in the current climatic conditions in the NHS may be difficult to support. The reality of today's NHS is that nurse shortages are reportedly reaching crisis point, establishment shortfall is nationally 20%, one third of all nurses are allocated no study time, and bed occupancy is running at 98% (Hall 2003). In such an environment, research records that NHS staff suffer considerably more stress than any other workforce with 28% recording levels above the symptom threshold (Wall *et al.* 1997). Further, few healthcare institutions can be described as learning organisations since in a system largely dominated by highly structured, hierarchical and historically determined professional demarcations, it is an infrequent occurrence that norms or assumptions are challenged or that the required unlearning or relearning takes place (Garside 1999). The task of managing these tensions and inspiring and motivating people to learn and contribute to the learning organisation in such a difficult, highly pressurised arena is one that I, as a transformational leader, recognise as a considerable challenge.

Senge (1990) writes that organisations learn only through individuals who learn. Individual learning alone does not guarantee organisational learning but without it no organisational learning occurs (Senge 1990). Truly excellent organisations are those that know how to tap people's commitment and capacity to learn at *all* levels of the organisation and therefore a crucial element of the learning organisation is that it pays attention to the role and development of every individual within it (Garside 1999; Senge 1990). This clearly suggests that the effective transformational leader should display a natural tendency to develop others and facilitate learning wherever staff members sit in the hierarchy of the NHS organisation. Good leadership can influence an organisation to act as an effective learning organisation, one that is responsive and adaptive to changes both from within and without to build an environment for better, safer health care (Moss 2001).

Malby (1996) suggests that reflection can lead to new mental models about how to do things differently and the development of the skill of reflective practice has certainly enabled me to know self more effectively, to frame and contextualise my own mental models and in a sense become more available to self. Johns (2002) writes that a core requirement is that the practitioner (i.e. myself) is available to work with others to realise desirable practice. In the context of leading, supporting and developing the learning organisation, I would argue that unless I am truly available and knowing to self, transference of such availability would be problematic. My developed ability to clarify my own personal perspectives on values and ethics through reflective practice combined with my understanding of the art and practice of the learning organisation has then implications for my transformational leadership capabilities within the context of organisational life and learning (Rippon 2001).

An organisation's capacity to learn can then be no greater than that of its members, and my role as clinical supervisor should enable me to facilitate such individual learning that contributes to the cultural transformation of the organisation into one that embraces learning as praxis (Senge 1990). As Johns identifies [see Chapter 3] clinical supervision explicitly intends to enable practitioners to realise, in collaboration with colleagues, each of the technologies that contribute to the learning organisation. The role of clinical supervision in the promotion of individual learning and the development of the learning organisation seems unquestionable, but many authors have written that its implementation may be fraught with difficulties. Cottrell (1999) notes that nurses' existing views of clinical supervision are all too often of a hostile, pseudoanalytic process of belittlement, criticism, shaming and the attribution of blame. The tensions between emancipatory and technical interests, particularly within bureaucratic cultures have also been suggested (Johns 2001a). Johns (2001a) opines that the emancipatory developmental and sustaining role of clinical supervision will be diminished in any interpretation of clinical supervision as a technical consumer protection methodology. A mandatory clinical supervision agenda within an organisation may suggest surveillance and lead to fear of retaliatory action from managers, and evidence suggests that some nurses covertly seek supervision outside the mandatory provision in these circumstances (Scanlon & Weir 1997). It seems then, that though widely espoused by governmental and professional bodies and achieving a form of hegemony among some managers of the nursing profession, clinical practitioners have not embraced the concept with a similar enthusiasm (Bond & Holland 1998; Gilbert 2001). Further, while some research evidence indicating its effectiveness exists, it seems that empirical validation is fraught with epistemological and conceptual problems (Burrow 1995; Goorapah 1997; Lyle 1998).

My role as clinical supervisor within this apparently confused, indeterminate and possibly hostile arena appears loaded with complication. It is here that my skills of transformational leadership need to be clearly demonstrated if the clinical supervision agenda is to contribute to the development of the learning organisation through therapeutic interaction with another. Johns (2001a) notes how the intent and emphasis of the supervisor can determine the nature of the supervisory experience. Working within a transformational paradigm, I am acutely aware that I need to take shared ownership of the clinical supervision sessions that I facilitate (alongside the supervisee) with the consequence that I (we) are in control of clinical supervision rather than being controlled by it. Without such customisation and ownership there is always the danger that clinical supervision and the intended learning may succumb to the transactional, manipulative, managerial and oppressive agenda that arguably constitutes the reality of the NHS today (Ghaye 2000a). Johns (2001a) poses a challenge when he asks whether clinical supervision can be accommodated to fit the existing culture or can the existing culture be shifted to the ideals of emancipatory supervision? For the transformational leader, a quite significant shift in the existing culture appears to be the desired state. My desire is to promote and liberate learning from experience within the clinical supervision relationship (the emancipatory element) rather than the production of a worker who can be monitored against specific criteria of what constitutes effectiveness (the technical element). This will hopefully contribute to the development of the learning organisation: one that is holistic, flexible, responsible, proactive and caring where contradictions between values and practices are identified and resolved (Johns 2003b; Senge 1990).

I have acted as clinical supervisor for almost two years within an advisory clinical supervision system in my current workplace. The organisation provides no formal training or support for clinical supervisors, which suggests that while it embraces the concept of clinical governance publicly, it may be covertly resisting the idea of clinical supervision as an emancipatory learning process for the organisation, since it may perceive it as a threat to established patterns of relating (Johns 2003). There seems no reciprocal agreement between the individual willing to learn through such supervision and the current organisational culture. While commitment is currently lacking and interpretation and introduction of clinical supervision in my own organisation is minimalist, future policy directives may mean that clinical supervision will become a 'must do' in the future (Bond & Holland 1998). My role as a transformational leader will be of critical importance once clinical supervision becomes mandatory within my organisation and I am hoping to influence the clinical supervision agenda, at least in my own work area toward the emancipatory rather than technical ideal. It is within this relatively unsupportive environment that, as Johns (2001a) noted, my own intent and emphasis determines the clinical supervision experience.

I have acted as clinical supervisor to Sarah, a junior staff nurse for six months. I am not Sarah's direct line manager nor do I work in the same clinical area; although our supervisor/supervisee relationship is mutually agreed and voluntary. The following discussion and illumination of recent clinical supervision sessions will explore my role in Sarah's learning and demonstrates my commitment to contribute to the emergence of the spirit of the learning organisation (Senge 1990). I had tacitly (and possibly naively) assumed that Sarah did not feel that I was monitoring her clinical perform-ance since we do not work together but reflected recently that Sarah and I have never discussed or clarified this aspect of our relationship. Perhaps this demonstrates my lack of knowledge at the time when we commenced the clinical relationship since I now recognise clearly the need to develop formal contracts with supervisees to clarify roles and meaning in the relationship if learning is to occur (Bond & Holland 1998). I remained undecided about the accuracy of my assumption regarding Sarah's perception (although I had intended to discuss it with her) until the following incident occurred.

It was the end of a clinical supervision session where a completely unre-lated issue concerning drug administration was discussed. As Sarah got up to leave the room she made some comments which, at the time, appeared almost inconsequential to her but which caused me deep reflection:

Sarah: "Well I had better get back to the ward now. It's not that I don't want to or that I don't care but I just find it so difficult to look after people like Mary with her dementia. She can't do anything for herself – she just lies there all day without doing anything or saying anything to anyone not even her husband or family. I never feed her – I can't bear it. I always get the health care assistants to do it. I can't help feeling that I don't like that sort of nursing. It's so unrewarding but I'd never tell anyone else that, it doesn't seem right does it?"

Sarah and I parted company without further comment being made. I was immediately concerned that, in six months of supervising Sarah, I had not encountered such a forthright expression of attitude from her that I instantly felt so uncomfortable with. I was, however, aware that the prevalence of negative attitudes toward the care of older people among the nursing pro-fession is widely reported (Courtney *et al*. 2000; Wade 1999). It seemed that although Sarah sensed a real tension between her professional role require-ment and her personal feelings she felt comfortable enough to express them to me. This signified that she did not see me in a surveillance role but my instant reaction was to feel transactional with the desire to confront Sarah about her poor performance and attitude, as I perceived it. However, I recognised that such a stance may change the nature of our supervisory rela-tionship and prove a stumbling block to learning in an unthreatening envir-onment in the future. A further concern of mine was that Sarah's honest expression perhaps signified that she felt I would have no concerns about her statement and possibly shared her opinions, which I did not. I considered previous clinical supervision sessions. Had Sarah and I suffered a learning bind where we had previously missed each other's meaning in the inter-pretation of our practice and values? Schön (1987) suggests that the ability to escape from such a learning bind depends on the supervisor's ability to reflect on the supervisor/supervisee dialogue and this I did extensively prior to the next session. Of necessity, the supervision sessions have not been described here in their entirety, although this has not distorted the essential nature of the reality of the interaction between myself and Sarah.

When Sarah arrived for her next supervision session I asked her if she would like to talk about Mary, since she seemed to find caring for her difficult. Sarah's immediate agreement signified that this was indeed something that she wished to share. At this point I was acutely aware that this situation leant itself clearly to a process of learning through guided reflective practice. Many authors write that reflective practice for both the supervisor and supervisee is intimately bound with the process of clinical supervision (Ghaye 2000b; Heath & Freshwater 2000; Power 1999). Johns (2003) describes guided reflection as a way of structuring the clinical supervision space and such reflective practice can aid the development of the learning organisation with great potential to lever quality and effective practice (Garside 1999).

I was acutely aware of the need to suspend my own values and assumptions in order to avoid a transactional, technical interest intent in the supervision sessions. I consciously worked hard to manage the creative tensions that existed for me between my own vision of what nursing should be and where I currently saw Sarah's practice and attitudes (Senge 1990). If we assume that the effective practitioner takes responsibility to ensure and monitor their own effectiveness then the role of the supervisor is not to sit in judgement but to enable the practitioner to make such judgements for herself (Johns 2001a). However, within clinical supervision there needs to be an element of challenge but this needs to be managed carefully to avoid a spiral of increasing challenge from the supervisor and resultant increasing resistance from the supervisee (Heath & Freshwater 2000; Smith 2000). I introduced Sarah to the Model of Structured Reflection as a way of focusing self challenge and to structure her deconstruction of her experiences in order to lead to new insights that could be applied to her practice. The model particularly lends itself to the development of the learning organisation described by Senge (1990) since it requires the reflector to embark on the journey toward personal mastery, surface mental models, explore vision, consider learning and knowledge of self and others (team learning) and examine how these disciplines fit into the whole system. Sarah and I discussed the issues at length and some of her comments were very illuminating:

Sarah: "Lots of old people get dementia don't they? I wonder what causes it and if it runs in families? My Grandma had it when I was little. She used to scare me and she didn't even seem to know who I was. I remember her wetting my Mum's settee one Christmas and my Dad got really cross and shouted at her. She ended up in a home and I don't remember seeing her after that. It's frightening to think anyone could end up like that."

Guided by the reflective model, Sarah and I discussed the origin and influence of her mental models at length and explored how they influenced her practice (Senge 1990). Johns' (2002) range of framing perspectives were also used within the guided reflective process and these served as cues to challenge Sarah to further explore her reflective learning potential. Sarah offered the opinion that she really felt she knew nothing significant about dementia but thought perhaps that she should and she asked if I could recommend anything for her to read. While mindful of the need to avoid the perception that I had greater skills or knowledge than Sarah (often detrimental in the clinical supervision relationship since it may suggest supervisor authority), I provided her with some relevant references without offering any opinion on their value (Power 1999). Sarah left the session professing a determination to think about our discussion and visit the library for more information:

When Sarah attended her next supervision session it quickly became obvious that she had reflected quite deeply on our session, undertaken some personal learning and reading and had applied this to her practice. She related her recent experience to me:

Sarah: "I've got to know Mary and Bill and they seem a really nice couple. Do you know Bill was telling me that during the war he didn't see Mary at all for three years. All that time she was looking after their little girl and working in a factory making aircraft parts and at night she did fire watching. That must have been so hard for her. Bill said Mary loved dancing and really missed it when the arthritis got so bad. I've seen photos of them in dance competitions and she looks lovely with her hair and make up all done."

Sarah continued with Mary and Bill's life story which signified that she now recognised and valued their person-hood. I asked Sarah if she felt more able to nurse Mary now and Sarah confirmed that she was happily taking a more active role in caring for Mary on a daily basis.

Sarah: "I think I was scared before because I didn't understand what was happening to Mary but I knew that I didn't feel right about the way I acted. Reading those articles you gave me and talking to my Mum about my own Grandma when she was young made me think that perhaps I'd missed something. It was only when I started to talk to Bill that I realised I'd been avoiding him and Mary. She had been a patient with us for two weeks and I knew nothing about her! I've noticed other people acting the same as I did and perhaps I can do something about that. I feel like a better nurse now and I've joined the Care of the Older Person Link Group. I might even go and do a course or something."

To me, Sarah's most significant statement came at the end of our session – again just as she was leaving the room:

Sarah: "Thanks a lot – I feel better about it all now and I've learnt a lot but I need to think about things a bit more don't I? I'm using that [reflective] model you gave me now and writing things down. See you next time!"

It seemed that for Sarah, real learning had occurred. Guided reflective practice had been used effectively within an emancipatory clinical supervision space and Freshwater notes that given the right environment even the neophyte nurse has the ability to reflect in depth and develop an increased capacity for autonomy and accountability (cited in Heath & Freshwater 2000). Through the learning process, Sarah had achieved some control of the creative tension that existed, where the current reality of her practice did not match the vision of her nursing care that she professed to hold. In this way, she had enhanced her own sense of personal mastery and now felt a 'better nurse' (Senge 1990). She had re-examined her vision for nursing and now felt she shared and lived the vision of nursing as a profession. Whether the vision of nursing as a profession matches that of the organisation with the performance versus process dilemma is an issue that would merit further examination. Sarah had surfaced and challenged the mental models that influenced her understanding of the issues through an engagement of self with self awareness and had accepted an internal locus of self control and responsibility for her own actions – the heart of professional practice (Heath & Freshwater 2000).

Sarah's personal learning had highlighted other learning needs within her team and she had resolved to join a group dedicated to learning about the care of older people and to share this with others. Senge (1990) describes such team learning as vital since teams, not individuals, are the fundamental learning unit in modern organisations. Finally, Sarah had learnt the importance of systems thinking and now seemed to understand the interaction between the other disciplines (personal mastery, shared vision, mental models and team thinking) and how they collectively create reality (Senge 1990).

Individual learning had occurred and an investment of my energies into the role of clinical supervisor had guided, rather than determined, the outcome. A transformational approach meant that I had avoided the transactional, technical interest intent of clinical supervision where monitoring, surveillance and a focus on role performance are evident. Rather, the transformational skills of effective communication, honesty and empathy, development of others and risk taking, experimentation and learning were all utilised to ensure that Sarah was guided on her own emancipatory learning journey of self awareness and discovery (Schuster 1994). I had introduced Sarah to a reflective model that I hoped would frame and inform her reflection in the future, particularly enhancing her learning in Schön's (1987) 'swampy lowlands' of nursing where situations are characterised by uncertainty but where the problems of greatest human concern occur. Sarah is clearly only one person in a very large organisation, one that is not currently particularly in tune with the concept of the learning organisation, and her learning may appear insignificant to some in the larger picture. Yet, organisations learn only through individuals who learn – people like Sarah, a junior staff nurse (Senge 1990).

The National Health Service has a long history of firmly established traditions and authoritarian practices. A cultural transformation will arguably be necessary if organisational learning which embraces new and expansive patterns of thinking, leading to real service wide quality improvements is to be developed (Senge 1990). It would seem that contributing to the emergence of a learning organisation from the current cultural stance poses a considerable challenge and requires real determination from the transformational health care practitioner/leader of today. For the transformational leader the spirit of learning and enquiry is an ever-present entity, and my contribution and commitment to the learning of both myself and others is a key aspect of my role, since the active force of any learning organisation must be the people who work there. Finally, my own sense of personal mastery has developed through this work, since I am aware that both Sarah and I have contributed to the learning organisation. We have created a more effective practice environment by working through an experience, identifying areas for growth, and generating the learning needed to achieve positive results.

Nurturing the learning organisation

On May 14 2003 I reflected with the second year masters in clinical leadership group, including Susan Brooks, on what factors might nurture the learning organisation as a whole and the discrete technologies that contributed to the whole. Reviewing each of Senge's technologies, vision is the fundamental technology that gives meaning and direction to practice. Hence the primary role of the leader is to constantly sharpen the focus of vision and engage colleagues to develop personal mastery. Clinical supervision provides the ideal learning milieu for personal mastery because it is grounded in both self and self's practice, as evidenced in Susan's essay, in Sarah's gradual realisation of herself in relation to Mary and Bill. In doing so she began to reveal to herself her mental models and systems that had reduced Mary and Bill into objects of despair.

Perhaps group clinical supervision might create the conditions for team learning; for Sarah to engage in guided dialogue with her colleagues about practice. Other opportunities include setting and reviewing standards of care, clinical audit, de-briefing (see Chapter 8) and shift reports (see Chapter 9). I have touched on the nature of dialogue at diverse points but its significance as the core condition for creating and sustaining the learning organisation cannot be overemphasised. Dialogue is the natural enactment of being mindful. Isaacs (1993) describes dialogue:

'as a movement towards creating a field of genuine meeting and inquiry where people can allow a *free flow of meaning* and vigorous exploration of the collective background of their thought, their personal pre-dispositions, the nature of their shared attention, and the rigid features of their individual and collective assumptions . . . as people learn to perceive, inquire into and allow transformation of the nature and shape of these fields, and the patterns of individual thinking and acting that inform them, they may discover entirely new levels of insight and forge substantive and, at times, dramatic changes in behaviour. As this happens, whole new possibilities for co-ordinated action develop.' (p. 25)

On an individual level this emergence of meaning and transformation happened for Sarah. However, the masters' cohort strongly believed that the initial focus should be on personal mastery so as to create the conditions for effective team learning. In other words, until the individual practitioner has accepted responsibility for her own practice and learning and developed a degree of personal mastery, she may be threatened by and resist team learning situations.

Teaching through reflective practice

Reflective practice is learning through experience towards realising self. As such, the student must consider what realising self means. I use the framing perspectives as lenses for the student to see self through (see Box 1.10). In particular, the philosophical and role-framing perspectives challenge the student to grasp a sense of what realising self might mean. As teaching is centred in the student's experience the teacher *must* create the conditions to enable the student to reveal self safely in group situations (see Chapter 3, clinical supervision). The teacher becomes a guide, guiding the students to learn through their experiences; shifting the milieu of the classroom from teacher-centred to student-centred. As such, reflective teaching is opening both the student and teacher to imagination, creativity and possibility, beyond the rational demand. The teacher must let go of the life raft of control to flow with what is unfolding, to surf the waves. It's okay to be thrown from time to time. Becoming a master requires practice, vulnerability, humility and courage. If we who teach ask this of our students then we must ask it of ourselves.

Camp fire teaching

On the Palliative Care courses I teach at Luton University, I dialogue with students by sitting with them around the *camp fire* where we share our stories of caring, seeking to learn through our shared experiences to transcend and expand the horizons of our understandings. My stories trigger their own stories; to capture meaning and evoke the imagination, and to take them deep within themselves. Sangharakshita (1993), in his book *The Drama of Cosmic Enlightenment*, tells the story of how Buddha taught through parable or story. He quotes the Buddha as saying, 'Through a parable, intelligent people reach understanding' (p. 70).

Sangharakshita continues by saying:

> 'Sometimes it is not easy to understand things when they are put in a dry abstract, conceptual manner, but with the help of a story much becomes clear.' (p. 70)

I need to access my own stories of caring because only if you have touched the essence of caring and continue to dwell in caring can you facilitate such ways of being with others. Teaching in this way inspires students to write their own stories and in doing so they become more aware of themselves within their practice and pay attention to the subtle nuances of caring that make the difference in effective palliative care. It is often the first time they have engaged themselves within the teaching process and addressed such issues as contemplating their own death and spirituality.

Sometimes I light a candle, especially if my stories concern someone who has died. Lighting the candle is a way of honouring the person and introducing ritual into the classroom. It is also symbolic of the camp fire – the fire that draws us together in a sacred space.

The mode of teaching is dialogue – listening to each other carefully, listening to the mystery of suffering and responding to suffering that the stories reveal. As Thomas Moore (1992) says:

> 'The basic intention in any caring is to alleviate suffering. But in relation to the symptom itself, observation means first of all listening and looking carefully at what is being revealed in the suffering.' (p. 10)

The process is valuable because it helps the student socialised into being busy and reactive pause to listen to herself – the way she is listening and responding to the stories. It makes her examine her own assumptions and feelings about herself and her practice. And when she returns to practice perhaps she will listen more carefully to her patients, her colleagues and herself.

> 'We must slow down or we will miss all that has meaning. Meaning is revealed only when you pause, when you stop, when you pay attention. Learn the lesson of tribal people. Put your busyness on pause, eliminate distractions, and allow the meaning of life and living return to you. Slow down in order to connect with the meaning of life.' (Blackwolf & Gina Jones 1996, p. 90)

As appropriate relevant readings from literature, for example the quotes from Thomas Moore and Blackwolf and Gina Jones, theories and research can be fed into the dialogue, weaving the voices as we construct knowing (Belenky *et al.* 1986 – see Chapter 1). The significance of the camp fire is reinforced by the fact that the students submit a portfolio of reflections as their assignment. Reflective teaching opens the door for the teacher's own learning: by listening to stories, the teacher must also reflect and consider the words in terms of his or her own experiences. Matthew (1995) says of St. John the Cross:

> 'John could create because he could learn; he was co-pupil not simply master.' (p. 14)

Matthew cites Francesca, a sister in the Bea community where St. John of the Cross worked:

> ' "It seemed as if every word we spoke to him opened a door for him".' (p. 14)

The moral is to listen not to lecture, to let go of knowing in order to be open to the learning possibilities within each moment.

Masters in clinical leadership

This innovative two year programme [see Box 10.4] is held together by the dissertation module in which the student researches self-being and becoming a clinical leader using guided reflection methodology. The remaining modules inform this process. As a consequence, the programme is constructed around this emerging journey of realising self as a transformational clinical leader. Along the journey, the hurdles that constrain the self's emergence are identified, understood and worked toward resolving. We have learnt quickly that moving from transactional to transformational leadership is not a smooth continuum but a radical creative tension between the reality of the organisation and transformational ideals. It is the cutting edge that creates the learning opportunity.

Hence the objective of the first semester is to enable the students to:

- understand health policy to grasp the edges of the shifting health care arena
- appreciate the leadership literature and positioning self within it, for example using Schuster's (1994) leadership model that outlines the range of skills needed to provide such leadership and support and guide others through the learning process from the transformational perspective (see Box 10.5 and consider the extent Sally and Susan, in exemplars 10.1 and 10.2 exhibit these characteristics within their reflective writing)
- manage conflict collaboratively in responding to conflict situations in congruent ways with transformational values. The 'managing conflict' module is constructed as a guided reflection group whereby the students are guided to learn through their stories of conflict – Sally's reflection is an example of this.

Box 10.4 Masters in clinical leadership programme

	Semester 1	Semester 2	Semester 3
Year 1	• Managing everyday conflict • Strategic policy development	• Alternative perspectives on leadership	• Research methodologies • Managing change and developing clinical practice
Year 2	• Clinical audit for clinical effectiveness • Creating and sustaining an effective practice environment • Work on dissertation	• Innovating the learning organisation • Work on dissertation	• Dissertation write up

The semester 2 module, 'Alternative perspectives on leadership' enables the student to observe and judge another leader within leadership frameworks (for example Schuster's characteristics of the transformational leader – see Box 10.5), and then to contrast with her own emerging leadership style. By now the student has a deeper understanding of the leadership literature juxtaposed with herself as leader. The module is constructed as an 'action learning set', whereby the students use the group as the resource to help them explore their experience and construct their 'report'. In doing so they develop the art of dialogue and a 'community of inquiry' essential to team learning processes and the course as a whole (Senge 1990).

In semester 3 the student writes a proposal for her dissertation, exploring the diverse philosophical influences and pragmatics involved. About this time the student draws a line under the first eight months on the programme, a making sense of the journey so far in focusing her dissertation work. The 'Managing change' module is very practical, focusing on leading a change project through its development, implementation, and evaluation phases. Central to the assignment work is a treatise on resistance, reinforcing the theme of self in context of the organisation.

In semester 4 the students undertake two modules, 'Clinical audit for clinical effectiveness' and 'Creating and sustaining the learning organisation'. The 'Clinical audit for clinical effectiveness' module is organised by the students drawing on their own resources to inform and dialogue with each other as an action learning set with teacher guidance at-a-distance. This arrangement intends to reinforce the students' own learning resources and responsibility to both contribute and deepen the 'community of inquiry'.

'Creating and sustaining the learning organisation' module, as Susan Brooks' reflection reveals, guides the student to focus on developing the learning organisation as a lived reality. To succeed in this enterprise is the transformational leader's primary aim. As with the other 'reflective' modules, the learning is grounded in understanding and developing the student's own practice; a work-based learning approach whereby the student can construct the assignment in ways that are most meaningful and practical whilst enabling a continuous dialogue between theoretical ideas and practice.

In semester 5 the students are taken on a journey into chaos theory, a process of letting go and being pulled away from the bonds that have wrapped the students in organisational spin. The course has unfolded through each semester to the brink of personal revelation and the understanding of chaos theory spirals them into the creative spaces necessary to pursue their dissertation and self-realisation as a clinical leader. It is an acknowledgement of the complex, unitary, contradictory, quantum, nature of practice whereby the illusionary Newtonian rules are exposed as deeply flawed and obstructive to transformational leadership. Control is achieved by embracing uncertainty as a creative flow not by trying to shut it down. The vibration of a butterfly's wings is deeply felt as a potential significant moment. It is as if the world is turned on its head.

Box 10.5   Schuster (1994): 13 qualities for the transformational leader to cultivate

	Characteristic	5	4	3	2	1
1	You hold a vision for the organisation that is intellectually rich, stimulating and rings true.					
2	You are honest and empathetic. People feel emotionally safe and trust that you have their interests at heart.					
3	Your character is well-developed, without the prominent dark side of ego power – your behaviour aligns with your words.					
4	You set aside your own interests in looking good and getting strokes, instead making others look good and giving others power and credit.					
5	You evince a concern for the whole (not just your organisation) reflected in your passionate and ethical voice being heard when necessary.					
6	Your natural tendency is to develop others to become engaged, deepen perspectives and be effective.					
7	You can share power with others – you believe sharing power is the best way to tap talent, engage others, and to get work done in optimal fashion.					
8	You risk, experiment and learn. Information is never complete.					
9	You have a true passion for work and the vision. That's evident in commitment of time, attention to detail, and ability to renew your energy.					
10	You effectively communicate, both listening and speaking.					
11	You understand and appreciate management and administration. They appreciate that – you move towards shared success without sacrifice.					
12	You celebrate the now. At meetings or wherever, you sincerely acknowledge accomplishment, staying in the moment before moving on.					
13	You persist in hard times. That means you have the courage to move ahead when you're tired, conflicted and getting mixed signals.					

Following semester 5, the students continue to work in guided group tutorials to develop their emerging dissertations. The course is an unfolding drama of creative tension with a loosely held agenda able to move in tune with the forces at play, itself tripping the fine line between negative feedback to ensure some order and positive feedback to create the creative space. In other words, the course is itself chaotic – as indeed it must be to succeed.

In summary, teaching through reflective practice can claim a number of advantages:

- it facilitates student-led practice
- it is grounded in the students' own practice – thus the course is both practical and meaningful
- it is more holistic, through the use of stories
- it is 'whole brain' teaching
- it introduces theory in relation to emerging issues – hence it is easier to relate to and assimilate within personal knowing
- it develops learning on an intuitive level and thus more suited to experienced and expert practitioners (see Chapter 1)
- it accesses the swampy lowlands where real issues lie rather than focus on hard high ground of abstract concepts
- it values and honours everyday practice
- it is values-based, constantly challenging and clarifying vision and purpose, pulling practitioners out of a predominantly 'doing' focus
- it is real-world-based, seeking understanding and meaning of why things are as they are
- it is problem solving, focusing on areas of contradiction, ethics, politics, tradition, power and change; enabling practitioners to become empowered and assertive
- it makes a difference to practice
- it is supportive, dynamic and engaging

Disadvantages?

- Perhaps some students may feel threatened by the intense gaze particularly if they lack commitment to practice or study. It is less prescriptive and therefore more 'adult' and requires more responsibility and self-direction.
- It is harder work than conventional learning, because it requires the critique and juxtaposition of theory with practice.
- The teacher or guide may not be good enough; stuck in traditional modes of teaching leading to issues of control or viewing reflection as an educational technology rather than an organic evolving process.

It is not good enough to tag reflection onto conventional programmes, it needs space to fulfil its learning potential. For example, on a pre-registration diploma or degree programme, I would have reflective practice as the core throughout the programme, at least 4 hours a week, to enable the students to reflect on clinical placements:

- understanding and working to resolve the contradictions and feelings that practice reveals
- as a way of integrating theory and practice
- as a supportive self development programme

Appendix 1

Clinical Supervision Evaluation Tool

This tool has been designed to enable you to reflect on the quality of your individual or group supervision. The information will facilitate giving feedback to your supervisor concerning the effectiveness of supervision.

How long have you been in supervision with your current supervisor?	
Is your supervisor (please circle)	Line manager Non-line manager within the organisation Outside the organisation
What is your grade?	
What is the grade/position of your supervisor?	
How frequently did you contract supervision?	Every................. days
How frequently (on average) do you actually have supervision?	Every............... days

Whilst completing the tool is perhaps time-consuming, please complete it carefully and honestly. *In particular please comment on your scores with specific examples.*

Mark along each scale the extent you agree with each statement:
5   most strongly agree
1   least agree

1	I felt safe to disclose my experiences	5 4 3 2 1

Comment

2	It was easy to identify experiences to reflect on	5 4 3 2 1

Comment

3	I always came to each session prepared to share an experience	5 4 3 2 1

Comment

4	I never cancelled sessions	5	4	3	2	1

Comment

5	The balance of challenge and support was excellent (I didn't feel too threatened or comfortable)	5	4	3	2	1

Comment

6	Supervision has inspired me	5	4	3	2	1

Comment

7	Supervision helped me clarify key issues and gain new insights into my practice	5	4	3	2	1

Comment

8	I have become very reflective	5	4	3	2	1

Comment

9	I have become more open and curious about my practice	5	4	3	2	1

Comment

10	I felt I was being moulded into becoming a 'supervisor' clone	5	4	3	2	1

Comment

11	I have become aware of the factors that influence the way I think, feel and respond within situations	5	4	3	2	1

Comment

12	I am more aware/focused on my role responsibility, authority, and autonomy	5	4	3	2	1

Comment

13	The input of theory was both relevant and substantial	5	4	3	2	1

Comment

14	Work has become more meaningful and interesting	5	4	3	2	1

Comment

15	Supervision picked me up when I felt overwhelmed	5	4	3	2	1

Comment

16	Reflection has helped me to express my ideas, opinions, and feelings	5	4	3	2	1

Comment

17	Supervision enabled me to tackle issues that I might otherwise would have avoided	5	4	3	2	1

Comment

18	Supervision helped me deal with negative emotions (such as anger, failure, outrage, guilt, distress, resentment)	5	4	3	2	1

Comment

19	I am more in control of 'who I am'	5	4	3	2	1

Comment

20	My supervisor really listened to me	5	4	3	2	1

Comment

21	I was happy with my supervisor	5	4	3	2	1

Comment

22	I never felt judged by my supervisor	5	4	3	2	1

Comment

23	We constantly reviewed the way supervision has helped me to develop and sustain my practice	5	4	3	2	1

Comment

| 24 | We always commenced each session by reviewing the previous session | 5 | 4 | 3 | 2 | 1 |

Comment

| 25 | Supervision sessions were never interrupted | 5 | 4 | 3 | 2 | 1 |

Comment

| 26 | I always knew what I needed to do at the end of each session | 5 | 4 | 3 | 2 | 1 |

Comment

| 27 | My supervisor always wanted 'to fix' the problem for me | 5 | 4 | 3 | 2 | 1 |

Comment

| 28 | My supervisor was overly parental and patronising | 5 | 4 | 3 | 2 | 1 |

Comment

| 29 | The environment for supervision was excellent | 5 | 4 | 3 | 2 | 1 |

Comment

Use this space to make any further comment

Appendix 2

Patients Enjoy a Nutritious Meal Scan Sheet

	The patient receives a meal:	3: yes 2: so-so 1: no score + comment
1	That he/she has chosen within limits	
2	In an amount he/she can enjoy	
3	That suits their dietary requirements	
4	At the correct temperature	
5	In an environment conducive to eating	
6	On a clean table	
7	With a drink within reach	
8	That they are not rushed to complete	
9	With assistance as required	
10	Where they are not interrupted	
11	They were prepared for	
12	Where any underlying symptom that might impair enjoyment has been adequately responded to: Constipation, diarrhoea, nausea, fatigue, pain etc	
13	Other factors: Please state:	

Appendix 3

List of Potential Standards in Complete Response to the National Care Standards Commission

No	Descriptor	Key worker[s]
1	Discharge & transfer	
2	Admission: 'what information do we need to know?'	
3	Patient rights are known and honoured	
3a	Patients with medical emergencies: Resuscitation	
4	Patients receive prescribed medications safely	
5	Patients can self medicate as appropriate safely	
6	Patient risk of infection is minimised	
7	Respite care	
	Patients feel their individuality, privacy and dignity is respected/involved in decision making (resuscitation)	
	Patients and their families received best care (to ease suffering) (in line with nationally respected best practice)	(this is a core standard that links the specific care standards together)
8	Oral hygiene (draft)	
9	Hygiene/skin needs (draft)	
10	Management of bowels (draft)	
11	Management of pain	
12	Breathlessness & fatigue	
13	Nausea and vomiting	

No	Descriptor	Key worker[s]
14	Sleep	
15	Patient emotional and spiritual needs	
16	Sedation and agitation (anxiety/fear)	
17	Nutrition	
18	Comfort/moving and handling	
19	Bereavement	
20	Relatives feel informed, involved and supported	
21	Creating a therapeutic and safe environment	
22	Complementary therapies/non-pharmacological approaches to care	
23	Wound care	
24	Laying out following death/after death care	
25	Staff responsibility/support/development	
26	Management & leadership	

References

Alexander, L. (1998) Writing in hospices. In *The Arts in Health Care: A Palette of Possibilities* (Kaye, C. & Blee, T., eds) Jessica Kingsley Publishers, London.

Alfano, G. (1971) Healing or caretaking – which will it be? *Nursing Clinics of North America* **6**(2); 273–80.

Argyris, C. & Schön, D. (1989) *Theory in Practice: Increasing Professional Effectiveness*, 2nd edn. Jossey-Bass, London.

Armitage, S. (1990) Research utilisation in practice. *Nurse Education Today* **10**: 10–15.

Atkinson, R. L., Atkinson, R. C. & Smith, E. (1990) *Introduction to Psychology*. Harcourt Brace, New York.

Autton, N. (1996) The use of touch in palliative care. *European Journal of Palliative Care* **3**(3): 121–4.

Batehup, L. & Evans, A. (1992) A new strategy. *Nursing Times* **88**(47): 40–41.

Batey, M. & Lewis, F. (1982) Clarifying autonomy and accountability in nursing service, part 1. *The Journal of Nursing Administration* **12**(9): 13–18

Begley, A-M. (1996) Literature and poetry: pleasure and practice. *International Journal of Nursing Practice* **2**: 182–8.

Belenky, M. F., Clinchy, B. M., Goldberger, N. R. & Tarule, J. M. (1986) *Women's Ways of Knowing: The Development of Self, Voice, and Mind*. Basic Books, New York.

Benjamin, M. & Curtis, J. (1986) *Ethics in Nursing*, 2nd edn. Oxford University Press, New York.

Benner, P. (1984) *From Novice to Expert*. Addison-Wesley, Menlo Park.

Benner, P., Tanner, C. & Chesla, C. (1996) *Expertise in Nursing Practice: Caring, Clinical Judgement, and Ethics*. Springer, New York.

Benner, P. & Wrubel, J. (1989) *The Primacy of Caring*. Addison-Wesley, Menlo Park.

Betz, M. & O'Connell, L. (1987) Primary nursing: panacea or problem? *Nursing and Health Care* **8**: 456–60.

Bohm, D. (1996) *On Dialogue* (Nichol, L., ed.) Routledge, London.

Bond, M. & Holland, S. (1998) *Skills of Clinical Supervision for Nurses*. Open University Press, Buckingham.

Boud, D., Keogh, R. & Walker, D. (1985) Promoting reflection in learning: a model. In *Reflection: Turning Experience into Learning* (Boud, D., Keogh, R. & Walker, D. eds) Kogan Page, London.

Boyd, E. & Fales, A. (1983) Reflective learning: key to learning from experience. *Journal of Humanistic Psychology* **23**(2): 99–117.

Breu, C. & Dracup, K. (1976) Implementing nursing research in a critical care setting. *Journal of Nursing Administration*. December.

Brodersen, L. (2001) Creatively capturing care: poetry and knowledge in nursing. *International Journal for Human Caring* **6**(1): 33–41.

Bruner, J. (1994) The remembered self. In *The Remembering Self: Construction and Accuracy in the Self Narrative* (Neisser, U. & Fivush, R., eds). Cambridge University Press, New York.

Buckenham, J. & McGrath, G. (1983) *The Social Reality of Nursing*. Adis, Sydney.

Burnard, P. & Morrison, P. (1991) Nurses' interpersonal skills: a study of nurses' perceptions. *Nurse Education Today* **11**: 24–9.

Burns, J. (1978) *Leadership*. Harper Row, New York.

Burrow, S. (1995) Supervision: Clinical Development or Managerial Control? *British Journal of Nursing* **4**: 879–82.

Burton, A. (2000) Reflection: nursing's practice and education panacea? *Journal of Advanced Nursing* **31**(5): 1009–17.

Butterfield, P. (1990) Thinking upstream: nurturing a conceptual understanding of the societal context of health behaviour. *Advances in Nursing Science* **12**(2): 1–8.

Callahan, S. (1988) The role of emotion in ethical decision making. *Hastings Center Report* **18**: 9–14.

Callanan, S. & Kelley, P. (1992) *Final Gifts*. Bantam Books, New York.

Campbell, J. (1988) *The Power of Myth*. Doubleday, New York.

Carmack, B. (1997) Balancing engagement and detachment in caregiving. *Image: Journal of Nursing Scholarship* **29**(2): 139–43.

Carp, F. & Carp, A. (1981) The validity, reliability and generalisability of diary data. *Experimental Aging Research* **7**(3): 281–96.

Carper, B. (1978) Fundamental patterns of knowing in nursing. *Advances in Nursing Science* **1**(1): 13–23.

Casement, P. (1985) *On Learning From the Patient*. Routledge, London.

Cavanagh, S. (1991) The conflict management style of staff nurses and nurse managers. *Journal of Advanced Nursing* **16**: 1254–60.

Chang, Ok Sung (2001) The conceptual structure of physical touch in caring. *Journal of Advanced Nursing* **33**(6): 820–27.

Chapman, G. (1983) Ritual and rational action in hospitals. *Journal of Advanced Nursing* **8**: 13–20.

Cherniss, G. (1980) *Professional Burn-out in Human Service Organisations*. Praeger, New York.

Cioffi, J. (1997) Heuristics, servants to intuition, in clinical decision making. *Journal of Advanced Nursing* **26**: 203–8.

Cixous, H. (1996) Sorties: Out and point: attacks/ways out/forays. In *The Newly Born Woman* (Cixous, H. & Clement, H. C.) Tauris, London.

Cochran, L. & Laub, L. (1994) *Becoming an Agent: Patterns and Dynamics for Shaping your Life*. State University of New York Press, Albany.

Coleman, P. (1986) *Ageing and Reminiscence Processes*. John Wiley, Chichester.

Cooper, M. (1991) Principle-oriented ethics and the ethic of care: a creative tension. *Advances in Nursing Science* **14**(2): 22–31.

Cope, M. (2001) *Lead Yourself: Be Where Others Will Follow*. Pearson Education, London.

Cotton, A. (2001) Private thoughts in public spheres: issues in reflection and reflective practices in nursing. *Journal of Advanced Nursing* **36**(4): 512–19.

Cottrell, S. (1999) Some current beliefs in the NHS and some consequences for implementing clinical supervision. Excerpt from conference address. http://www.clinical-supervision.com (accessed 18/03/03).

Courtney, M., Tong, S. & Walsh, A. (2000) Acute Care Nurses' Attitudes Towards Older People: A Literature Review. *International Journal of Nursing Practice* **6**: 62–9.

Cowling, W. R. (2000) Healing as appreciating wholeness. *Advances in Nursing Science* **22**(3): 16–32.

Cox, H., Hickson, P. & Taylor, B. (1991) Exploring reflection: knowing and constructing practice. In *Towards a Discipline of Nursing* (Gray, G. & Pratt, R., eds) pp. 373–90. Churchill Livingstone, Melbourne.

Davidhizar, R. & Giger, J. (1997) When touch is not the best approach. *Journal of Clinical Nursing* **6**(3): 203–6.

Dawson, J. (1987) Evaluation of a community based night sitter service. In *Research in the Nursing Care of the Elderly* (Fielding, P., ed). John Wiley, Chichester.

Day, C. (1993) Reflection: a necessary but not sufficient condition for professional development. *British Educational Research Journal* **19**(1): 83–93.

De Hennezel, M. (1997) *Intimate Death: How the Dying Teach us to Live* (trans. C. Janeway) Warner Books, London.

De La Cuesta, C. (1983) The nursing process: from development to implementation. *Journal of Advanced Nursing* **8**: 365–71.

Department of Health (1990) *National Health Service and Community Care Act*. HMSO, London.

Department of Health (1996) *Clinical Audit in the NHS*. HMSO, London.

Department of Health (1999) *Making A Difference*. The Stationery Office, London.

Department of Health & Social Security (1972) *Report of the Committee on Nursing* (Chairperson Professor Asa Briggs). HMSO, London.

DeSalvo, L. (1999) *Writing as a Way of Healing: How Telling Our Stories Transform Our Lives*. The Women's Press, London.

Deutsch, M. (1971) Towards an understanding of conflict. *International Journal of Group Tensions* **1**: 42–54.

Dewey, J. (1933) *How We Think*. J. C. Heath, Boston.

Dickson, A. (1982) *A Woman In Your Own Right*. Quartet Books, London.

Donaldson, L. J. (2001) Safe High Quality Health Care: Investing in Tomorrow's Leaders. *Quality in Health Care* **10**: 8–12.

Dreyfus, H. & Dreyfus, S. (1986) *Mind Over Machine*. Free Press, New York.

Dunham, J. & Klafehn, K. (1990) Transformational leadership and the nurse executive. *Journal of Advanced Nursing* **20**(4): 28–33.

Edwards, S. (1998) An anthropological interpretation of nurses' and patients' perceptions of the use of space and touch. *Journal of Advanced Nursing* **28**: 809–17.

Eifried, S., Riley-Giomariso, O. & Voight, G. (2000) Learning to care amid suffering: how art and narrative give voice to the student experience. *International Journal for Human Caring* **5**(2): 42–51.

Estabrooks, C. & Morse, J. (1992) Toward a theory of touch: the touching process and acquiring a touching style. *Journal of Advanced Nursing* **17**: 448–56.

Farrar, M. (1992) How much do they want to know? *Professional Nurse* **7**(9): 606–10.

Faugier, J. & Butterworth, T. (undated) *Clinical Supervision: A Position Paper*. School of Nursing Studies, University of Manchester.

Fay, B. (1987) *Critical Social Science*. Polity Press, Cambridge.

Foucault, M. (1979) *Discipline and Punish: The Birth of the Prison*. (trans. A. Sheridan) Vintage/Random House, New York.

Frank, A. (2002) Relations of caring: demoralization and remoralization in the clinic. *International Journal of Human Caring* **6**(2): 13–19.

Fredriksson, L. (1999) Modes of relating in a caring conversation: a research synthesis on presence, touch and listening. *Journal of Advanced Nursing* **30**(5): 1167–76.

Freire, P. (1979) *Pedagogy of the Oppressed*. Penguin Books, London.

French, J. & Raven, B. (1968) The bases of social power. In *Group Dynamics* (Cartwright, D. & Zander, A. eds) pp. 150–67. Row Peterson, Evanston, Illinois.

Friedson, E. (1970) *Professional Dominance*. Aldine Atherton, Chicago.

Gadamer, H-G. (1975) *Truth and Method*. Seabury Press, New York.

Gadow, S. (1980) Existential advocacy. In *Nursing: Image and Ideals* (Spickler, S. & Gadow, S., eds) pp. 79–101. Springer, New York.

Garside, P. (1999) The learning organisation: a necessary setting for improving care? *Quality in Health Care* **8**: 211.

Ghaye, T. (2000a) Colleague-centred care: the reframing of clinical supervision. In *Effective Clinical Supervision* (Ghaye, T. & Lillyman, S., eds). Mark Allen Publishers, Dinton.

Ghaye, T. (2000b) The role of reflection in nurturing clinical conversations. In *Effective Clinical Supervision* (Ghaye, T. & Lillyman, S., eds). Mark Allen Publishers, Dinton.

Gibbs, G. (1988) *Learning by Doing: A Guide to Teaching and Learning Methods.* Further Education Unit, Oxford Polytechnic, now Oxford Brookes University.

Gilbert, T. (2001) Reflective practice and clinical supervision: meticulous rituals of the confessional. *Journal of Advanced Nursing* **36**(2): 199–205.

Gilligan, C. (1982) *In a Different Voice.* Harvard University Press.

Goorapah, D. (1997) Clinical Supervision. *Journal of Clinical Nursing* **6**(3): 173–78.

Gray, G. & Forsstrom, S. (1991) Generating theory from practice: the reflective technique. In *Towards A Discipline of Nursing* (Gray, G. & Pratt, R., eds) p. 3. Churchill Livingstone. Melbourne.

Hall, C. (2003) Nurse Shortage in NHS is Near to Crisis Point. *Daily Telegraph* 29 April 2003.

Hall, L. (1964) Nursing – what is it? *Canadian Nurse* **60**(2): 150–54.

Halldórsdóttir, S. (1996) *Caring and Uncaring Encounters in Nursing and Health Care – Developing a Theory.* Linkoping University Medical Dissertations No. 493. Department of Caring Sciences. Linkoping University, Sweden.

Halligan, A. & Donaldson, L. J. (2001) Implementing clinical governance: turning vision into reality. *British Medical Journal* **322**(7299): 1413–17.

Hampe, S. (1975) The needs of the grieving spouse in a hospital setting. *Nursing Research* **24**(2): 113–20.

Hawkins, P. & Shohet, R. (1989) *Supervision for the Helping Professions.* Open University Press, Buckingham.

Hayes, J. & Cox, C. (2000) Immediate effects of a five-minute foot massage on patients in critical care. *Complementary Therapies in Nursing and Midwifery* **6**(1): 9–13.

Heath, H. & Freshwater, D. (2000) Clinical supervision as an emancipatory process: avoiding inappropriate intent. *Journal of Advanced Nursing* **32**: 1298–1306.

Heidegger, M. (1962) *Being and Time* (trans. Macquarrie, J. & Robinson, E.) Harper & Row, New York.

Heron, J. (1975) *Six-category Intervention Analysis.* Human Potential Resource Group, University of Surrey, Guildford.

Hickman, P. & Holmes, C. (1994) Nursing the post-modern body: a touching case. *Nursing Inquiry* **1**: 3–14.

Holly, M. L. (1989) Reflective writing and the spirit of inquiry. *Cambridge Journal of Education* **19**(1): 71–80.

Howse, E. & Bailey, J. (1992) Resistance to documentation – a nursing research issue. *International Journal of Nursing Studies* **29**(4): 371–80.

Hughes, C., Blackburn, F. & Walgo, M. (1986) On masking among clients. *Topics in Clinical Nursing* **3**(1): 83–9.

Hunt, J. (1981) Indicators for nursing practice: the use of research findings. *Journal of Advanced Nursing* **6**: 189–94.

Isaacs, W. (1993) Taking flight: dialogue, collective thinking, and organizational learning. *Centre for Organizational Learning's Dialogue Project.* MIT, Massachusetts.

James, N. (1989) Emotional Labour: Skill and Work in the Social Regulation of Feelings. *Sociological Review* **37**(1): 15–42.

Johns, C. (1989a) *The Impact of Introducing Primary Nursing on the Culture of a Community Hospital.* Master of Nursing dissertation, University of Wales College of Medicine, Cardiff.

Johns, C. (1989b) To whom it may concern. *Nursing Times* **85**(39): 60–61.

Johns, C. (1992) Ownership and the harmonious team: barriers to developing the therapeutic team in primary nursing. *Journal of Clinical Nursing* **1**: 89–94.

Johns, C. (1993) On becoming effective in taking ethical action. *Journal of Clinical Nursing* **2**: 301–12.

Johns, C. (1994) *The Burford NDU Model: Caring in Practice.* Blackwell Publishing, Oxford.

Johns, C. (1995a) Framing learning through reflection within Carper's fundamental ways of knowing. *Journal of Advanced Nursing* **22**: 226–34.

Johns, C. (1995b) Time to care? Time for reflection. *International Journal of Nursing Practice* **1**: 37–42.

Johns, C. (1996a) Visualising and realising caring in practice through guided reflection. *Journal of Advanced Nursing* **24**: 1135–43.

Johns, C. (1996b) Understanding and managing interpersonal conflict as a therapeutic nursing activity. *International Journal of Nursing Practice* **2**: 194–200.

Johns, C. (1998a) *Becoming a Reflective Practitioner through Guided Reflection.* PhD thesis. The Open University.

Johns, C. (1998b) Unravelling the dilemmas of everyday nursing practice. *Nursing Ethics* **6**: 287–98.

Johns C. (1998c) Caring through a reflective lens: giving meaning to being a reflective practitioner. *Nursing Inquiry* **5**: 18–24.

Johns, C. (1999) Caring connections: knowing self within caring relationships through reflection. *International Journal for Human Caring* **3**(2): 31–8.

Johns, C. (2000) Working with Alice: a reflection. *Complementary Therapies in Nursing and Midwifery* **6**: 199–203.

Johns, C. (2001a) Depending on the intent and emphasis of the supervisor, clinical supervision can be a different experience. *Journal of Nursing Management* **9**: 139–145.

Johns, C. (2001b) The caring dance. *Complementary Therapies in Nursing and Midwifery* **7**(1): 8–12.

Johns, C. (2002) *Guided Reflection: Advancing Practice.* Blackwell Publishing, Oxford.

Johns, C. (2003) Clinical supervision as a model for clinical leadership. *Journal of Nursing Management* **11**: 25–34.

Johns, C. (2004) *Being Mindful, Easing Suffering: Reflections on Palliative Care.* Jessica Kingsley Publishers, London.

Johns, C. & Graham, J (1996) Using a reflective model of nursing and guided reflection. *Nursing Standard* **11**(2): 34–8.

Johns, C. & Hardy, H. (1998) Voice as a metaphor for transformation through reflection. In *Transforming Nursing Through Reflective Practice* (Johns, C. & Freshwater, D., eds.) Blackwell Science, Oxford.

Johns, C. & McCormack, B. (1998) Unfolding the conditions where the transformative potential of guided reflection (clinical supervision) might flourish or flounder. In *Transforming Nursing Through Reflective Practice* (Johns, & C. Freshwater, D., eds), Blackwell Science, Oxford.

Johnson, D. (1974) Development of theory: a requisite for nursing as a primary health profession. *Nursing Research* **23**(5): 373–7.

Jones, Blackwolf & Jones, G. (1996) *Earth Dance Drum*. Commune-E-Key, Salt Lake City.

Jourard, S. (1971) *The Transparent Self*. Van Nostrand, Newark.

Kearney, M. (1996) *Mortally Wounded*. Touchstone, New York.

Kemmis, S. (1985) Action research and the politics of reflection. In *Reflection: Turning Experience into Learning* (Boud, D., Keogh, R. & Walker, D., eds) Kogan Page, New York.

Kermode (1966) Cited in Mattingly, C. (1994).

Kerfoot, K. (1996) World Class Excellence. *Dermatology Nursing* **8**(6): 433–34

Kieffer, C. (1984) Citizen empowerment: a developmental perspective. *Prevention in Human Services* **84**(3): 9–36.

Kikuchi, J. (1992) Nursing questions that science cannot answer. In *Philosophic Inquiry in Nursing* (Kikuchi, J. & Simmons, H., eds) Sage, Newberry Park.

King, L. & Appleton, J. (1997) Intuition: a critical review of the research and rhetoric. *Journal of Advanced Nursing* **26**: 194–202.

Kitson, A. (1989) *A Framework for Quality: A Patient-centred Approach to Quality Assurance in Health Care*. Scutari Press, Middlesex.

Klakovich, M. (1994) Connective leadership for the 21st century: a historical perspective and future directions. *Advanced Nursing Science* **16**(4): 42–54.

Klein, D. (1968) *Community Dynamics and Mental Health*. John Wiley, New York.

Knopf, M. (1994) Treatment options for early stage breast cancer. *MEDSURG Nursing* **3**: 249–57.

Kübler-Ross, E. (1969) *On Death and Dying*. Tavistock, London.

Larson, P. (1987) Comparison of cancer patients' and professional nurses' perceptions of important nurse caring behaviours. *Heart and Lung* **16**(2): 187–93.

Latimer, J. (1995) The nursing process re-examined: enrolment and translation. *Journal of Advanced Nursing* **22**: 213–20.

Lawler, J. (1991) *Behind the Scenes: Nursing, Somology and the Problems of the Body*. Churchill Livingstone, Melbourne.

Levine, S. (1986) *Who dies? An investigation of Conscious Living and Conscious Dying*. Gateway Books, Bath.

Lewin, K. (1951) *Field theory in Social Science*. Harper & Row, New York.

Lieberman, A. (1989) *Staff Development in Culture Building, Curriculum and Teaching: The Next 50 Years*. Teachers' College Press, Columbia University, New York.

Lyle, D. (1998) Opinion: is clinical supervision the answer to quality care? *Nursing Management* **5**(6): 3.

Mackintosh, C. (1998) Reflection: a flawed strategy for the nursing profession. *Nurse Education Today* **18**: 553–7.

Macleod, M. (1994) 'It's the little things that count': the hidden complexity of everyday clinical nursing practice. *Journal of Clinical Nursing* **3**(6): 361–8.

Madrid, M. (1990) The Participating Process of Human Filed Patterning in an Acute Care Environment. In *Visions of Rogers's Science-based Nursing* (Barrett, E., ed.) pp. 93–104. National League for Nursing, New York.

Malby, R. (1996) The need for nursing leadership. *British Journal of Healthcare Management* **2**: 3.

Margolis, H. (1993) *Paradigm and Barriers: How Habits of Mind Govern Scientific Beliefs*. University of Chicago Press, Chicago.

Marris, P. (1986) *Loss and Change*. Routledge & Kegan Paul, London.

Maslach, C. (1976) Burned-out. *Human Behaviour* **5**: 16–22.

Matthew, I. (1995) *The Impact of God: Soundings from St John of the Cross*. Hodder & Stoughton, London.

Mattingly, C. (1994) The concept of therapeutic 'employment'. *Social Sciences and Medicine* **38**(6): 811–22.

Mayer, D. (1986) Cancer patients' and their families' perceptions of nurse caring behaviours. *Topics in Clinical Nursing* **8**(2): 30–36.

Mayeroff, M. (1971) *On Caring*. Harper Perennial, New York.

Mayo, S. (1996) Symbol, metaphor and story: the function of group art therapy in palliative care. *Palliative Medicine* **10**: 209–16.

McCaffery, M. (1983) *Nursing the Patient in Pain*. Harper & Row, London.

McElroy, A., Corben, V. & McLeish, K. (1995) Developing care plan documentation: an action research project. *Journal of Nursing Management* **3**: 193–9.

McNeeley, R. (1983) Organizational patterns and work satisfaction in a comprehensive human service agency: an empirical test. *Human Relations* **36**(10): 957–72.

McNiff, S. (1992) *Art as Medicine: Creating a Therapy of the Imagination*. Shambhala, Boston.

McSherry, W. (1996) Raising the spirit. *Nursing Times* **92**(3): 48–9.

Menzies-Lyth, I. (1988) A case study in the functioning of social systems as a defence against anxiety. In *Containing Anxiety in Institutions: Selected Essays*. Free Association Books, London.

Mezirow, J. (1981) A critical theory of adult learning and education. *Adult Education* **32**(1): 3–24.

Milne, A. A. (1926) *Winnie the Pooh*. Methuen, London.

Moore, T. (1992) *Care of the Soul*. HarperCollins, New York.

Morse, J. (1991) Negotiating commitment and involvement in the nurse-patient relationship. *Journal of Advanced Nursing* **16**: 552–8.

Morse, J., Bottorff, J., Anderson, G., O'Brien, B. & Solberg, S. (1992) Beyond empathy: expanding expressions of caring. *Journal of Advanced Nursing* **17**: 809–21.

Moss, F. (2001) Leadership and Learning: Building the Environment for Better, Safer Health Care. *Quality in Health Care* **10** (Suppl 2): 1–2.

Munley, A. (1986) Sources of hospice staff stress and how to cope with it. *Nursing Clinics of North America* **20**(2): 343–55.

National Health Service Management Executive (N.H.S.M.E.) (1993) *A Vision for The Future*. Department of Health, London.

Nehring, V. & Geach, B. (1973) Why they don't complain: patient's evaluation of their care. *Nursing Outlook* **21**(5): 317–21.

Newell, M. (1992) Anxiety, accuracy, and reflection: the limits of professional development. *Journal of Advanced Nursing* **17**: 1326–33.

Newman, M. (1994) Health as expanded consciousness. *National League for Nursing*, New York.

Newman, M. (1999) The rhythm of relating in a paradigm of wholeness. *Image: Journal of Nursing Scholarship* **31**(3): 227–30.

Nicklin, P. (1987) Violence to the spirit. *Senior Nurse* **6**(5): 10–12.

Noddings, N. (1984) *Caring – A Feminine Approach to Ethics and Moral Education*. University of California Press, Berkeley.

Nolan, M. & Grant, G. (1989) Addressing the needs of informal carers: a neglect area of nursing practice. *Journal of Advanced Nursing* **14**: 950–61.

Northouse, L. L., Jeffs, M., Cracchiolo-Caraway, A., Lampman, L. & Dorris, G. (1995) Emotional distress reported by women and husbands prior to breast biopsy. *Nursing Research* **44**: 196–201.

Novelestsky-Rosenthal, H. & Solomon, K. (2001) Reflections on the use of Johns' model of structured reflection in nurse-practitioner education. *International Journal for Human Caring* **5**(2): 21–6.

Nursing and Midwifery Council (2002) Code of Professional Conduct. Nursing and Midwifery Council, London.

Oakley, A. (1984) The importance of being a nurse. *Nursing Times* **83**(50): 24–7.

Ochs, L. (2001) This nurse suggests asking before you touch. *RN* **64**(4): 10.

O'Donohue, J. (1997) *Anam Cara: Spiritual Wisdom from the Celtic World*. Bantam Press, London.

Ottaway, R. (1978) A change strategy to implement new norms, new styles and new environment in the work organization. *Personnel Review* **5**(1): 13–18.

Parker, M. (2002) Aesthetic ways in day-to-day nursing. In *Therapeutic Nursing* (Freshwater, D., ed.) Sage, London.

Parker, R. (1990) Nurses' stories: the search for a relational ethic of care. *Advances in Nursing Science* **13**(1): 31–40.

Parse, R. R. (1987) Parse's Man-Living-Health theory of nursing. In *Nursing Science: Major Paradigms, Theories and Critiques* (Parse, R. R., ed.) W. B. Saunders, Philadelphia.

Pearson, A. (1983) *The Clinical Nursing Unit*. Heinemann Medical Books, London.

Pennebaker, J. (1989) Confession, inhibition and disease. *Advances in Experimental Social Psychology* **22**: 211–44.

Pennebaker, J., Hughes, C. & O'Heeron, R. (1987) The pyschophysiology of confession: linking inhibitory and psychosomatic processes. *Journal of Personality and Social Psychology* **52**: 781–93.

Pennebaker, J., Colder, M. & Sharp, L. (1990) Accelerating the coping process. *Journal of Personality and Social Psychology* **58**: 528–37.

Pennebaker, J., Mayne, T. & Francis, M. (1997) Linguistic predictors of adaptive bereavement. *Journal of Personality and Social Psychology* **72**: 863–71.

Picard, C., Sickul, C. & Natale, S. (1999) Healing reflections: the transformative mirror. *International Journal for Human Caring* **2**(2): 40–47.

Pike, A. (1991) Moral outrage and moral discourse in nurse-physician collaboration. *Journal of Professional Nursing* **7**(6): 351–63.

Plager, K. (1994) Hermeneutic phenomenology: a methodology for family health and health promotion study in nursing. In *Interpretive Phenomenology* (Benner, P., ed.). Sage, Thousand Oaks.

Platzer, H., Blake, D. & Ashford, D. (2000) Barriers to learning from reflection; a study of the use of groupwork with post-registration nurses. *Journal of Advanced Nursing* **31**(5): 1001–8.

Polanyi, M. (1958) *Personal Knowledge: Towards a Post Critical Philosophy*. Routledge and Kegan Paul, London.

Polkingthorne, D. (1996) Transformative narratives: from victimic to agentic life plots. *The American Journal of Occupational Therapy* **50**(4): 299–305.

Powell, J. (1989) The reflective practitioner in nursing. *Journal of Advanced Nursing* **14**: 824–32.

Power, S. (1999) *Nursing Supervision: A Guide for Clinical Practice*. Sage Publications, London.

Proctor, B. (1988) Supervision: a working alliance. Videotape training manual. Alexa Publications, St Leonards-on-Sea.

Ramos, M. (1992) The nurse-patient relationship: Themes and variations. *Journal of Advanced Nursing* **17**: 496–506.

Rawnsley, M. (1990) Of human bonding: the context of nursing as caring. *Advances in Nursing Science* **13**: 41–8.

Ray, M. (1989) The theory of bureaucratic caring for nursing practice in the organizational culture. *Nursing Administrative Quarterly* **13**(2) 31–42.

Reiman, D. (1986) Non-caring and caring in the clinical setting: patients' descriptions. *Topics in Clinical Nursing* **8**(2): 30–36.

Reissetter, K. & Thomas, B. (1986) Nursing care of the dying: its relationship to selected nurse characteristics. *International Journal of Nursing Studies* **23**: 39–50.

Remen, R. (1996) *Kitchen Table Wisdom*. Riverhead Books, New York.

Reverby, S. (1987) A caring dilemma: womanhood and nursing in historical perspective. *Nursing Research* **36**(1): 5–11.

Richardson, A. (1994) The health diary: an examination of its use as a data collection method. *Journal of Advanced Nursing* **19**: 782–91.

Richmond, J. (1995) The spirit of nursing and its healing art: a Jungian perspective. *Nursing Inquiry* **2**: 215–20.

Rinpoche, S. (1992) *The Tibetan Book of Living and Dying*. Rider, London.

Rippon, S. (2001) Nurturing nurse leadership: how does your garden grow? *Nursing Management* **8**(7): 11–15.

Roach, S. (1992) *The Human Act of Caring*. Canadian Hospital Association Press, Ottawa.

Roberts, S. (1983) Oppressed group behaviour: implications for nursing. *Advances in Nursing Science* **5**(4): 21–30.

Robinson, S. & Thorne, C. (1984) Strengthening family interference. *Journal of Advanced Nursing* **9**: 597–602.

Rogers, C. (1969) *Freedom to Learn: A View of what Education Might be*. Merrill, Columbus, OH.

Rogers, M. (1986) Science of unitary human beings. In *Explorations of Martha Rogers's Science of Unitary Human Beings* (Malinski, V., ed.), Appleton-Century-Crofts, Norwalk.

Roper, N., Logan, W. & Tierney, A. (1980) *The Elements of Nursing*. Churchill Livingstone, Edinburgh.

Sacks, O. (1976) *Awakenings*. Pelican Books, London.

Sangharakshita (1993) *The Drama of Cosmic Enlightenment*. Windhorse, Birmingham.

Saunders, C. (1996) Foreword in *Mortally Wounded: Stories of Soul Pain, Death & Healing* (Kearney, M.). Touchstone, New York.

Scanlon, C. & Weir, W. S. (1997) Learning from practice? Mental health nurses' perceptions and experiences of clinical supervision. *Journal of Advanced Nursing* **26**: 295–303.

Schön, D. (1983) *The Reflective Practitioner*. Avebury, Aldershot.

Schön, D. (1987) *Educating the Reflective Practitioner*. Jossey-Bass, San Francisco.

Schuster, J. (1994) Transforming your leadership style. *Leadership* 39–43.

Seden, J. (2003) Managers And Their Organisations. In *Managing Care In Context* (Henderson, J. & Atkinson, D., eds) Cromwell Press, London.

Seedhouse, D. (1988) *Ethics: The Heart of Health Care*. Wiley, Chichester.

Senge, P. (1990) *The Fifth Discipline: The Art and Practice of the Learning Organisation*. Century Business, London.

Sinha, L. & Scherera, K. (1987) Ask the patient. *Nursing Times* **83**(45): 40–42.

Sloan, G. & Watson, H. (2001) John Heron's six-category intervention analysis: towards understanding interpersonal relations and progressing the delivery of clinical supervision for mental health nursing in the United Kingdom. *Journal of Advanced Nursing* **36**(2): 206–14.

Smith, G. (2000) Friendship within clinical supervision: a model for the NHS? http://www.clinical-supervision.com. Accessed 18 March 2003.

Smith, M. & Liehr, P. (1999) Attentively embracing story: a middle range theory with practice and research implications. *Scholarly Inquiry for Nursing Practice* **13**(3): 3–27.

Smyth, J. (1998) Written emotional expression: effect sizes, outcome types and moderating variables. *Journal of Consulting and Clinical Psychology* **66**(1): 174–84.

Smyth, J., Stone, A., Hurewitz, A. & Kaell, A. (1999) Effects of writing about stressful experiences on symptom reduction in patients with asthma or rheumatoid arthritis. *Journal of the American Medical Association* **281**: 1304–9.

Smyth, W. J. (1987) *A Rationale for Teachers' Critical Pedagogy*. Deakin University Press, Melbourne.

Stewart, I. & Joines, V. (1987) *TA Today: A New Introduction to Transactional Analysis*. Lifespace Publishing, Nottingham & Chapel Hill.

Street, A. (1992) *Inside Nursing: A Critical Ethnography of Clinical Nursing*. State University of New York Press, Albany.

Suzuki, S. (2002) *Not Always So: Practicing the True Spirit of Zen*. Harper Collins, New York.

Sutherland, L. (1994) Caring as mutual empowerment: working with the BNDU model at Burford. In *The Burford NDU Model: Caring in Practice* (Johns, C., ed.). Blackwell Science, Oxford.

Talton, C. (1995) Complementary therapies: touch-of-all-kinds is therapeutic. *RN* **58**(2): 61–4.

Taylor, B. (1992) From helper to human: a reconceptualisation of the nurse as a person. *Journal of Advanced Nursing* **17**: 1042–9.

Taylor, D. & Singer, E. (1983) *New Organisation From Old*. IPM Management Publications, London.

Thomas, K. & Kilmann, R. (1974) *Thomas Kilmann Conflict Mode Instrument*. Xicom, Toledo.

Tschudin, V. (1993) *Ethics In Nursing* 2nd edn Butterworth Heinemann, Oxford.

Turton, P. (1989) Touch me, feel me, heal me. *Nursing Times* **85**(19): 42–44.

Tversky, A. & Khaneman, D. (1974) Judgement under uncertainty: heuristics and biases. *Science* **185**: 1124–31.

Tyler, J. (1998) Nonverbal communication and the use of art in the care of the dying. *Palliative Medicine* **12**: 123–6.

UKCC (1987) *Advisory paper: Confidentiality – an elaboration of clause 9*. UKCC, London.

Vachon, M. (1988) Battle fatigue in hospice/palliative care. In *A Safer Death* (Gilmore, A. & Gilmore, S., eds). Plenum Publishing, New York.

Van Manen, M. (1990) *Researching Lived Experience*. State University of New York Press, New York.

Vaught-Alexander, K. (1994) The personal journal for nurses: writing for delivery and healing. In *Caring as Healing: Renewal Through Hope* (Gaut, D. & Boykin, A., eds). National league for Nursing Press, New York.

Visinstainer, M. (1986) The nature of knowledge and theory in nursing. *Image: The Journal of Nursing Scholarship* **18**: 32–8.

Wade, S. (1999) Promoting quality of care for older people: Developing positive attitudes to working with older people. *Journal of Nursing Management* **7**: 339–47.

Wagner, L. (1999) Within the circle of death: transpersonal poetic reflections on nurses' stories about the quality of the dying process. *International Journal for Human Caring* **3**(2): 21–30.

Wainwright, P. (2000) Towards an aesthetics of nursing. *Journal of Advanced Nursing* **32**(3): 750–55.

Wall, T. D., Bolden, R. I. & Borril, C. S. (1997) Minor psychiatric disturbance in NHS Trust staff. *British Journal of Psychiatry* **171**: 519–23.

Ward, K. (1988) Not just the patient in bed three. *Nursing Times* **84**(78): 39–50.

Watson, J. (1988) *Nursing: Human Science and Human Care. A Theory of Nursing*. National League for Nursing, New York.

Watson, J. (1990) The moral failure of the hierarchy. *Nursing Outlook* **38**(2): 62–6.

White, A. (1993) The nursing process: a constraint on expert practice. *Journal of Nursing Management* **1**: 245–52.

Wilber, K. (1991) *No Boundary. Eastern and Western Approaches to Personal Growth.* Shambhala, Boston.

Wilber, K. (1998) *The Eye of Spirit: An Integral Vision for a World gone Slightly Mad.* Shambhala, Boston.

Wilkinson, J. (1988) Moral distress in nursing practice: experience and effect. *Nursing Forum* **23**(1): 16–29.

Wolf, Z. (1986) Nurses' work: the sacred and the profane. *Holistic Nursing Practice* **1**(1): 29–35.

Woolf, V. (1945) *A Room of One's Own*. Penguin Books, London.

Woodward, V. (1998) Caring, patient autonomy and the stigma of paternalism. *Journal of Advanced Nursing* **28**: 1046–52.

Woodward, V. & Webb, C. (2001) Women's anxieties surrounding breast disorders: a systematic review of the literature. *Journal of Advanced Nursing* **33**(1): 29–41.

Wyshcogrod, E. (1981) Empathy and Sympathy as Tactile Encounter. *Journal of Medical Philosophy* **6**(1): 25–43.

Younger, J. (1995) The alienation of the sufferer. *Advances in Nursing Science* **17**(4): 53–72.

Index